# SURGICAL RECALL
## 5TH EDITION

# SURGICAL RECALL
## 5TH EDITION

Recall Series Editor and Senior Editor

**Lorne H. Blackbourne, M.D., F.A.C.S.**
Trauma, Burn, and Critical Care Surgeon
San Antonio, Texas

"In the operating room we can save more lives, cure more cancer, restore more function, and relieve more suffering than anywhere else in the hospital."

—R. Scott Jones, M.D.

Wolters Kluwer | Lippincott Williams & Wilkins
Health

Philadelphia · Baltimore · New York · London
Buenos Aires · Hong Kong · Sydney · Tokyo

*Acquisitions Editor:* Donna M. Balado
*Developmental Editor:* Kathleen H. Scogna
*Managing Editor:* Kelley Squazzo
*Associate Production Manager:* Kevin P. Johnson
*Marketing Manager:* Emilie Moyer
*Design Coordinator:* Holly McLaughlin
*Artist:* Holly Fischer, M.F.A.
*Compositor:* International Typesetting and Composition

*Printed in the United States of America*

First Edition, 1994
Second Edition, 1998
Third Edition, 2002
Fourth Edition, 2006

**Library of Congress Cataloging-in-Publication Data**

Surgical recall / senior editor, Lorne H. Blackbourne. — 5th ed.
    p. ; cm. — (Recall series)
  Includes bibliographical references and index.
  ISBN-13: 978-0-7817-7076-7
  ISBN-10: 0-7817-7076-9
 1. Surgery—Examinations, questions, etc.  I. Blackbourne, Lorne H.  II. Series.
  [DNLM:  1. Surgical Procedures, Operative—Examination Questions.
  WO 18.2 S9618 2008]
  RD37.2.S9748 2008
  617.0076—dc22

                                 2007041347

# Dedication

This manual is dedicated to the memory of Leslie E. Rudolf, Professor of Surgery and Vice-Chairman of the Department of Surgery at the University of Virginia. Dr. Rudolf was born on November 12, 1927, in New Rochelle, New York. He served in the U.S. Army Counter-Intelligence Corps in Europe after World War II.

He graduated from Union College in 1951 and attended Cornell Medical College, where he graduated in 1955. He then entered his surgical residency at Peter Brigham Hospital in Boston, Massachusetts, and completed his residency there, serving as Chief Resident Surgeon in 1961.

Dr. Rudolf came to Charlottesville, Virginia as an Assistant Professor of Surgery in 1963. He rapidly rose through the ranks, becoming Professor of Surgery and Vice-Chairman of the Department in 1974 and a Markle Scholar in Academic Medicine from 1966 until 1971. His research interests included organ and tissue transplantation and preservation. Dr. Rudolf was instrumental in initiating the Kidney Transplant Program at the University of Virginia Health Sciences Center. His active involvement in service to the Charlottesville community is particularly exemplified by his early work with the Charlottesville/ Albemarle Rescue Squad, and he received the Governor's Citation for the Commonwealth of Virginia Emergency Medical Services in 1980.

His colleagues at the University of Virginia Health Sciences Center, including faculty and residents, recognized his keen interests in teaching medical students, evaluating and teaching residents, and helping the young surgical faculty. He took a serious interest in medical student education, and he would have strongly approved of this teaching manual, affectionately known as the "Rudolf" guide, as an extension of ward rounds and textbook reading.

In addition to his distinguished academic accomplishments, Dr. Rudolf was a talented person with many diverse scholarly pursuits and hobbies. His advice and counsel on topics ranging from Chinese cooking to orchid raising were sought by a wide spectrum of friends and admirers.

This manual is a logical extension of Dr. Rudolf's interests in teaching. No one book, operation, or set of rounds can begin to answer all questions of surgical disease processes; however, in a constellation of learning endeavors, this effort would certainly have pleased him.

*John B. Hanks, M.D.*
*Professor of Surgery*
*University of Virginia*
*Charlottesville, Virginia*

# Editors and Contributors

**ADVISOR:**

**CURTIS G. TRIBBLE, M.D.**
Professor and Vice Chairman
Department of Surgery
Chief of Thoracic and
    Cardiovascular Surgery
University of Florida College
    of Medicine
Gainesville, Florida

**EDITOR:**

**C. SUZANNE CUTTER, M.D.**
Chief Resident in General
    Surgery
New York Hospital Queens
Flushing, New York

**PAST EDITORS AND
    CONTRIBUTORS:**

**EDITORS:**

**BRUCE CROOKES, M.D.**
**ALFA O. DIALLO, M.D.**
**MATTHEW EDWARDS, M.D.**
**ARA J. FIENSTEIN, M.D.**
**E. WILLIAM JOHNSON, M.D.**
**PETER LOPEZ, M.D.**
**MARTIN I. NEWMAN, M.D.**
**CARL SCHULMAN, M.D.**
**DAVID SHATZ, M.D.**

**ASSOCIATE EDITORS:**

**NICHOLAS R. ALVEREZ, B.S.**
**JOS AMORTEQUI, M.D.**
**JOSHUA I. BLEIER, M.D.**
**ANDREW CAMERON, M.D.**
**DIANE DIESEN, M.D.**
**GLADYS L. GIRON, M.D.**
**LAWERENCE V. GULOTTA, M.D.**
**FAHIM HABIB, M.D.**
**JENNIFER HALL, M.D.**
**DAVID KING, M.D.**
**JOSEPH MICHAELS V, M.D.**
**RUPEN G. MODI, M.B.A.**
**PAYMANN MOIN, B.S.**
**TODD M. MORGAN, M.D.**
**ANDREW NEWMAN, B.S.**
**LOUIS PIZANO, M.D.**
**DIMITRIS G. PLACANTONAKIS,
    M.D. PH.D.**
**JUSTIN YOVINO, M.D.**

**CONTRIBUTORS:**

**ESTEBAN AMBRAD-CHALELA, M.D.**
**DAVID CHESSIN, M.D.**
**OWEN JOHNSON, B.S.**
**PETER T. KENNEALY, M.D.**
**GEOFFERY LAM, M.D.**
**GARRETT NASH, M.D.**
**INDERPAL SARKARIA, M.D.**
**ALYSANDRA SCHWARZ, M.D.**
**ALI VAFA, M.D.**
**NABIL WASIF, M.D.**

## INTERNATIONAL EDITORS:

### HEYTHEM A. ALZAMEL, M.D.
General Surgery, Trauma, and
   Critical Care
King Fahad National Guard
   Hospital
Riyadh, Saudi Arabia

### MOHAMMAD AZFAR, M.B.B.S., F.R.C.S.
General Surgeon
Kuwait City, Kuwait

### MUDR. JA'N BEREC, M.D.
Trauma and Orthopedic
   Surgery
Bratislava, Slovak Republic

### DROR SOFFER, M.D.
Trauma Surgeon
Tel Aviv University
Tel Aviv, Israel

### STEPHEN WASHINGTON, M.B.CH.B.
Department of Surgery
University of Manchester
Manchester, United Kingdom

### NIZAR YAMANI, M.D.
Department of Surgery,
   Division of Thoracic Surgery
King Fahad National Guard
   Hospital
Riyadh, Saudi Arabia

# Foreword

*Surgical Recall* represents the culmination of several years' effort by Lorne Blackbourne and his friends, who began the project when they were third-year medical students. Lorne, who completed his residency in General Surgery at the University of Virginia, has involved other surgical residents and medical students to provide annual updates and revisions.

This reflects the interest, enthusiasm, and true dedication to learning and teaching that permeates the medical school classes and surgical residencies in our institution. It is an honor, privilege, and a continuing stimulus to work in the midst of this group of dedicated young people. I congratulate all the students and residents involved in this project and also acknowledge the leadership of the surgical faculty. The professor's ultimate satisfaction occurs when all the learners assume ownership of learning and teaching.

This book encompasses the essential information in general surgery and surgical specialties usually imparted to students in our surgical clerkship and reviewed and developed further in electives. Developed from the learner's standpoint, the text includes fundamental information such as a description of the diseases, signs, symptoms, essentials of pathophysiology, treatments, and possible outcomes. The unique format of this study guide uses the Socratic method by employing a list of questions or problems posed along the left side of the page with answers or responses on the right. In addition, the guide includes numerous practical tips for students and junior residents to facilitate comprehensive and effective management of patients. This material is essential for students in the core course of surgery and for those taking senior electives.

In this fifth edition, the authors have expanded the existing chapters for a fuller and more complete coverage of all subjects, including new subjects. We hope you find this expanded version of this work stimulating and easy to use.

*R. Scott Jones, M.D.*
*University of Virginia*
*Charlottesville, Virginia*

# Preface

*Surgical Recall* began as a source of surgical facts during my Surgery Clerkship when I was a third-year medical student at the University of Virginia. My goal has been to provide concise information that every third-year surgical student should know in a "rapid fire," two-column format.

The format of *Surgical Recall* is conducive to the recall of basic surgical facts because it relies on repetition and positive feedback. As one repeats the question-and-answer format, one gains success.

This new fifth edition includes completely updated information, new acronyms and mnemonics, new illustrations, and more streamlined rapid-fire answers, as well as a Rapid-Fire Power Review: Top 100 Clinical Surgical Microvignettes. We have combed the textbooks and have come up with the facts you need to know.

We have dedicated our work to the living memory of Professor Leslie Rudolf. It is our hope that those who knew Dr. Rudolf will remember him and those who did not will ask.

*Lorne H. Blackbourne, M.D., F.A.C.S*
*Trauma, Burn, and Critical Care Surgeon*
*San Antonio, Texas*

P.S. We would like to hear from you if you have any corrections, acronyms, and classic ward or operating room questions (all contributors will be credited). You can reach me via e-mail in care of Lippincott Williams & Wilkins at book_comments@lww.com.

# Contents

Dedication...................................................................................................v
Editors and Contributors.....................................................................vii
Foreword...............................................................................................ix
Preface..................................................................................................xi

**SECTION I**
**OVERVIEW AND BACKGROUND SURGICAL**
**INFORMATION**

1.  Introduction........................................................................................1
    Surgical Notes.....................................................................................9
    Common Abbreviations You Should Know.....................................15
    Glossary of Surgical Terms You Should Know...............................18
    Surgery Signs, Triads, etc., You Should Know................................25
2.  Surgical Syndromes............................................................................32
3.  Surgical Most Commons...................................................................35
4.  Surgical Percentages..........................................................................38
5.  Surgical History..................................................................................40
6.  Surgical Instruments..........................................................................42
7.  Sutures and Stitches..........................................................................52
8.  Surgical Knot Tying...........................................................................60
9.  Procedures for the Surgical Ward and Clinic.................................65
10. Incisions..............................................................................................72
11. Surgical Positions...............................................................................77
12. Surgical Speak....................................................................................78
13. Preoperative 101...............................................................................79
14. Surgical Operations You Should Know.............................................81
15. Wounds...............................................................................................90
16. Drains and Tubes...............................................................................91
17. Surgical Anatomy Pearls..................................................................102
18. Fluids and Electrolytes.....................................................................106
19. Blood and Blood Products..............................................................122
20. Surgical Hemostasis.........................................................................127
21. Common Surgical Medications.......................................................129
22. Complications...................................................................................137
23. Common Causes of Ward Emergencies.........................................155
24. Surgical Respiratory Care...............................................................157

25. Surgical Nutrition........................................................................................159
26. Shock.........................................................................................................164
27. Surgical Infection.......................................................................................169
28. Fever..........................................................................................................180
29. Surgical Prophylaxis...................................................................................182
30. Surgical Radiology......................................................................................183
31. Anesthesia..................................................................................................190
32. Surgical Ulcers...........................................................................................195
33. Surgical Oncology......................................................................................197

# SECTION II
# GENERAL SURGERY

34. GI Hormones and Physiology......................................................................199
35. Acute Abdomen and Referred Pain...........................................................203
36. Hernias.......................................................................................................209
37. Laparoscopy...............................................................................................223
38. Trauma........................................................................................................226
39. Burns..........................................................................................................246
40. Upper GI Bleeding.....................................................................................254
41. The Stomach..............................................................................................270
42. Bariatric Surgery........................................................................................280
43. Ostomies....................................................................................................282
44. Small Intestine...........................................................................................284
45. The Appendix.............................................................................................292
46. Carcinoid Tumors.......................................................................................300
47. Fistulas.......................................................................................................304
48. Colon and Rectum......................................................................................307
49. The Anus....................................................................................................325
50. Lower GI Bleeding.....................................................................................334
51. Inflammatory Bowel Disease (IBD):
     Crohn's Disease and Ulcerative Colitis....................................................338
52. Liver...........................................................................................................345
53. Portal Hypertension...................................................................................357
54. Biliary Tract...............................................................................................364
55. Pancreas.....................................................................................................383
56. The Breast..................................................................................................400
57. Endocrine...................................................................................................419
58. Thyroid Gland............................................................................................439
59. Parathyroid.................................................................................................453
60. Spleen and Splenectomy............................................................................459

61. Surgically Correctable HTN ................................................................................ 464
62. Soft Tissue Sarcomas and Lymphomas ......................................................... 465
63. Skin Lesions .......................................................................................................... 471
64. Melanoma ............................................................................................................... 473
65. Surgical Intensive Care ..................................................................................... 480
66. Vascular Surgery .................................................................................................. 493

# SECTION III
# SUBSPECIALTY SURGERY

67. Pediatric Surgery ................................................................................................. 521
68. Plastic Surgery ..................................................................................................... 579
69. Hand Surgery ........................................................................................................ 585
70. Otolaryngology: Head and Neck Surgery ................................................... 593
71. Thoracic Surgery ................................................................................................. 629
72. Cardiovascular Surgery ..................................................................................... 656
73. Transplant Surgery .............................................................................................. 680
74. Orthopaedic Surgery .......................................................................................... 699
75. Neurosurgery ........................................................................................................ 729
76. Urology ................................................................................................................... 752

    Rapid Fire Power Review ...................................................................................... 776
    Figure Credits ......................................................................................................... 784
    Index ......................................................................................................................... 785

# Section I

## Overview and Background Surgical Information

# Chapter 1

## Introduction

### PREPARING FOR THE SURGERY CLERKSHIP

#### USING THE STUDY GUIDE

This study guide was written to accompany the surgical clerkship. It has evolved over the years through student feedback and continued updating. In this regard, we welcome any feedback (both positive and negative) or suggestions for improvement. The objective of the guide is to provide a rapid overview of common surgical topics. The guide is organized in a self-study/quiz format. By covering the information/answers on the right with the bookmark, you can attempt to answer the questions on the left to assess your understanding of the information. Keep the guide with you at all times, and when you have even a few spare minutes (e.g., between cases) hammer out a page or at least a few questions. Many students read this book as a primer before the clerkship even begins!

Your study objectives in surgery should include the following four points:
1. OR question-and-answer periods
2. Ward questioning
3. Oral exam
4. Written exam

The optimal plan of action would include daily reading in a text, anatomy review prior to each OR case, and *Surgical Recall*. But remember, this guide helps you recall basic facts about surgical topics. Reading should be done daily! The advanced student should read *Advanced Surgical Recall*.

To facilitate learning a surgical topic, first break down each topic into the following categories and, in turn, master each category:

1. What is it?
2. Incidence
3. Risk factors
4. Signs and symptoms
5. Laboratory and radiologic tests
6. Diagnostic criteria
7. Differential diagnoses
8. Medical and surgical treatment
9. Postoperative care
10. Complications
11. Stages and prognosis

Granted, it is hard to read after a full day in the OR. For a change, go to sleep right away and wake up a few hours early the next day and read **before** going to the hospital. It sounds crazy, but it does work.

°Remember–REPETITION is the key to learning for most adults.

## APPEARANCE

| | |
|---|---|
| **Why is your appearance so important?** | The patient sees only the wound dressing, the skin closure, and you. You can wear whatever you want, **but you best look clean. Do not wear religious or political buttons because this is not fair to your patients with different beliefs!** |

## WHAT THE PERFECT SURGICAL STUDENT CARRIES IN HER COAT

Stethoscope
Penlight
Scissors
Minibook on medications (e.g., trade names, doses)
Tape/4 × 4s
Sutures to practice tying
Pen/notepad/small notebook to write down pearls
Notebook or clipboard with patient's data (always write down chores with a box next to them so you can check off the box when the chore is completed)
Small calculator
List of commonly used telephone numbers (e.g., radiology)
(Oh, and of course, *Surgical Recall!*)

## THE PERFECT PREPARATION FOR ROUNDS

Interview your patient (e.g., problems, pain, wishes).

Talk with your patient's nurse (e.g., "Were there any events during the last shift?").

Examine patient (e.g., cor/pulm/abd/**wound**).

Record vital signs (e.g., $T_{max}$).

Record input (e.g., IVF, PO).

Record output (e.g., urine, drains).

Check labs.

Check microbiology (e.g., culture reports, Gram stains).

Check x-rays.

Check pathology reports.

Know the patient's allergies.

Check allied health updates (e.g., PT, OT).

Read chart.

Check medication (don't forget $H_2$ blocker in the hyperalimentation).

Check nutrition.

Always check with the intern for chores, updates, or insider information **before** rounds.

## PRESENTING ON ROUNDS

Your presentation on rounds should be like an iceberg. State important points about your patient (the tip of the iceberg visible above the ocean), but know **everything** else about your patient that your chief might ask about (that part of the iceberg under the ocean). Always include:

Name

Postoperative day s/p-procedure

A concise overall assessment of how the patient is doing

Vital signs/temp status/antibiotics day

Input/output-urine, drains, PO intake, IVF

Change in physical examination

Any complaints (not yours—the patient's)

Plan

Your presentation should be concise, with good eye contact (you should not simply read from a clipboard). The intangible element of confidence cannot be overemphasized; if you do not know the answer to a question about a patient, however, the correct response should be "I do not know, but I will find out." Never lie or hedge on an answer because it will only serve to make the remainder of your surgical rotation less than desirable. Furthermore, do your best to be enthusiastic and motivated. **Never, ever whine.** And remember to be a **team player.** Never make your fellow students look bad! Residents pick up on this immediately and will slam you.

## THE PERFECT SURGERY STUDENT

Never whines

Never pimps his residents or fellow students (or attendings)

Never complains

Is never hungry, thirsty, or tired

Is always enthusiastic

Loves to do scut work and can never get enough

Never makes a fellow student look bad

Is always clean (a patient sees only you and the wound dressing)

Is never late

Smiles a lot and has a good sense of humor

Makes things happen

Is not a "know-it-all"

Never corrects anyone **during** rounds unless it will affect patient care

Makes the intern/resident/chief look good at all times, if at all possible

**Knows more about her patients than anyone else**

Loves the OR

Never wants to leave the hospital

Takes correction, direction, and instruction very well

Says "Sir" and "Ma'am" to the scrub nurses (and to the attending,
    unless corrected)

Never asks questions he can look up for himself

Knows the patient's disease, surgery, indication for surgery, and the anatomy
    before going to the OR

Is the first one to arrive at clinic and the last one to leave

Always places x-rays up in the OR

Reads from a surgery text **every day**

Is a team player

Asks for feedback

Never has a chip on her shoulder

Loves to suture

Is honest and always admits fault and errors

Knows when his patient is going to the OR (e.g., by calling)

Is confident but **not** cocky

Has a **"Can-Do"** attitude and can figure out things on her own

Is not afraid to get help when needed

Never says **"No"** or **"Maybe"** to involvement in patient care

Treats everyone (e.g., nurses, fellow students) with respect

Follows the chain of command

Praises others when appropriate

Checks with the intern beforehand for information for rounds
    (test results/surprises)

**RUNS** for materials, lab values, test results, etc., during rounds before any
    house officer

Gives credit where credit is due
Dresses and undresses wounds on rounds
Has a steel bladder, a cast-iron stomach, and a heart of gold
Always writes the op note without question
Always checks with the intern after rounds for chores
Always makes sure there is a medical student in every case
Always follows the patient to the recovery room
In the OR, always asks permission to ask a question
Always reviews anatomy prior to going to the OR
Does what the intern asks (i.e., the chief will get feedback from the intern)
Is a high-speed, low-drag, hardcore **HAMMERHEAD**

**Define HAMMERHEAD.**    A hammerhead is an individual who places his head to the ground and **hammers** through any and all obstacles to get a job done and then asks for more work. One who gives 110% and never complains. One who **desires** work.

## OPERATING ROOM

Your job in the OR will be to retract (water-skiing) and answer questions posed by the attending physicians and residents. Retracting is basically idiot-proof. Many students emphasize anticipating the surgeon's next move, but stick to following the surgeon's request. More than 75% of the questions asked in the OR deal with anatomy; therefore, read about the anatomy and pathophysiology of the case, which will reduce the "I don't knows."

Never argue with the scrub nurses—they are always right. They are the selfless warriors of the operating suite's sterile field, and arguing with one will only **make matters worse.**

**Never** touch or take instruments from the Mayo tray (tray with instruments on it over the patient's feet) unless given explicit permission to do so. Every day when you approach the OR suite door **STOP** and ask yourself if you have on scrubs, shoe covers, a cap, and a mask to avoid the embarrassing situation of being yelled at by the OR staff (A.K.A. the 3 strikes test: strike 1 = no mask, strike 2 = no headcover, strike 3 = no shoe covers . . . any strikes and you are outta here—place a mental stop sign outside of the OR with the 3 strikes rule on it)! Always wear eye protection. When entering the OR, first introduce yourself to the scrub nurse and ask if you can get your gloves or gown. If you have questions in the OR, first **ask** if you can ask a question because it may be a bad time and this way it will not appear as though you are pimping the resident/attending.

Other thoughts on the OR:

If you feel faint, ask if you can sit down (try to eat prior to going to the OR). If your feet swell in the OR, try wearing support hose socks. If your back hurts, try taking some ibuprofen (with a meal) **prior** to the case. Also, sit-ups or abdominal crunches help to relieve back pain by strengthening the abdominal muscles. At the end of the case, ask the scrub nurse for some left-over ties (clean ones) to practice tying knots with and, if there is time, start writing your OP Note.

## OPERATING ROOM FAQS

| | |
|---|---|
| **What if I have to sneeze?** | Back up STRAIGHT back. Do not turn your head, as the sneeze exits through the sides of your mask! |
| **What if I feel faint?** | Do not be a hero. Say, "I feel faint. May I sit down?" This is no big deal and is very common. (However, it helps to always eat before going to the OR.) |
| **What should I say when I first enter the OR?** | Introduce yourself as a student. State that you are going to scrub and ask if you need to get out your gloves and/or gown. |
| **Should I wear my ID tag into the OR?** | Yes |
| **Can I wear nail polish?** | Yes, as long as it is not chipped. |
| **Can I wear my rings and my watch when scrubbed in the OR?** | No |
| **Can I wear earrings?** | No |
| **When scrubbed, is my back sterile?** | No |
| **When in the surgical gown, are my underarms sterile?** | No. Do not put your hands under your arms. |
| **How far down my gown is considered part of the sterile field?** | Just to your waist |
| **How far up my gown is considered sterile?** | Up to your nipples |

**How do I stand if I am waiting for the case to start?**

Hands together in front above your waist

**Can I button up a surgical gown (when I am not scrubbed!) with bare hands?**

Yes. Remember, the back of the gown is NOT sterile.

**How many pairs of gloves should I wear when scrubbed?**

2 (2 layers)

**What is the normal order of sizes of gloves: small pair, then larger pair?**

No. Usually the order is a larger size followed by a smaller size (e.g., most men wear a size #8 covered by a size #7.5; most women wear a size #7 covered by a size #6.5)

**What is a "scrub nurse" versus a "circulating nurse"?**

The scrub nurse is "scrubbed" and hands the surgeon sutures, instruments, and so forth. This person is often an Operating Technician (A.K.A. "Scrub Tech"). The circulating nurse "circulates" and gets everything needed before and during the procedure.

**What items comprise the sterile field in the operating room?**

The instrument table, the Mayo tray, and the anterior drapes on the patient.

**What is the tray with the instruments called?**

Mayo tray

**Can I grab things off the Mayo tray?**

No. Ask the scrub nurse/tech; they may give you permission.

**How do you remove blood with a laparotomy pad ("lap pad")?**

*Dab.* Do not wipe, because wiping removes platelet plugs.

**Can you grab the skin with DeBakey pickups?**

NO. Pickups for the skin must have teeth (e.g., Adson, Rat-tooth) as it is "better to cut the skin than crush it."

**How should you cut the sutures after tying a knot?**

1. Rest the cutting hand on the noncutting hand.
2. Slip the scissors down to the knot and then cant the scissors at 45 degrees so you do not cut the knot itself.

| What should you do when you are scrubbed and someone is tying a suture? | Ask the scrub nurse for a pair of scissors, so you are ready if you are asked to cut the sutures. |
|---|---|
| Why always wipe the Betadine® (povidone-iodine) off your patient at the end of the procedure? | The Betadine® can become very irritating and itchy. |

## SURGICAL NOTES

### HISTORY AND PHYSICAL REPORT

The history and physical examination report, better known as the H & P, can make the difference between life and death. You should take this responsibility very **seriously.** Fatal errors can be made in the H & P, including the incorrect diagnosis, the wrong side, the wrong medications, the wrong allergies, and the wrong past surgical history. Operative reports of the patient's past surgical procedures are invaluable! The surgical H & P needs to be both accurate and **concise.** To save space, use − for a negative sign/symptom and + for a positive sign/symptom.

| What are the two words most commonly misspelled in a surgical history note? | 1. guaiac<br>2. abscess |
|---|---|

#### Favorite Trick Questions

| What is the most common intra-operative bladder "tumor"? | Foley catheter |
|---|---|
| Describe a stool with melena. | Melenic—not melanotic |
| Is amylase part of Ranson's criteria? | Amylase is NOT part of Ranson's criteria! |
| Can a patient in shock have "STABLE" vital signs? | Yes—stable vital signs are any vital signs that are not changing! Always say "normal" vital signs, not "stable!" |
| What is the most commonly pimped, yet the rarest, cause of pancreatitis? | Pancreatitis from a scorpion bite (scorpion found on island of Trinidad) |
| Where can you go to obtain an abdominal CT scan on a 600-pound, morbidly obese patient? | The ZOO (used in the past but now is rarely used due to liability) |

## Example H & P (very brief—for illustrative purposes only—see below or next section for abbreviation key):

Mr. Smith is a 22-year-old white man who was in his normal state of excellent health until he noted the onset of periumbilical pain 1 day prior to admission. This pain was followed approximately 4 hours later by pain in his right lower quadrant that any movement exacerbated. + vomiting, anorexia. − fever, urinary tract symptoms, change in bowel habits, constipation, BRBPR, hematemesis, or diarrhea.

Medications: Ibuprofen prn headaches

Allergies: NKDA

PMH: none

PSH: none

SH: ETOH, tobacco

FH: − CA

ROS: − resp disease, − cardiac disease, − renal disease

PE:

HEENT ncat, tms clear

cor nsr, − m,r,g

pulm clear b/l

abd nondistended, + bs, + tender RLQ, + rebound RLQ

rectal guaiac − nl tone, − mass

ext nt, − c,c,e

neuro wnl

LABS: urinalysis (ua) normal. chem 7, PT/PTT, CBC pending

X-RAYS: none

ASSESSMENT: 22 y.o. wm with hx and physical findings of right lower quadrant peritoneal signs consistent with (c/w) appendicitis.

Plan:

Consent

IVF with Lactated Ringer's

IV cefoxitin

To OR for appendectomy

Wilson Tyler cc III/

NKDA = no known drug allergies; PMH = past medical history; PSH = past surgical history; SH = social history; FH = family history; ROS = review of systems, ncat = normocephalic atraumatic; tms = tympanic membranes; cor = heart; m, r, g = murmur, rub, gallop; NSR = normal sinus rhythm; b/l = bilateral; bs = bowel sounds; ext = extremity; nt = nontender; c, c, e = cyanosis, clubbing, or erythema; wnl = within normal limits; cc III = clinical clerk, third year

## PREOP NOTE

The preop note is written in the progress notes the day before the operation.
*Example:*

| | |
|---|---|
| Preop Dx: | Colon CA |
| Labs: | CBC, chem 7, PT/PTT |
| CXR: | − infiltrate |
| Blood: | T & C × 2 units |
| ECG: | NSR, wnl |
| Anesthesia: | Preop completed |
| Consent: | Signed and on front of chart |
| Orders: | |

1. Void OCTOR
2. 1 gm cefoxitin OCTOR
3. Hibiclens scrub this p.m.
4. Bowel prep today
5. NPO p̄ MN

NPO = nothing by mouth; OCTOR = on call to OR; p̄ = after;
MN = midnight

## OP NOTE

The op note is written in the progress note section of the chart in the OR
before the patient is in the PACU (or recovery room).
*Example:*

| | |
|---|---|
| Preop Dx: | Acute appendicitis |
| Postop Dx: | Same |
| Procedure: | Appendectomy |
| | |
| Surgeon: | Halsted |
| Assistants: | Harvey Cushing, Curt Tribble |
| Op findings: | No perforation |
| Anesthesia: | GET |
| °I/O: | 1000 mL LR/uo 600 mL |
| °EBL: | 50 mL |
| Specimen: | Appendix to pathology |
| Drains: | None |
| Complications: | None (if there are complications, ask what you should write) |

To PACU in stable condition

GET = general endotracheal; I/O = ins and outs; EBL = estimated blood
loss; PACU = postanesthesia care unit
°Ask the anesthesiologist or Certified Registered Nurse Anesthetist (CRNA)
for this information.

| | |
|---|---|
| **How do I remember what is in the op note when I am in the OR?** | Remember the acronym PPP SAFE DISC:<br>**P**reop dx<br>**P**ostop dx<br>**P**rocedure<br><br>**S**urgeon (and assistants)<br>**A**nesthesia<br>**F**luids<br>**E**stimated blood loss (EBL)<br><br>**D**rains<br>**IV** Fluids<br>**S**pecimen<br>**C**omplications |

## POSTOP NOTE

The postop note is written on the day of the operation in the progress notes.
*Example:*

| | |
|---|---|
| Procedure: | Appendectomy |
| Neuro: | A and O × 3 |
| V/S: | Stable/afebrile |
| I/O: | 1 L LR/uo 600 mL (urine output) |
| Labs: | postop Hct: 36 |
| PE: | cor RRR |
| | pulm CTA |
| | abd drsg dry & intact |
| Drains: | JP 30 mL serosanguinous fluid |
| Assess: | Stable postop |
| Plan: | |

1. IV hydration
2. 1 g cefoxitin q 8 hr

A and O × 3 = alert and oriented times 3; V/S = vital signs; Hct = hematocrit; RRR = regular rhythm and rate; JP = Jackson-Pratt

## ADMISSION ORDERS

The admission orders are written in the physician orders section of the patient's chart on admission, transfer, or postop.
*Example:*
Admit to 5E Dr. DeBakey

| | |
|---|---|
| Dx: | AAA |
| Condition: | Stable |
| V/S: | q 4 hr or q shift; if postop, q 15 min × 2 hr, then q 1 hr × 4, then q 4 hr |

| | |
|---|---|
| Allergies: | NKDA |
| Activity: | Bedrest or OOB to chair |
| Nursing: | Daily wgt; I/O; change drsg q shift |
| Call HO for: | Temp > 38.5 |
| | UO < 30 mL/hr |
| | SBP > 180 < 90 |
| | DBP > 100 |
| | HR < 60 > 110 |
| Diet: | NPO |
| IVF: | D5 1/2 NS c̄ 20 KCL |
| Drugs: | ANCEF |
| Labs: | CBC |

OOB = out of bed; I/O = ins and outs; HO = House Officer; SBP = systolic blood pressure; DBP = diastolic blood pressure, HR = heart rate; KCL = potassium chloride

## ADMISSION ORDERS/POSTOP ORDERS

AC/DC AVA PAIN DUD

**A**dmit to 5E
**C**are Provider
**D**iagnosis
**C**ondition

**A**llergies
**V**itals
**A**ctivity

**P**ain meds
**A**ntibiotics
**IV**F/Incentive Spirometry
**N**ursing (Drains, etc.)

**D**VT prophylaxis
**U**lcer prophylaxis
**D**iet

## DAILY NOTE—PROGRESS NOTE

Basically a SOAP note, but it is not necessary to write out SOAP. For many reasons, make your notes very OBJECTIVE and, as a student, do not mention discharge because this leads to confusion.
*Example:*
10/1/90 Blue Surgery
POD #4 s/p appendectomy
Day #5 cefoxitin

Pt without c/o
V/S: 120/80 76 12 afebrile (Tmax 38)
I/O: 1000/600
Drains: JP #1 60 last shift
PE:   cor RRR-no m, g, r
       pulm CTA
       abd +BS, +flatus, −rigidity
       ext nt, −cyanosis, −erythema
ASSESS: Stable POD #4 on IV antibiotics
PLAN:
1. Increase PO intake.
2. Increase ambulation.
3. Follow cultures.
Grayson Stuart, cc III/
°°Always date, time, and sign your notes and leave the room for them to be cosigned!
POD = Postop day (The day after operation is POD 1. The day of operation is the operative day. °°But note: antibiotic day #1 is the day the antibiotics were started.)
nt = nontender
cc III = clinical clerk, third year
The following is an acronym for what should be checked on your patient daily before rounding with the surgical team: "AVOID WTE":
**A**ppearance—any subjective complaints
**V**ital signs
**O**utput—urine/drains
**I**ntake—IV/PO
**D**rains—# of/output/character

**W**ound/dressing/weight
**T**emperature
**E**xam—cor, pulm, abd, etc.

## INTENSIVE CARE NOTE

*The note is by systems:*
Neurologic (GCS, MAE)
Pulmonary (vent settings, etc.)
CVS (pressors, swann numbers, etc.)
Heme (CBC)
F.E.N. (Chem 10, nutrition, etc.)
Renal (urine output, BUN, Cr, etc.)
I.D. (Tmax, WBC, antibiotics, etc.)
Assessment
Plan

(CVS = current vital signs; F.E.N. = fluids, electrolytes, nutrition; BUN = blood urea nitrogen; Cr = creatinine; I.D. = incision and drainage)
PE, labs, radiology studies, etc. are included in each section. This is also an excellent way to write progress notes for the very complicated floor patient.

## CLINIC NOTE

Often the clinic note is a letter to the referring doctor. It should always include:
1. Patient name, history #, date
2. Brief hx, current complaints/symptoms
3. PE, labs, x-rays
4. Assessment
5. Plan

**How is a medication prescription written?**

Tylenol® 500 mg tablet
Disp (dispense): 100 tablets
*sig:* 1–2 P.O. q 4 hrs PRN pain

## COMMON ABBREVIATIONS YOU SHOULD KNOW

(Check with *your* hospital for approved abbreviations!)

| | |
|---|---|
| **ā** | Before |
| **AAA** | Abdominal aortic aneurysm, "triple A" |
| **ABD** | Army battle dressing |
| **ABG** | Arterial blood gas |
| **ABI** | Ankle to brachial index |
| **AKA** | Above the knee amputation |
| **A.K.A.** | Also known as |
| **Ao** | Aorta |
| **APR** | Abdominoperineal resection |
| **ARDS** | Acute respiratory distress syndrome |
| **ASA** | Aspirin |
| **AXR** | Abdominal x-ray |
| **B1** | Billroth 1 gastroduodenostomy |
| **B2** | Billroth 2 gastrojejunostomy |
| **BCP** | Birth control pill |
| **BE** | Barium enema |
| **BIH** | Bilateral inguinal hernia |
| **BKA** | Below the knee amputation |
| **BRBPR** | Bright red blood per rectum |
| **BS** | Bowel sounds, breath sounds, blood sugar |
| **BSE** | Breast self-examination |
| **c̄** | With |
| **CA** | Cancer |
| **CABG** | Coronary artery bypass graft ("CABBAGE") |
| **CBC** | Complete blood cell count |

| | |
|---|---|
| **CBD** | Common bile duct |
| **C/O** | Complains of |
| **COPD** | Chronic obstructive pulmonary disease |
| **CP** | Chest pain |
| **CTA** | Clear to auscultation, CT angiogram |
| **CVA** | Cerebral vascular accident, costovertebral angle |
| **CVP** | Central venous pressure |
| **CXR** | Chest x-ray |
| **Dx** | Diagnosis |
| **DDx** | Differential diagnosis |
| **DI** | Diabetes insipidus |
| **DP** | Dorsalis pedalis |
| **DPL** | Diagnostic peritoneal lavage |
| **DPC** | Delayed primary closure |
| **DT** | Delirium tremens |
| **DVT** | Deep venous thrombosis |
| **EBL** | Estimated blood loss |
| **ECG** | Electrocardiogram (also EKG) |
| **ECMO** | Extracorporeal membrane oxygenation |
| **EGD** | Esophagogastroduodenoscopy (UGI scope) |
| **ELAP** | Exploratory laparotomy |
| **EOMI** | Extraocular muscles intact |
| **ERCP** | Endoscopic retrograde cholangiopancreatography |
| **ETOH** | Alcohol |
| **EUA** | Exam under anesthesia |
| **EX LAP** | Exploratory laparotomy |
| **FAP** | Familial adenomatous polyposis |
| **FAST** | Focused abdominal sonogram for trauma |
| **FEN** | Fluids, electrolytes, nutrition |
| **FNA** | Fine needle aspiration |
| **FOBT** | Fecal occult blood test |
| **GCS** | Glasgow Coma Scale |
| **GERD** | Gastroesophageal reflux disease |
| **GET(A)** | General endotracheal (anesthesia) |
| **GU** | Genitourinary |
| **HCT** | Hematocrit |
| **HEENT** | Head, Eyes, Ears, Nose, and Throat |
| **HO** | House officer |
| **IABP** | Intra-aortic balloon pump |
| **IBD** | Inflammatory bowel disease |
| **ICU** | Intensive care unit |
| **I & D** | Incision and drainage |
| **I & O** | Ins and outs, in and out |
| **IMV** | Intermittent mandatory ventilation |
| **IVC** | Inferior vena cava |

| | |
|---|---|
| **IVF** | Intravenous fluids |
| **IVP** | Intravenous pyelography |
| **IVPB** | Intravenous piggyback |
| **JVD** | Jugular venous distention |
| Ⓛ | Left |
| **LAP APPY** | Laparoscopic appendectomy |
| **LAP CHOLE** | Laparoscopic cholecystectomy |
| **LE** | Lower extremity |
| **LES** | Lower esophageal sphincter |
| **LIH** | Left inguinal hernia |
| **LLQ** | Left lower quadrant |
| **LR** | Lactated Ringer's |
| **LUQ** | Left upper quadrant |
| **MAE** | Moving all extremities |
| **MAST** | Military antishock trousers |
| **MEN** | Multiple endocrine neoplasia |
| **MI** | Myocardial infarction |
| **MSO4** | Morphine sulfate |
| **NGT** | Nasogastric tube |
| **NPO** | Nothing per os |
| **NS** | Normal saline |
| **OBR** | Ortho bowel routine |
| **OCTOR** | On call to OR |
| **OOB** | Out of bed |
| **ORIF** | Open reduction internal fixation |
| **p̄** | After |
| **PCWP** | Pulmonary capillary wedge pressure |
| **PE** | Pulmonary embolism, Physical examination |
| **PEEP** | Positive end-expiratory pressure |
| **PEG** | Percutaneous endoscopic gastrostomy (via EGD and skin incision) |
| **PERRL** | Pupils equal and react to light |
| **PFT** | Pulmonary function tests |
| **PICC** | Peripherally inserted central catheter |
| **PGV** | Proximal gastric vagotomy (i.e., leaves fibers to pylorus intact to preserve emptying) |
| **PID** | Pelvic inflammatory disease |
| **PO** | Per os (by mouth) |
| **POD** | Postoperative day |
| **PR** | Per rectum |
| **PRN** | As needed: literally "pro re nata" |
| **PT** | Physical therapy, Patient, Posterior tibial |
| **PTC** | Percutaneous transhepatic cholangiogram (dye injected via a catheter through skin and into dilated intrahepatic bile duct) |

| | |
|---|---|
| **PTCA** | Percutaneous transluminal coronary angioplasty |
| **PTX** | pneumothorax |
| $\overline{\mathbf{q}}$ | Every |
| **®** | Right |
| **RIH** | Right inguinal hernia |
| **RLQ** | Right lower quadrant |
| **Rx** | Treatment |
| **RTC** | Return to clinic |
| $\overline{\mathbf{S}}$ | Without |
| **SBO** | Small bowel obstruction |
| **SCD** | Sequential compression device |
| **SIADH** | Syndrome of inappropriate antidiuretic hormone |
| **SICU** | Surgical intensive care unit |
| **SOAP** | Subjective, objective, assessment, and plan |
| **S/P** | Status post |
| **STSG** | Split thickness skin graft |
| **SVC** | Superior vena cava |
| **Sx** | Symptoms |
| **TEE** | Transesophageal echocardiography |
| **T & C** | Type and cross |
| **T & S** | Type and screen |
| **Tmax** | Maximal temperature |
| **TPN** | Total parenteral nutrition |
| **TURP** | Transurethral resection of the prostate |
| **UE** | Upper extremity |
| **UGI** | Upper gastrointestinal |
| **UO** | Urine output |
| **U/S** | Ultrasound |
| **UTI** | Urinary tract infection |
| **VAD** | Ventricular assist device |
| **VOCTOR** | Void on call to OR |
| **W→D** | Wet-to-dry dressing |
| **XRT** | X-ray therapy |
| **ZE** | Zollinger-Ellison syndrome |
| − | No, negative |
| + | Yes, positive |
| ↑ | Increase, more |
| ↓ | Decrease, less |
| < | Less than |
| > | Greater than |

## GLOSSARY OF SURGICAL TERMS YOU SHOULD KNOW

| | |
|---|---|
| **Abscess** | Localized collection of pus anywhere in the body, surrounded and walled off by damaged and inflamed tissues |

| | |
|---|---|
| **Achlorhydria** | Absence of hydrochloric acid in the stomach |
| **Acholic stool** | Light-colored stool as a result of decreased bile content |
| **Adeno-** | Prefix denoting gland or glands |
| **Adhesion** | Union of two normally separate surfaces |
| **Adnexa** | Adjoining parts; usually means ovary/fallopian tube |
| **Adventitia** | Outer coat of the wall of a vein or artery (composed of loose connective tissue) |
| **Afferent** | Toward |
| **-algia** | Suffix denoting pain |
| **Amaurosis fugax** | Transient visual loss in one eye |
| **Ampulla** | Enlarged or dilated ending of a tube or canal |
| **Analgesic** | Drug that prevents pain |
| **Anastomosis** | Connection between two tubular organs or parts |
| **Anergy** | Lack of response to a specific antigen |
| **Angio-** | Prefix denoting blood or lymph vessels |
| **Anomaly** | Any deviation from the normal (i.e., congenital or developmental defect) |
| **Apnea** | Cessation of breathing |
| **Atelectasis** | Collapse of alveoli |
| **Bariatric** | Weight reduction; bariatric surgery is performed on morbidly obese patients to effect weight loss |

| | |
|---|---|
| **Beta** | β-HCG (pregnancy test) |
| **Bifurcation** | Point at which division into two branches occurs |
| **Bile salts** | Alkaline salts of bile necessary for the emulsification of fats |
| **Bili-** | Prefix denoting bile |
| **Boil** | Tender inflamed area of the skin containing pus |
| **Bovie** | Electrocautery |
| **Calculus** | Stone |
| **Carbuncle** | A collection of boils (furuncle) with multiple drainage channels (CARbuncle = car = big) |
| **Cauterization** | Destruction of tissue by direct application of heat |
| **Celiotomy** | Surgical incision into the peritoneal cavity (laparotomy = celiotomy) |
| **Cephal-** | Prefix denoting the head |
| **Chole-** | Prefix denoting bile |
| **Cholecyst-** | Prefix denoting gallbladder |
| **Choledocho-** | Prefix denoting the common bile duct |
| **Chyme** | Semiliquid mass of food that passes from the stomach to the duodenum |
| **Cleido-** | Prefix denoting the clavicle |
| **Colic** | Intermittent abdominal pain usually indicating pathology in a tubular organ (e.g., small bowel) |

| | |
|---|---|
| **Colloid** | Serum proteins, albumin |
| **Colonoscopy** | Endoscopic examination of the colon |
| **Colostomy** | Surgical operation in which part of the colon is brought through the abdominal wall |
| **Constipation** | Infrequent or difficult passage of stool |
| **Cor pulmonale** | Enlargement of the right ventricle caused by lung disease and resultant pulmonary hypertension |
| **Curettage** | Scraping of the internal surface of an organ or body cavity by means of a spoon-shaped instrument |
| **Cyst** | Abnormal sac or closed cavity lined with epithelium and filled with fluid or semisolid material |
| **Direct bilirubin** | Conjugated bilirubin (indirect = unconjugated) |
| **-dynia** | Suffix denoting pain |
| **Dys-** | Prefix: difficult/painful/abnormal |
| **Dyspareunia** | Painful sexual intercourse |
| **Dysphagia** | Difficulty in swallowing |
| **Ecchymosis** | Bruise |
| **-ectomy** | Suffix denoting the surgical removal of a part or all of an organ (e.g., gastrectomy) |
| **Efferent** | Away from |
| **Endarterectomy** | Surgical removal of an atheroma and the inner part of the vessel wall to relieve an obstruction (carotid endarterectomy = CEA) |

**Enteritis** — Inflammation of the small intestine, usually causing diarrhea

**Enterolysis** — Lysis of peritoneal adhesions; not to be confused with enteroclysis, which is a contrast study of the small bowel

**Eschar** — Scab produced by the action of heat or a corrosive substance on the skin

**Excisional biopsy** — Biopsy with removal of entire tumor (think: Excisional = Entire removal)

**Fascia** — Sheet of strong connective tissue

**Fistula** — Abnormal communication between two hollow, epithelialized organs or between a hollow organ and the exterior (skin)

**Foley** — Bladder catheter

**Frequency** — Abnormally increased frequency (e.g., urinary frequency)

**Furuncle** — Boil, small subcutaneous staphylococcal infection of follicle (think furuncle = follicle < car = carbuncle)

**Gastropexy** — Surgical attachment of the stomach to the abdominal wall

**Hemangioma** — Benign tumor of blood vessels

**Hematemesis** — Vomiting of blood

**Hematoma** — Accumulation of blood within the tissues, which clots to form a solid swelling

**Hemoptysis** — Coughing up blood

**Hemothorax** — Blood in the pleural cavity

**Hepato-** — Prefix denoting the liver

**Herniorrhaphy** — Surgical repair of a hernia

| | |
|---|---|
| **Hesitancy** | Difficulty in initiating urination |
| **Hiatus** | Opening or aperture |
| **Hidradenitis** | Inflammation of the apocrine glands, usually caused by blockage of the glands |
| **Icterus** | Jaundice |
| **Ileostomy** | Surgical connection between the lumen of the ileum and the skin of the abdominal wall |
| **Ileus** | Abnormal intestinal motility (usually paralytic) |
| **Incisional biopsy** | Biopsy with only a "slice" of tumor removed |
| **Induration** | Abnormal hardening of a tissue or organ |
| **Inspissated** | Hard |
| **Intussusception** | Telescoping of one part of the bowel into another |
| **-itis** | Suffix denoting inflammation of an organ, tissue, etc. (e.g., gastritis) |
| **Lap appy** | Appendectomy via laparoscopy |
| **Laparoscopy** | Visualization of the peritoneal cavity via a laparoscope |
| **Laparotomy** | Surgical incision into the abdominal cavity (laparotomy = celiotomy) |
| **Lap chole** | Cholecystectomy via laparoscopy |
| **Leiomyoma** | Benign tumor of smooth muscle |
| **Leiomyosarcoma** | Malignant tumor of smooth muscle |
| **Lieno-** | Denoting the spleen |
| **Melena** | Black tarry stool (melenic, not melanotic stools) |

| | |
|---|---|
| **Necrotic** | Dead |
| **Obstipation** | Failure to pass flatus or stool |
| **Odynophagia** | Painful swallowing |
| **-orraphy** | Surgical repair (e.g., herniorrhaphy) |
| **-ostomy** | General term referring to any operation in which an artificial opening is created between two hollow organs or between one viscera and the abdominal wall for drainage purposes (e.g., colostomy) or for feeding (e.g., gastrostomy) |
| **-otomy** | Suffix denoting surgical incision into an organ |
| **Percutaneous** | Performed through the skin |
| **-pexy** | Suffix denoting fixation |
| **Phleb-** | Prefix denoting vein or relating to veins |
| **Phlebolith** | Calcification in a vein—a vein stone |
| **Phlegmon** | Diffuse inflammation of soft tissue, resulting in a swollen mass of tissue (most commonly seen with pancreatic tissue) |
| **Plica** | Fold or ridge |
| **Plicae circulares** | Circular (complete circles) folds in the lumen of the small intestine (A.K.A. valvulae conniventes) |
| **Plicae semilunares** | Folds (semicircular) into lumen of the large intestine |
| **Pneumaturia** | Passage of urine containing air |
| **Pneumothorax** | Collapse of lung with air in pleural space |
| **Pseudocyst** | Fluid-filled cavity resembling a true cyst, but **not** lined with epithelium |

| | |
|---|---|
| **Pus** | Liquid product of inflammation, consisting of dying leukocytes and other fluids from the inflammatory response |
| **Rubor** | Redness; a classic sign of inflammation |
| **Steatorrhea** | Fatty stools as a result of decreased fat absorption |
| **Stenosis** | Abnormal narrowing of a passage or opening |
| **Sterile field** | Area covered by sterile drapes or prepped in sterile fashion using antiseptics (e.g., Betadine) |
| **Succus** | Fluid (e.g., succus entericus is fluid from the bowel lumen) |
| **Tenesmus** | Urge to defecate with ineffectual (and often painful) straining |
| **Thoracotomy** | Surgical opening of the chest cavity |
| **Transect** | To divide transversely (to cut in half) |
| **Trendelenburg** | Patient posture with pelvis higher than the head, inclined about 45° (A.K.A. "Headdownenburg") |
| **Urgency** | Sudden strong urge to urinate; often seen with a UTI |
| **Wet-to-dry dressing** | Damp gauze dressing placed on a wound and removed after the dressing dries to the wound, providing microdébridement |

## SURGERY SIGNS, TRIADS, ETC., YOU SHOULD KNOW

| | |
|---|---|
| **What are the A, B, C, Ds of melanoma?** | Signs of melanoma: **A**symmetric **B**order irregularities **C**olor variation **D**iameter > 0.6 cm **and D**ark black color |

**What is the Allen's test?**

Test for patency of ulnar artery prior to placing a radial arterial line or performing an ABG. Simply stated, occlude both ulnar and radial arteries with the examiner's fingers with the patient's hand in a fist; open fist and release ulnar artery occlusion and assess blood flow to hand

**Define the following terms:**

**Ballance's sign**

Constant dullness to percussion in the left flank/LUQ and resonance to percussion in the right flank seen with splenic rupture/hematoma

**Barrett's esophagus**

Columnar metaplasia of the distal esophagus (GERD related)

**Battle's sign**

Ecchymosis over the mastoid process in patients with basilar skull fractures

**Beck's triad**

Seen in patients with cardiac tamponade:
1. JVD
2. Decreased or muffled heart sounds
3. Decreased blood pressure

**Bergman's triad**

Seen with fat emboli syndrome:
1. Mental status changes
2. Petechiae (often in the axilla/thorax)
3. Dyspnea

**Blumer's shelf**

Metastatic disease to the rectouterine (pouch of Douglas) or rectovesical pouch creating a "shelf" that is palpable on rectal examination

**Boas' sign**

Right subscapular pain resulting from cholelithiasis

**Borchardt's triad**

Seen with gastric volvulus:
1. Emesis followed by no emesis
2. Epigastric distention
3. Failure to pass an NgT

**Carcinoid triad**

Seen with carcinoid syndrome:
1. Flushing
2. Diarrhea
3. Right-sided heart failure (FDR)

**Charcot's triad**

Seen with cholangitis:
1. Fever (chills)
2. Jaundice
3. Right upper quadrant pain
(Pronounced "char-cows")

**Chvostek's sign**

Twitching of facial muscles upon tapping the facial nerve in patients with hypocalcemia (think: **Ch**vostek's = **Ch**eek)

**Courvoisier's law**

An enlarged nontender gallbladder seen with obstruction of the common bile duct, most commonly with pancreatic cancer

**Note:** not seen with acute cholecystitis because the gallbladder is scarred secondary to chronic cholelithiasis. (pronounced "koor-vwah-ze-ay")

**Cullen's sign**     Bluish discoloration of the periumbilical area due to retroperitoneal hemorrhage tracking around to the anterior abdominal wall through fascial planes (e.g., acute hemorrhagic pancreatitis)

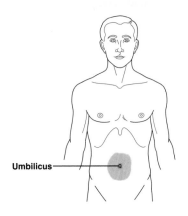

Umbilicus

**Cushing's triad**     Signs of increased intracranial pressure:
1. Hypertension
2. Bradycardia
3. Irregular respirations

**Dance's sign**     Empty right lower quadrant in children with ileocecal intussusception

**Fothergill's sign**     Used to differentiate an intra-abdominal mass from one in the abdominal wall; if mass is felt while there is tension on the musculature, then it is in the wall (i.e., sitting halfway upright)

**Fox's sign**     Ecchymosis of inguinal ligament seen with retroperitoneal bleeding

**Goodsall's rule**     Anal fistulae course in a straight path anteriorly and a curved path posteriorly from midline (think of a dog with a straight anterior nose and a curved posterior tail)

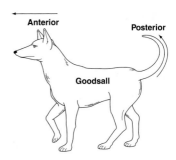

**Grey Turner's sign**   Ecchymosis or discoloration of the flank in patients with retroperitoneal hemorrhage as a result of dissecting blood from the retroperitoneum (think: turn side-to-side = flank)

**Hamman's sign/crunch**   Crunching sound on auscultation of the heart resulting from emphysematous mediastinum, seen with Boerhaave's syndrome, pneumomediastinum, etc.

**Homans' sign**   Calf pain on forced dorsiflexion of the foot in patients with DVT

**Howship-Romberg sign**   Pain along the inner aspect of the thigh; seen with an obturator hernia as the result of nerve compression

**Kehr's sign**   Severe left shoulder pain in patients with splenic rupture (as a result of referred pain from diaphragmatic irritation)

**Kelly's sign**   Visible peristalsis of the ureter in response to squeezing or retraction; used to identify the ureter during surgery

**Krukenberg tumor**   Metastatic tumor to the ovary (classically from gastric cancer)

**Laplace's law**   Wall tension = pressure × radius (thus, the colon perforates preferentially at the cecum because of the increased radius and resultant increased wall tension)

| | |
|---|---|
| **McBurney's point** | One-third the distance from the anterior iliac spine to the umbilicus on a line connecting the two |
| **McBurney's sign** | Tenderness at McBurney's point in patients with appendicitis |
| **Meckel's diverticulum rule of 2s** | Two percent of the population have a Meckel's diverticulum, 2 of those are symptomatic, and they occur within approximately 2 feet of the ileocecal valve |
| **Mittelschmerz** | Lower quadrant pain due to ovulation |
| **Murphy's sign** | Cessation of inspiration while palpating under the right costal margin; the patient cannot continue to inspire deeply because it brings an inflamed gallbladder under pressure (seen in acute cholecystitis) |
| **Obturator sign** | Pain upon internal rotation of the leg with the hip and knee flexed; seen in patients with appendicitis/pelvic abscess |

| | |
|---|---|
| **Pheochromocytoma SYMPTOMS triad** | Think of the first three letters in the word pheochromocytoma—"P-H-E": **P**alpitations **H**eadache **E**pisodic diaphoresis |
| **Pheochromocytoma rule of 10s** | 10% bilateral, 10% malignant, 10% in children, 10% extra-adrenal, 10% have multiple tumors |

**Psoas sign**

Pain elicited by extending the hip with the knee in full extension, seen with appendicitis and psoas inflammation

**Raccoon eyes**

Bilateral black eyes as a result of basilar skull fracture

**Reynold's pentad**

1. Fever
2. Jaundice
3. Right upper quadrant pain
4. Mental status changes
5. Shock/sepsis

Thus, Charcot's triad plus # 4 and # 5; seen in patients with **suppurative** cholangitis

**Rovsing's sign**

Palpation of the left lower quadrant resulting in pain in the right lower quadrant; seen in appendicitis

**Saint's triad**

1. Cholelithiasis
2. Hiatal hernia
3. Diverticular disease

**Silk glove sign**

Indirect hernia sac in the pediatric patient; the sac feels like a finger of a silk glove when rolled under the examining finger

| | |
|---|---|
| **Sister Mary Joseph's sign (A.K.A. Sister Mary Joseph's node)** | Metastatic tumor to umbilical lymph node(s) |
| **Virchow's node** | Metastatic tumor to left supraclavicular node (classically due to gastric cancer) |
| **Virchow's triad** | Risk factors for thrombosis: <br> 1. Stasis <br> 2. Abnormal endothelium <br> 3. Hypercoagulability |
| **Trousseau's sign** | Carpal spasm after occlusion of blood to the forearm with a BP cuff in patients with hypocalcemia |
| **Valentino's sign** | Right lower quadrant pain from a perforated peptic ulcer due to succus/pus draining into the RLQ |
| **Westermark's sign** | Decreased pulmonary vascular markings on CXR in a patient with pulmonary embolus |
| **Whipple's triad** | Evidence for insulinoma: <br> 1. Hypoglycemia (< 50) <br> 2. CNS and vasomotor symptoms (e.g., syncope, diaphoresis) <br> 3. Relief of symptoms with administration of glucose |

---

# Chapter 2

# Surgical Syndromes

| | |
|---|---|
| **What is afferent loop syndrome?** | Obstruction of the afferent loop of a Billroth II gastrojejunostomy |
| **What does ARDS stand for?** | **A**cute **R**espiratory **D**istress **S**yndrome (poor oxygenation caused by leaky capillaries) |

**What is blind loop syndrome?**

Bacterial overgrowth of intestine caused by stasis

**What is Boerhaave's syndrome?**

Esophageal perforation

**What is Budd-Chiari syndrome?**

Thrombosis of hepatic veins

**What is carcinoid syndrome?**

Syndrome of "B FDR":
**B**ronchospasm
**F**lushing
**D**iarrhea
**R**ight-sided heart failure (caused by factors released by carcinoid tumor)

**What is compartment syndrome?**

Compartmental hypertension caused by edema, resulting in muscle necrosis of the lower extremity, seen in the calf; patient may have a distal pulse

**What is Cushing's syndrome?**

Excessive cortisol production

**What is dumping syndrome?**

Delivery of a large amount of hyperosmolar chyme into the small bowel, usually after vagotomy and a gastric drainage procedure (pyloroplasty/gastrojejunostomy); results in autonomic instability, abdominal pain, and diarrhea

**What is Fitz-Hugh-Curtis syndrome?**

Perihepatic gonorrhea infection

**What is Gardner's syndrome?**

GI polyps and associated findings of **S**ebaceous cysts, **O**steomas, and **D**esmoid tumors (**SOD**); polyps have high malignancy potential (think: a Gardner plants **SOD**)

**What is HITT syndrome?**

**H**eparin-**I**nduced **T**hrombocytopenic **T**hrombosis syndrome: Heparin-induced platelet antibodies cause platelets to thrombose vessels, often resulting in loss of limb or life (also known as "white clot syndrome").

| | |
|---|---|
| **What is Leriche's syndrome?** | **C**laudication of buttocks, thighs, **I**mpotence, **A**trophy of legs (seen with iliac occlusive disease) (Think: **CIA**) |
| **What is Mallory-Weiss syndrome?** | Post emesis/retching tears in the gastric mucosa (near gastroesophageal junction) |
| **What is Mendelson's syndrome?** | Chemical pneumonitis after aspiration of gastric contents |
| **What is Mirizzi's syndrome?** | Extrinsic obstruction of the common hepatic bile duct from a cystic duct gallstone |
| **What is Munchausen syndrome?** | Self-induced illness |
| **What is Ogilvie's syndrome?** | Massive **nonobstructive** colonic dilatation |
| **What is Peutz-Jeghers syndrome?** | Benign GI polyps and buccal pigmentation (think: **P**eutz = **P**igmentation) |
| **What is Plummer-Vinson syndrome?** | Syndrome of: 1. Esophageal web 2. Iron-deficiency anemia 3. Dysphagia 4. Spoon-shaped nails 5. Atrophic oral and tongue mucosa Usually occurs in elderly women; 10% develop squamous cell carcinoma |
| **What is RED reaction syndrome?** | Syndrome of rapid vancomycin infusion, resulting in skin erythema |
| **What is refeeding syndrome?** | Hypokalemia, hypomagnesemia, and hypophosphatemia after refeeding a starved patient |
| **What is Rendu-Osler-Weber (ROW) syndrome?** | Syndrome of GI tract telangiectasia/A-V malformations |
| **What is short-gut syndrome?** | Malnutrition resulting from less than 100 cm of viable small bowel |
| **What is SIADH?** | **S**yndrome of **I**nappropriate **A**nti**D**iuretic **H**ormone (think: **I**nappropriately **I**ncreased ADH) |

| | |
|---|---|
| **What is another name for Sipple's syndrome?** | MEN II |
| **What is superior vena cava (SVC) syndrome?** | Obstruction of the SVC (e.g., by tumor, thrombosis) |
| **What is thoracic outlet syndrome?** | Compression of the structures exiting from the thoracic outlet |
| **What is Tietze's syndrome?** | Costochondritis of rib cartilage; aseptic (treat with NSAIDs) |
| **What is toxic shock syndrome?** | *Staphylococcus aureus* toxin-induced syndrome marked by fever, hypotension, organ failure, and **rash** (desquamation—especially palms and soles) |
| **What is Trousseau's syndrome?** | Syndrome of deep venous thrombosis (DVT) associated with carcinoma |
| **What is another name for Wermer's syndrome?** | MEN I |
| **What is Zollinger-Ellison syndrome?** | Gastrinoma and PUD |

# Chapter 3

# Surgical Most Commons

| | |
|---|---|
| **What is the most common:** | |
| **Indication for surgery with Crohn's disease?** | Small bowel obstruction (SBO) |
| **Type of melanoma?** | Superficial spreading |
| **Type of breast cancer?** | Infiltrating ductal |
| **Site of breast cancer?** | Upper outer quadrant |

| | |
|---|---|
| **Vessel involved with a bleeding duodenal ulcer?** | Gastroduodenal artery |
| **Cause of common bile duct obstruction?** | Choledocholithiasis |
| **Cause of cholangitis?** | Bile duct obstruction resulting from choledocholithiasis |
| **Cause of pancreatitis?** | EtOH |
| **Bacteria in stool?** | *Bacteroides fragilis* ("B. frag") |
| **Cause of SBO in adults in the United States?** | Adhesions |
| **Cause of SBO in children?** | Hernias |
| **Cause of emergency abdominal surgery in the United States?** | Acute appendicitis |
| **Site of GI carcinoids?** | Appendix |
| **Abdominal x-ray (AXR) finding with SBO?** | Air-fluid levels |
| **Electrolyte deficiency causing ileus?** | Hypokalemia |
| **Cause of transfusion hemolysis?** | Clerical error |
| **Cause of blood transfusion resulting in death?** | Clerical error (wrong blood types) |
| **Site of distant metastasis of sarcoma?** | Lungs |
| **Cause of shock in a surgical patient?** | Hypovolemia |
| **Cause of esophageal perforation?** | Iatrogenic |

| | |
|---|---|
| **Position of anal fissure?** | Posterior |
| **Cause of large bowel obstruction?** | Colon cancer |
| **Type of colonic volvulus?** | Sigmoid volvulus |
| **Cause of fever <48 post-operative hours?** | Atelectasis |
| **Bacterial cause of urinary tract infection (UTI)?** | *Escherichia coli* |
| **Chest x-ray (CXR) finding with traumatic thoracic aortic injury?** | Widened mediastinum |
| **Abdominal organ injured in blunt abdominal trauma?** | Liver (not the spleen, as noted in recent studies!) |
| **Abdominal organ injured in penetrating abdominal trauma?** | Small bowel |
| **Benign tumor of the liver?** | Hemangioma |
| **Malignancy of the liver?** | Mets |
| **Pneumonia in the ICU?** | Gram-negative bacteria |
| **Cause of epidural hematoma?** | Middle meningeal artery injury |
| **Cause of lower GI bleeding?** | Upper GI bleeding |
| **Hernia?** | Inguinal hernia (right > left) |
| **Cause of esophageal laceration?** | Iatrogenic instrumentation (e.g., EGD) |
| **Cancer in females?** | Lung cancer |
| **Cancer in males?** | Prostate cancer |

| | |
|---|---|
| **Type of cancer causing DEATH in males and females?** | LUNG cancer |
| **Cause of free peritoneal air?** | Perforated PUD |
| **Symptom with gastric cancer?** | Weight loss |
| **Site of colon cancer hematogenous mets?** | Liver |

---

# Chapter 4

# Surgical Percentages

| | |
|---|---|
| **What percentage of people in the United States will develop acute appendicitis?** | Approximately 7% |
| **What is the acceptable percentage of normal appendices removed with the preoperative diagnosis of appendicitis?** | Up to 20%; it is better to remove some normal appendices than to miss a case of acute appendicitis, which could result in a ruptured appendix |
| **In what percentage of cases can ultrasound diagnose cholelithiasis?** | 98% |
| **In what percentage of cases does a lower GI bleed stop spontaneously?** | Approximately 90% |
| **In what percentage of cases does a UGI bleed stop spontaneously?** | Approximately 80% |

| | |
|---|---|
| **What percentage of patients undergoing laparotomy develop a postoperative small bowel obstruction at some time later?** | Approximately 5% |
| **What percentage of American women develop breast cancer?** | 10% |
| **What percentage of patients with acute appendicitis will have a radiopaque fecalith on abdominal x-ray (AXR)?** | Only about 5% |
| **What percentage of patients with gallstones will have radi-opaque gallstones on AXR?** | Approximately 10% |
| **What percentage of kidney stones are radiopaque on AXR?** | Approximately 90% |
| **At 6 weeks, wounds have achieved what percentage of their total tensile strength?** | Approximately 90% |
| **What percentage of patients with ARDS will die?** | Approximately 40% |
| **What percentage of the population has a Meckel's diverticulum?** | 2% |
| **What is the risk of appendiceal rupture 24 hours after the onset of symptoms?** | Approximately 25% |
| **What percentage of colonic villous adenomas contain cancer?** | Approximately 40% (think: VILLous = VILLain) |
| **One unit of packed RBCs increases the hematocrit by how much?** | 3% |

| | |
|---|---|
| **Additional 1 liter by nasal cannula increases FIO$_2$ by how much?** | 3% |
| **What percentage of porcelain gallbladders will contain cancer?** | Approximately 50% |
| **What percentage of patients with gastric ulcers have cancer on biopsy?** | 10% |

---

# Chapter 5     Surgical History

**Identify the following:**

| | |
|---|---|
| **First to use antiseptic (carbolic acid)** | Lister (British surgeon) |
| **First to advocate surgical gloves** | Halsted (made by GOODYEAR®) |
| **Father of antiseptic surgery** | Lister (1827–1912) |
| **Father of American neurosurgery** | Harvey Cushing |
| **Developer of vascular grafts** | DeBakey (his wife hand sewed them!) |
| **Developed electrocautery for surgery with Dr. Cushing** | Bovie (1928) |
| **The Mayo Brothers' scrub nurse** | Sister Joseph (of St. Mary's hospital) |

| | |
|---|---|
| **Developed the cardio-pulmonary bypass** | Gibbon |

**Identify the year the following procedures were first performed and the physician who performed them:**

| | |
|---|---|
| **Renal transplant** | 1954; Murray |
| **CABG** | 1962; Sabiston |
| **CEA** | 1953; DeBakey |
| **Heart transplant** | 1967; Barnard |
| **Artificial heart valve** | 1960; Starr |
| **Liver transplant** | 1963; Starzl |
| **Total parenteral nutrition (TPN)** | 1968; Rhoades |
| **Vascular anastomosis** | 1902; Carrel |
| **Lung transplant** | 1964; Hardy |
| **Pancreatic transplant** | 1966; Najarian |
| **Heart-lung transplant** | 1982; Reitz |
| **AAA rx** | 1951; Dubost |
| **First lap chole** | 1987; Mouret and Dubois in France |
| **First appendectomy** | 1848; Hancock |
| **First gastric resection** | 1881; Billroth |
| **First lap appy** | 1983; Semm (GYN DOCTOR!) |
| **Who was the only surgeon to win the Pulitzer Prize?** | Cushing (for his biography on Osler) |

| Which surgeons have won the Nobel Prize? (9) | Kocher 1909 (thyroid surgery)<br>Gullstrand 1911 (ophthalmology)<br>Carrel 1912 (transplantation/vascular anastomosis)<br>Bárány 1914 (inner ear disease-vestibular disease)<br>Banting 1922 (insulin)<br>Hess 1949 (brain physiology)<br>Forssman 1956 (cardiac catheterization)<br>Huggins 1966 (oncology)<br>Murray 1990 (kidney transplant) |
|---|---|
| When was the Dakin solution developed? | World War I; Dakin developed the solution to treat dirty combat wounds |

# Chapter 6

# Surgical Instruments

| How should a pair of scissors/needle-driver/clamp be held? | With the thumb and **fourth** finger, using the index finger to steady |
|---|---|

| Is it better to hold the skin with a DeBakey or an Adson, or toothed, forcep? | Better to use an Adson, or toothed, pickup as it is better to cut the skin rather than crush it! |
|---|---|
| What helps steady the scissor- or Bovie-hand? | Resting it on the opposite hand |

| What can be done to guarantee that you do not cut the knot when cutting sutures? | Slide the scissors down to the knot, then turn the scissors at a 45° angle, and cut. |
|---|---|

**How should a pair of forceps be held?**

Like a pencil

**What are forceps also known as?**

"Pickups"

**Identify the following instruments:**

Forcep

DeBakey pickup

Adson pickup

Iris scissors

Bandage scissors

Needle-driver

Right-angle clamp

Kelly clamp

Babcock clamp

Tonsil clamp

Metzenbaum scissors

Mayo scissors (heavy scissors)

**Straight**          **Curved**

GIA stapler

**What does "GIA" stand for?**    **G**astro **I**ntestinal **A**nastomosis

TA stapler

**What does "TA" stand for?**    **T**horaco **A**bdominal

EEA stapler

**What does "EEA" stand for?**     End-to-End Anastomosis

Pott's scissors

Allis clamp

Kocher clamp, for very thick tissue
(e.g., fascia)

**Define the following scalpel
blades:**

Number 10

Number 11

Number 15

**Bovie electrocautery**

**Yankauer suction (sucker)**

## RETRACTORS (YOU WILL GET TO KNOW THEM WELL!)

**What does it mean to "toe in" the retractor?**

To angle the tip of the retractor in by angling the retractor handle up

Deaver retractor

Sweetheart retractor (Harrington)

Army–Navy retractor

**Weitlaner** retractor also known as a "WHEATY" (self-retaining retractor; sorry, operates without a student!)

Richardson retractor also known as a "RICH"

**What is a "malleable" retractor?**

A metal retractor that can be bent to customize to the situation at hand

# Chapter 7

# Sutures and Stitches

## SUTURE MATERIALS

### GENERAL INFORMATION

**What is a suture?**

Any strand of material used to ligate blood vessels or to approximate tissues

**How are sutures sized?**

By diameter; stated as a number of O's: the higher the number of O's, the smaller the diameter (e.g., 2-O suture has a larger diameter than 5-O suture)

| | |
|---|---|
| **Which is thicker, 1-O suture or 3-O suture?** | 1-O suture (pronounced "one oh") |

## CLASSIFICATION

| | |
|---|---|
| **What are the two most basic suture types?** | Absorbable and nonabsorbable |
| **What is an absorbable suture?** | The suture is completely broken down by the body (dissolving suture). |
| **What is a nonabsorbable suture?** | The suture is not broken down (permanent suture). |

## SUTURES

### Catgut

| | |
|---|---|
| **What are "catgut" sutures made of?** | Purified collagen fibers from the intestines of healthy cows or sheep (sorry, no cats) |
| **What are the two types of gut sutures?** | Plain and chromic |
| **What is the difference between plain and chromic gut?** | Chromic gut is treated with chromium salts (chromium trioxide), which results in more collagen crosslinks, making the suture more resistant to breakdown by the body. |

### Vicryl® Suture

| | |
|---|---|
| **What is it?** | Absorbable, braided, multifilamentous copolymer of lactide and glycoside |
| **How long does it retain its strength?** | 60% at 2 weeks, 8% at 4 weeks |
| **Should you ever use PURPLE-colored Vicryl® for skin closure?** | NO—it may cause purple tattooing. |

### PDS®

| | |
|---|---|
| **What is it?** | Absorbable, monofilament polymer of polydioxanone (absorbable fishing line) |
| **How long does it maintain its tensile strength?** | 70% to 74% at 2 weeks, 50% to 58% at 4 weeks, 25% to 41% at 6 weeks |

| | |
|---|---|
| **How long does it take to complete absorption?** | 180 days (6 months) |
| **What is silk?** | Braided protein filaments spun by the silkworm larva; known as a nonabsorbable suture |
| **What is Prolene?** | Nonabsorbable suture (used for vascular anastomoses, hernias, abdominal fascial closure) |
| **What is nylon?** | Nonabsorbable "fishing line" |
| **What is monocryl?** | **Ab**sorbable monofilament |

## WOUND CLOSURE

### GENERAL INFORMATION

| | |
|---|---|
| **What is the purpose of a suture closure?** | To approximate divided tissues to enhance wound healing |
| **What are the three types of wound healing?** | 1. Primary closure (intention) 2. Secondary intention 3. Tertiary intention (**D**elayed **P**rimary **C**losure = DPC) |
| **What is primary intention?** | When the edges of a clean wound are closed in some manner immediately (e.g., suture, Steri-Strips®, staples) |
| **What is secondary intention?** | When a wound is allowed to remain open and heal by granulation, epithelization, and contraction—used for dirty wounds, otherwise an abscess can form |
| **What is tertiary intention?** | When a wound is allowed to remain open for a time and then closed, allowing for debridement and other wound care to reduce bacterial counts prior to closure (i.e., delayed primary closure) |
| **What is another term for tertiary intention?** | DPC = **D**elayed **P**rimary **C**losure |

**Classic time to wait before closing an open abdominal wound by DPC?**

5 days

**What rule is constantly told to medical students about wound closure?**

"Approximate, don't strangulate!" Translation: If sutures are pulled too tight, then the tissue becomes ischemic as the blood supply is decreased, resulting in necrosis, infection, or both.

## SUTURE TECHNIQUES

**What is a taper-point needle?**

Round body, leaves a round hole in tissue (spreads without cutting tissue)

**What is it used for?**

Suturing of soft tissues other than skin (e.g., GI tract, muscle, nerve, peritoneum, fascia)

**What is a conventional cutting needle?**

Triangular body with the sharp edge toward the inner circumference; leaves a triangular hole in tissue

**What are its uses?**

Suturing of **skin**

**What is a simple interrupted stitch?**

| | |
|---|---|
| **What is a vertical mattress stitch?** | A simple stitch is made, the needle is reversed, and a small bite is taken from each wound edge; the knot ends up on one side of the wound. |

| | |
|---|---|
| **What is the vertical mattress stitch also known as?** | Far-far, near-near stitch—oriented perpendicular to wound |
| **What is it used for?** | Difficult-to-approximate skin edges; everts tissue well |
| **What is a horizontal mattress stitch?** | A simple stitch is made, the needle is reversed, and the same size bite is taken again—oriented parallel to wound. |

| | |
|---|---|
| **What is a simple running (continuous) stitch?** | Stitches made in succession without knotting each stitch |

**What is a subcuticular stitch?**

A stitch (usually running) placed just underneath the epidermis, can be either absorbable or nonabsorbable (pull-out stitch if nonabsorbable)

**What is a pursestring suture?**

A stitch that encircles a tube perforating a hollow viscus (e.g., gastrostomy tube), allowing the hole to be drawn tight and thus preventing leakage

**What are metallic skin staples?**

**What is a staple removal device?**

**What is a gastrointestinal anastomosis (GIA) device?**

A stapling device that lays two rows of small staples in a hemostatic row and **automatically cuts** in between them

**What is a suture ligature (A.K.A. stick tie)?**

The suture is anchored by passing it through the vessel **on a needle** before wrapping it around and occluding the vessel; it prevents slippage of knot-use on larger vessels.

**What is a retention suture?**

A large suture (No. 2) that is full thickness through the entire abdominal wall except the peritoneum. It is used to buttress an abdominal wound at risk for dehiscence.

**What is a pop-off suture?**

A suture that is not permanently swaged to the needle, allowing the surgeon to "pop" off the needle from the suture without cutting the suture

# Chapter 8

# Surgical Knot Tying

## KNOTS AND EARS

**What is the basic surgical knot?**

The square knot

**What is the first knot that should be mastered?**

Instrument knot

**What is a "surgeon's knot"?**

A double-wrap throw followed by single square knot throws

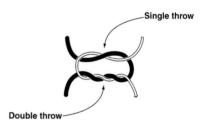

Single throw

Double throw

**How many (correct) throws are necessary to ensure that your knots do not slip?**

As many as the attending surgeon wants

**What are the guidelines for the number of minimal throws needed?**

Depends on the suture material
**Silk**—3
**Gut**—4
**Vicryl®, Dexon®, other braided synthetics**—4
**Nylon, polyester, polypropylene, PDS, Maxon**—6

**How long should the ears of the knot be cut?**

Some guidelines are:
**Silk vessel ties**—1 to 2 mm
**Abdominal fascia closure**—5 mm

**Skin sutures, drain sutures**—5 to 10 mm (makes them easier to find and remove)

**When should skin sutures be removed?**

As soon as the wound has healed enough to withstand expected mechanical trauma

Any stitch left in more than approximately 10 days will leave a scar

Guidelines are:

**Face**—3 to 5 days

**Extremities**—10 days

**Joints**—10–14 days

**Back**—14 days

**Abdomen**—7 days

**How can strength be added to an incision during and after suture removal?**

With Steri-Strips®

**In general, in which group of patients should skin sutures be left in longer than normal?**

Patients on steroids

**How should the sutures be cut?**

Use the tips of the scissors to avoid cutting other tissues.

Try to remove the cut ends (less foreign material decreases risk of infection).

Rest the scissor-hand on the non-scissor-hand to steady.

**How is an instrument knot tied?**

Always start with a double wrap, known as a "surgeon's knot" and then use a single wrap, pulling the suture in the opposite directions after every "throw."

**Does a student need to know a one-hand tie?**

No! Master the two-hand tie and the instrument tie.

## Instrument Tie

Then continue with single throws.

## TWO-HAND TIE

**What is the basic position for the two-hand tie?**

The "C" position, formed by the thumb and index finger; the suture will **alternate** over the thumb and then the index finger for each throw

**How is a two-hand knot tied?**

First, use the index finger to lead.

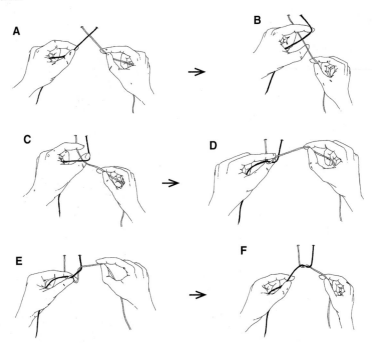

Then use thumb to lead:

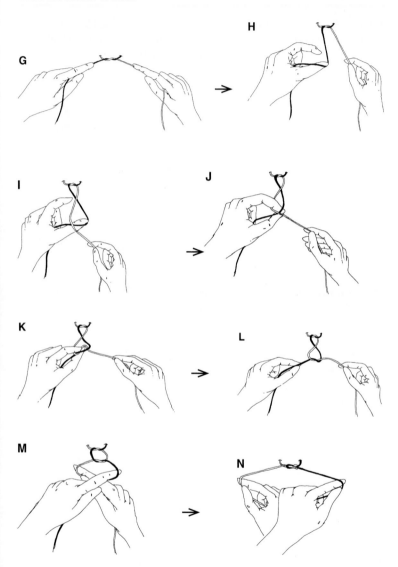

Ask a resident or intern to help you after you have tried for awhile.

# Chapter 9

# Procedures for the Surgical Ward and Clinic

## COMMON PROCEDURES

**How do you place a peripheral intravenous (IV) catheter?**

1. Place a tourniquet above the site.
2. Use alcohol antiseptic.
3. Place IV into vein with "flash" of blood.
4. Remove inner needle while advancing IV catheter.
5. Secure with tape.

**How do you draw blood from the femoral vein?**

Remember **NAVEL.** In the lateral to medial direction—**N**erve, **A**rtery, **V**ein, **E**mpty space, **L**ymphatics—and thus place needle medial to the femoral pulse.

Femoral nerve
Femoral artery
Femoral vein
Saphenous vein

**How do you remove staples?**

Use a staple remover (see Chapter 7), then place Steri-Strips®.

**How do you remove stitches?**

1. Cut the suture next to the knot.
2. Pull end of suture out by holding onto the knot.
3. Place Steri-Strips®.

**How do you place Steri-Strips®?**

1. Dry the skin edges of the wound.
2. Place adhesive (e.g., benzoin).
3. With the Adson pickup or with your fingers, place strips to gently appose epidermis (avoid any tension or blisters will appear!).

HRF '04

**How do you place a Foley catheter?**

1. Stay sterile.
2. Apply Betadine® to the urethral opening (meatus).
3. Lubricate the catheter.
4. Place catheter into urethra.
5. As soon as urine returns, inflate balloon with saline (balloon size is given in cc on the catheter).

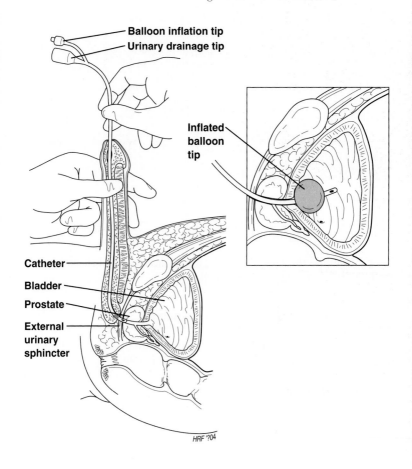

Balloon inflation tip
Urinary drainage tip
Inflated balloon tip
Catheter
Bladder
Prostate
External urinary sphincter

HRF '04

**How do you find the urethra in females?**

First find the clitoris and clitoral hood. The urethra is just below these structures. Wiping a Betadine®-soaked sponge over this area will often result in having the urethra "wink" open.

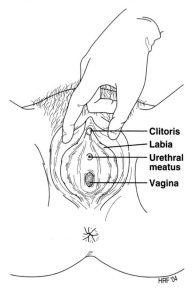

- Clitoris
- Labia
- Urethral meatus
- Vagina

HRF '04

**Can you inflate the Foley balloon before you get urine return?**

No, you might blow up a balloon in the urethra!

## NASOGASTRIC TUBE (NGT) PROCEDURES

**How do you determine how much of the NGT should be advanced into the body for the correct position?**

A rough guide: from nose, around ear, to 5 cm below the xiphoid

**How do you place the NGT in a nare?**

First place lubrication (e.g., Surgilube®) then place NGT straight back—not up or down!

**What is the best neck position for advancing the NGT?**

Neck FLEXED! Also have the patient drink some water (using a straw).

**What if there is 3 liters/24 hours drainage from an NGT?**

Think DUODENUM—the NGT may be in the duodenum and not the stomach! Check an x-ray.

**How can you clinically confirm that an NGT is in the stomach?**

Use a Toomey syringe to "inject" air while listening over the stomach with a stethoscope. You will hear the "swish" if the NGT is in place.

**How do you tape an NGT?**

**What MUST you obtain and examine before using an NGT for feeding?**

A LOWER chest/upper abdominal x-ray to absolutely verify placement into the stomach and NOT the LUNG—patients have died from pulmonary tube feeding!

**How do you draw a radial arterial blood gas (ABG)?**

Feel for the pulse and advance directly into the artery. ABG syringes do not have to have the plunger withdrawn manually.

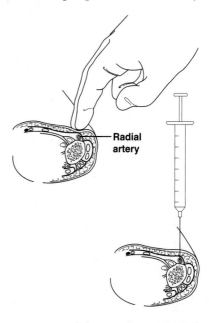

**How do you drain an abscess?**

By incision and drainage (or an "I & D"). After using local anesthetic, use a number 11 blade to incise and then open the abscess pocket. Large abscesses are best drained with a cruciate incision or removal of a piece of skin. Pack the open wound.

**How do you remove an epidermal cyst or sebaceous cyst?**

1. Administer local anesthetic.
2. Remove the ellipse of skin overlying the cyst, including the pore.
3. Remove the cyst with the encompassing sac lining.

# Chapter 10      **Incisions**

**If a patient has an old incision, is it best to make a subsequent incision next to or through the old incision?**

Through the old incision, or excise the old incision, because it has scar tissue that limits the amount of collaterals that would be needed to heal an incision placed next to it

**What is used to incise the epidermis?**

Scalpel blade

**What is used to incise the dermis?**

Scalpel or electrocautery

**Describe the following incisions:**

**Kocher**

Right subcostal incision for open cholecystectomy:

**Midline laparotomy**

Incision down the middle of abdomen along and through the linea alba:

**McBurney's**

Small, oblique right lower quadrant incision for an appendectomy through McBurney's point (one-third from the anterior superior iliac spine to the umbilicus):

**Rocky-Davis**
Like a McBurney's incision except transverse (straight across):

**Pfannenstiel**
Low transverse abdominal incision with retraction of the rectus muscles laterally; most often used for gynecologic procedures:

**Kidney transplant**
Lower quadrant; kidney placed extraperitoneally:

**Liver transplant**

Chevron or Mercedes-Benz® incision in the upper abdomen:

**Median sternotomy**

Midline sternotomy incision for heart procedures; less painful than a lateral thoracotomy:

**Thoracotomy**

Usually through the fourth or fifth intercostal space; may be anterior or posterior lateral incisions
Very painful, but many are performed with muscle sparing (muscle retraction and not muscle transection):

**CEA (carotid endarterectomy)**

Incision down anterior border of the sternocleidomastoid muscle to expose the carotid:

**Inguinal hernia repair (open)**

**Laparoscopic cholecystectomy**

Four trocar incisions:

# Chapter 11

# Surgical Positions

**Define the following positions:**

**Supine**  Patient lying flat, face up

**Prone**  Patient lying flat, face down

**Left lateral decubitus**  Patient lying down on his left side (think: left lateral decubitus = left side down)

**Right lateral decubitus**  Patient lying down on his right side (think: "right lateral decubitus = right side down")

**Lithotomy**  Patient lying supine with legs spread

| | |
|---|---|
| **Trendelenburg** | Patient supine with head lowered (A.K.A. "headdownenburg"—used during placement of a subclavian vein catheter as the veins distend with blood from gravity flow) |

| | |
|---|---|
| **Reverse Trendelenburg** | Patient supine with head elevated (usual position for laparoscopic cholecystectomy to make the intestines fall away from the operative field) |

# Chapter 12    Surgical Speak

The language of surgery is quite simple if you master a few suffixes.

**Define the suffix:**

| | |
|---|---|
| **-ectomy** | To surgically **remove** part of or an entire structure/organ |
| **-orraphy** | Surgical **repair** |
| **-otomy** | Surgical **incision into** an organ |
| **-ostomy** | Surgically created **opening** between two organs or organ and skin |
| **-plasty** | Surgical "shaping" or formation |

**Now test your knowledge of surgical speak:**

| | |
|---|---|
| **Word for the surgical repair of a hernia** | Herniorrhaphy |
| **Word for the surgical removal of the stomach** | Gastrectomy |
| **Word for the surgical creation of an opening between the colon and the skin** | Colostomy |
| **Word for the surgical formation of a "new" pylorus** | Pyloroplasty |
| **Word for the surgical opening of the stomach** | Gastrotomy |
| **Surgical creation of an opening (anastomosis) between the common bile duct and jejunum** | Choledochojejunostomy |
| **Surgical creation of an opening (anastomosis) between the stomach and jejunum** | Gastrojejunostomy |

# Chapter 13

# Preoperative 101

**When can a patient eat prior to major surgery?**

The patient should be NPO after midnight the night before or at least for 8 hours before surgery.

**What risks should be discussed with all patients and documented on the consent form for a surgical procedure?**

Bleeding, infection, anesthesia, scar; other risks are specific to the individual procedure (also MI, CVA, and death if cardiovascular disease is present)

| | |
|---|---|
| **If a patient is on antihypertensive medications, should the patient take them on the day of the procedure?** | Yes, (remember clonidine "rebound") |
| **If a patient is on an oral hypoglycemic agent (OHA), should the patient take the OHA on the day of surgery?** | Not if the patient is to be NPO on the day of surgery |
| **If a patient is taking insulin, should the patient take it on the day of surgery?** | No, only half of a long-acting insulin (e.g., lente) and start D5 NS IV; check glucose levels often preoperatively, operatively, and postoperatively |
| **Should a patient who smokes cigarettes stop before an operation?** | Yes, improvement is seen in just 2 to 4 weeks after smoking cessation. |
| **What laboratory test must all women of childbearing age have before entering the OR?** | Beta-HCG and CBC because of the possibility of pregnancy and anemia from menses |
| **What preoperative procedures should be performed before colon surgery?** | Bowel prep with colon cathartic (e.g., GoLYTELY), oral antibiotics (neomycin and erythromycin base), and IV antibiotic before incision (most surgeons) |
| **What preoperative medication can decrease postoperative cardiac events and death?** | Beta-blockers! |
| **What must you always order preoperatively for your patient undergoing a major operation?** | 1. NPO/IVF<br>2. Preoperative antibiotics<br>3. Type and cross blood (PRBCs) |
| **What electrolyte must you check preoperatively if a patient is on hemodialysis?** | Potassium |
| **Who gets a preoperative ECG?** | Patients older than 40 years of age |

# Chapter 14

# Surgical Operations You Should Know

**Define the following procedures:**
  **Billroth I**

Antrectomy with gastroduodenostomy

  **Billroth II**

Antrectomy with gastrojejunostomy

**How do you remember the difference between a Billroth I and a Billroth II?**

Billroth 1 has one limb; Billroth 2 has two limbs.

**Describe the following procedures:**

**Roux-en-Y limb**

Jejunojejunostomy forming a Y-shaped figure of small bowel; the free end can then be anastomosed to a second hollow structure (e.g., esophagojejunostomy)

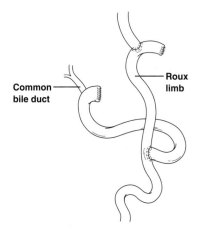

**Brooke ileostomy**

Standard ileostomy that is **folded on itself** to protrude from the abdomen approximately 2 cm to allow easy appliance placement and collection of succus

**CEA**

**C**arotid **E**nd**A**rterectomy; removal of atherosclerotic plaque from a carotid artery

**Bassini herniorrhaphy**

Repair of inguinal hernia by approximating transversus abdominis aponeurosis and the conjoint tendon to the reflection of **Poupart's** (inguinal) ligament

**McVay herniorrhaphy**

Repair of inguinal hernia by approximating the transversus abdominis aponeurosis and the conjoint tendon to **Cooper's** ligament (which is basically the superior pubic bone periosteum)

| | |
|---|---|
| **Lichtenstein herniorrhaphy** | "Tension-free" inguinal hernia repair using onlay mesh (**synthetic** graft material) |
| **Shouldice herniorrhaphy** | Repair of inguinal hernia by **imbrication** of the transversalis fascia, transversus abdominis aponeurosis, and the conjoint tendon and approximation of the transversus abdominis aponeurosis and the conjoint tendon to the inguinal ligament |
| **Plug and patch hernia RX** | Prosthetic plug pushes hernia sac in and then is covered with a prosthetic patch to repair inguinal hernias. |
| **APR** | **A**bdomino**P**erineal **R**esection; removal of the rectum and sigmoid colon through abdominal and perineal incisions (patient is left with a colostomy); used for low rectal cancers less than 8 cm from the anal verge |
| **LAR** | **L**ow **A**nterior **R**esection; **resection** of **low** rectal tumors through an **anterior** abdominal incision |
| **Hartmann's procedure** | 1. Proximal colostomy<br>2. Distal stapled-off colon or rectum that is left in peritoneal cavity |
| **Mucus fistula** | Distal end of the colon is brought to the abdominal skin as a stoma (proximal end is brought up to skin as an end colostomy). |
| **Kocher maneuver** | Dissection of the duodenum from the right-sided peritoneal attachment to allow mobilization and visualization of the back of the duodenum/pancreas |
| **Seldinger technique** | Placement of a central line by first placing a wire in the vein, followed by placing the catheter over the wire |
| **Cricothyroidotomy** | Emergent surgical airway through the cricoid membrane |
| **Hepaticojejunostomy** | Anastomosis between a jejunal roux limb and the hepatic ducts |

**Puestow procedure**

Side-to-side anastomosis of the pancreas and jejunum (pancreatic duct is filleted open)

**Stamm gastrostomy**

Gastrostomy placed by open surgical incision and tacked to the abdominal wall

**Highly selective vagotomy**

Transection of vagal fibers to the body of the stomach without interruption of fibers to the pylorus (does not need pyloroplasty or other drainage procedure because the pylorus should still function)

| | |
|---|---|
| **Enterolysis** | Lysis of peritoneal adhesions |
| **LOA** | **L**ysis **O**f **A**dhesions (enterolysis) |
| **Appendectomy** | Removal of the appendix |
| **Lap appy** | Laparoscopic removal of the appendix |
| **Cholecystectomy** | Removal of the gallbladder |
| **Lap chole** | Laparoscopic removal of the gallbladder |
| **Nissen** | Nissen fundoplication; 360° wrap of the stomach by the fundus of the stomach around the distal esophagus to prevent reflux |

| | |
|---|---|
| **LAP Nissen** | Nissen fundoplication with laparoscopy |
| **Simple mastectomy** | Removal of breast and nipple without removal of nodes |
| **Choledochojejunostomy** | Anastomosis of the common bile duct to the jejunum (end to side) |
| **Graham patch** | Placement of omentum with stitches over a gastric or duodenal perforation (i.e., omentum is used to plug the hole) |

**Heineke-Mikulicz pyloroplasty**

Longitudinal incision through all layers of the pylorus, sewing closed in a transverse direction to make the pylorus non-functional (used after truncal vagotomy)

**Pringle maneuver**

Temporary occlusion of the porta hepatis (for temporary control of liver blood flow when liver parenchyma is actively bleeding)

**Modified radical mastectomy**

Removal of the breast, nipple, **and axillary lymph nodes** (no muscle is removed)

**Lumpectomy and radiation**

Removal of breast mass and axillary lymph nodes; normal surrounding breast tissue is spared; patient then undergoes postoperative radiation treatments

**I and D**

**I**ncision and **D**rainage of pus; the wound is then packed open

**PEG**

**P**ercutaneous **E**ndoscopic **G**astrostomy; the endoscope is placed in the stomach, which is then inflated with air. A needle is passed into the stomach percutaneously, wire is passed through the needle traversing the abdominal wall, and gastrostomy is then placed by using the Seldinger technique over the wire.

**Exploratory laparotomy**    Laparotomy to explore the peritoneal cavity looking for the cause of pain, peritoneal signs, obstruction, hemorrhage, etc.

**TURP**    **T**rans**U**rethral **R**esection of the **P**rostate; removal of obstructing prostatic tissue via scope in the urethral lumen

**Fem pop bypass**    **Fem**oral artery to **pop**liteal artery bypass using synthetic graft or saphenous vein; used to bypass blockage in the femoral artery

Bypass graft

**AX FEM**

Long prosthetic graft tunneled under the skin placed from the **AX**illary artery to the **FEM**oral artery

**Triple A repair**

Repair of an AAA (**A**bdominal **A**ortic **A**neurysm). Open aneurysm and place prosthetic graft. Then close old aneurysm sac around graft.

**CABG**

**C**oronary **A**rtery **B**ypass **G**rafting; via saphenous vein graft or internal mammary artery bypass grafts to coronary arteries from aorta (cardiac revascularization)

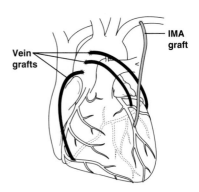

**Hartmann's pouch**

Oversewing of a rectal stump (or distal colonic stump) after resection of a colonic segment; patient is left with a proximal colostomy

**Ileoanal pull-through**    Anastomosis of the ileum to the anus after total proctocolectomy

**Hemicolectomy**    Removal of a colonic segment (i.e., partial colectomy)

**Truncal vagotomy**    Transection of the vagus nerve trunks; must provide drainage procedure to stomach (e.g., gastrojejunostomy or pyloroplasty) because after truncal vagotomy, the **pylorus does not relax**

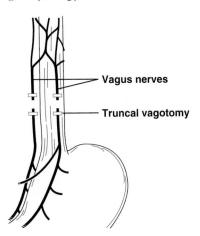

Vagus nerves

Truncal vagotomy

**Antrectomy**    Removal of stomach antrum

**Whipple procedure**    Pancreaticoduodenectomy:
    Cholecystectomy
    Truncal vagotomy
    Pancreaticoduodenectomy—removal of the head of the pancreas and duodenum
    Choledochojejunostomy
    Pancreaticojejunostomy (anastomosis of distal pancreas remnant to the jejunum)
    Gastrojejunostomy (anastomosis of stomach to jejunum)

**Excisional biopsy**      Biopsy with complete excision of all suspect tissue (mass)

**Incisional biopsy**      Biopsy with incomplete removal of suspect tissue (incises tissue from mass)

**Tracheostomy**      Placement of airway tube into trachea surgically or percutaneously

# Chapter 15

# Wounds

**Define the following terms:**

**Primary wound closure**      Suture wound closes immediately (A.K.A. first intention).

**Secondary wound closure**      Wound is left open and heals over time **without sutures;** it heals by granulation, contraction, and epithelialization over weeks (leaves a larger scar).

**Delayed primary closure (DPC)**      Suture wound closes 3 to 5 days AFTER incision (classically 5 days).

**How long until a sutured wound epithelializes?**      24–48 hours

**After a primary closure, when should the dressing be removed?**

Postoperative day 2

**When can a patient take a shower after a primary closure?**

Anytime after postoperative day 2 (after wound epithelializes)

**What is a wet-to-dry dressing?**

A damp (not wet) gauze dressing placed over a granulating wound and then allowed to dry to the wound; removal allows for "microdebridement" of the wound

**What inhibits wound healing?**

Infection, ischemia, diabetes mellitus, malnutrition, anemia, steroids, cancer, radiation

**What reverses the deleterious effects of steroids on wound healing?**

Vitamin A

**What is an abdominal wound dehiscence?**

Opening of the fascial closure (not skin); treat by returning to the OR for immediate fascial reclosure

**What is Dakin solution?**

Dilute sodium hypochlorite (**bleach**) used in contaminated wounds

# Chapter 16

# Drains and Tubes

**What is the purpose of drains?**

1. Withdrawal of fluids
2. Apposition of tissues to remove a potential space by suction

**What is a Jackson-Pratt (JP) drain?**

A closed drainage system attached to a suction bulb ("grenade")

**What are the "three S's" of Jackson-Pratt drain removal?**

1. **S**titch removal
2. **S**uction discontinuation
3. **S**low, steady pull

**What is a Penrose drain?**

An open drainage system composed of a thin rubber hose; associated with increased infection rate in clean wounds

**Define the following terms:**

**G-tube**

Gastrostomy tube; used for drainage or feeding

**J-tube**

Jejunostomy tube; used for feeding; may be a small-needle catheter (remember to flush after use or it will clog) or a large, red rubber catheter

**Cholecystostomy tube**

Tube placed surgically or percutaneously with ultrasound guidance to drain the gallbladder

**T-tube**

A tube placed in the common bile duct with an ascending and descending limb that forms a "T"

Drains percutaneously; usually placed after common bile duct exploration

## CHEST TUBES

**What is a thoracostomy tube?**

Chest tube

**What is the purpose of a chest tube?**

To appose the parietal and visceral pleura by draining blood, pus, fluid, chyle, or air

**How is a chest tube inserted?**

1. Administer local anesthetic.
2. Incise skin in the fourth or fifth intercostal space between the mid- and anterior-axillary lines.
3. Perform blunt Kelly-clamp dissection **over** the rib into the pleural space.
4. Perform finger exploration to confirm intrapleural placement.
5. Place tube posteriorly and superiorly.

**Is the chest tube placed under or over the rib?**

**Over** to avoid the vessels and nerves

**What are the goals of chest tube insertion?**

**Drain** the pleural cavity
**Appose** parietal and visceral pleura to
    seal any visceral pleural holes

**In most cases, where should the chest tube be positioned?**

Posteriorly into the apex

**How can you tell on CXR if the last hole on the chest tube is in the pleural cavity?**

The last hole is cut through the radiopaque line in the chest tube and is seen
on CXR as a break in the line, which
should be within the pleural cavity.

**What are the cm measurements on a chest tube?**

The centimeters from the last hole on the
chest tube

**What is the chest tube connected to?**

A Pleuravac® (three-chambered box)

**What are the three chambers of the Pleuravac®?**

1. Collection chamber
2. Water seal
3. Suction control

**Describe how each chamber of the Pleuravac® box works as the old three-bottle system:**
   **Collection chamber**

Collects fluid, pus, blood, or chyle and measures the amount; connects to the water seal bottle and to the chest tube

**Water-seal chamber**

One-way valve—allows air to be removed from the pleural space; does not allow air to enter pleural cavity; connects to the suction control bottle and to the collection chamber

**Suction-control chamber**

Controls the amount of suction by the height of the water column; sucking in room air releases excessive suction; connects to wall suction and to the water seal bottle

**Give a good example of a water seal.**

Place a straw in a cup of water—you can blow air out but if you suck in, the straw fills with water and thus forms a one-way valve for air just like the chest tube water seal.

**How is a chest tube placed on water seal?**

By removing the suction; a tension pneumothorax (PTX) cannot form because the one-way valve (water seal) allows release of air buildup

**Should a chest tube ever be clamped off?**

No, except to "run the system" **momentarily**

**What does it mean to "run the system" of a chest tube?**

To see if the air leak is from a leak in the pleural cavity (e.g., hole in lung) or from a leak in the tubing

**Momentarily** occlude the chest tube and if the air leak is still present, it is from the tubing or tubing connection, not from the chest.

**How can you tell if the chest tube is "tidling"?**

Take the Pleuravac® off of suction and look at the water seal chamber. The fluid should move with respiration/ventilation. This is called "tidling." This decreases and ceases if the pleura seals off the chest tube.

**How can you check for an air leak?**

Look at the water seal chamber on suction; if bubbles pass through the water seal fluid, a large air leak (i.e., air leaking into chest tube) is present. If no air leak is evident on suction, remove suction and ask the patient to cough. If air bubbles through the water seal, a small air leak is present.

**What is the usual course for removing a chest tube placed for a PTX?**

1. Suction until the PTX resolves and the air leak is gone.
2. Water seal for 24 hours.
3. Remove the chest tube if no PTX or air leak is present after 24 hours of water seal.

**How fast is a small, stable PTX absorbed?**

Approximately 1% daily; therefore, a 10% PTX by volume will absorb in approximatily 10 days

**How should a chest tube be removed?**

1. Cut the stitch.
2. Ask the patient to exhale or inhale maximally.
3. Rapidly remove the tube (split second) and at same time, place petroleum jelly gauze covered by 4 × 4's and then tape.
4. Obtain a CXR.

**What is a Heimlich valve?**

A one-way flutter valve for a chest tube

Direction of flow

## NASOGASTRIC TUBES (NGT)

**How should an NGT be placed?**

1. Use lubrication and have suction up on the bed.
2. Use anesthetic to numb nose.
3. Place head in flexion.
4. Ask patient to drink a small amount of water when the tube is in the back of the throat and to swallow the tube; if the patient can talk without difficulty and succus returns, the tube should be in the stomach. (Get an x-ray if there is any question.)

**How should an NGT be removed?**

Give patient a tissue, discontinue suction, untape nose, remove quickly, and tell patient to blow nose.

**What test should be performed before feeding via any tube?**

High abdominal x-ray to confirm placement into the GI tract and NOT the lung!

**How does an NGT work?**

**Sump pump,** dual lumen tube—the large clear tube is hooked to suction and the small blue tube allows for air sump (i.e., circuit sump pump with air in the blue tube and air and succus sucked out through the large clear lumen)

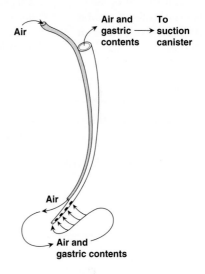

**How can you check to see if the NGT is working?**

The blue port will make a sucking noise. Always keep the blue port opening above the stomach.

**Should an NGT be placed on continuous or intermittent suction?**

Continuous low suction—side holes disengage if they are against mucosa because of the sump mechanism and multiple holes

**What happens if the NGT is clogged?**

The tube will not decompress the stomach and will keep the low esophageal sphincter (LES) open (i.e., a setup for aspiration).

**How should an NGT be unclogged?**

Saline-flush the clear port, reconnect to suction, and flush air down the blue sump port.

**What is a common cause of excessive NGT drainage?**

The tip of the NGT is inadvertently placed in the duodenum and drains the pancreatic fluid and bile; an x-ray should be taken and the tube repositioned into the stomach.

**What is the difference between a feeding tube (Dobbhoff tube) and an NGT?**

A feeding tube is a thin tube weighted at the end that is not a sump pump but a simple catheter. It is usually placed past the pylorus, which is facilitated by the weighted end and peristalsis.

## FOLEY CATHETER

**What is a Foley catheter?**

Catheter into the bladder, allowing accurate urine output determination

**What is a coudé catheter?**

A Foley catheter with a small, curved tip to help maneuver around a large prostate

**Coudé catheter**

**If a Foley catheter cannot be inserted, what are the next steps?**

1. Anesthetize the urethra with a sterile local anesthetic (e.g., lidocaine jelly).
2. Try a **larger** Foley catheter.

**What if a patient has a urethral injury and a Foley cannot be placed?**

A suprapubic catheter will need to be placed.

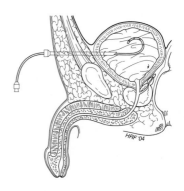

## CENTRAL LINES

**What are they?**

Catheters placed into the major veins (central veins) via subclavian, internal jugular, or femoral vein approaches

**What major complications result from placement?**

PTX (always obtain postplacement CXR), bleeding, malposition (e.g., into the neck from subclavian approach), dysrhythmias

**In long-term central lines, what does the "cuff" do?**

Allows ingrowth of fibrous tissue, which:
    Holds the line in place
    Forms a barrier to the advance of
        bacteria

**What is a Hickman® or Hickman-type catheter?**

External central line tunneled under the skin with a "cuff"

**What is a Port-A-Cath®?**

Central line that has a port buried under the skin that must be accessed through the skin (percutaneously)

**What is a "cordis"?**

Large central line catheter; used for massive fluid resuscitation or for placing a Swan-Ganz catheter

**If you try to place a subclavian central line unsuccessfully, what must you do before trying the other side?**

Get a CXR—a bilateral pneumothorax can be fatal!

**MISCELLANEOUS**

| | |
|---|---|
| **How can diameter in mm be determined from a French measurement?** | Divide the French size by pi or 3.14 (e.g., a 15 French tube has a diameter of 5 mm). |
| **How can needle-gauge size be determined?** | A 14-gauge needle is 1/14 of an inch (and thus a 14-gauge needle is larger than a 21-gauge needle). |
| **What is a Tenckhoff catheter?** | Catheter placed into the peritoneal cavity for peritoneal dialysis |

# Chapter 17

# Surgical Anatomy Pearls

| | |
|---|---|
| **What is the drainage of the left testicular vein?** | Left renal vein |
| **What is the drainage of the right testicular vein?** | IVC |
| **What is Gerota's fascia?** | Fascia surrounding the kidney |
| **What are the prominent collateral circulations seen in portal hypertension?** | Esophageal varices, hemorrhoids (inferior hemorrhoidal vein to internal iliac vein), patent umbilical vein (caput medusa), and retroperitoneal vein via lumbar tributaries |
| **What parts of the GI tract are retroperitoneal?** | Most of the duodenum, the ascending colon, the descending colon, and the pancreas |
| **What is the gubernaculum?** | Embryologic structure that adheres the testes to the scrotal sac; used to help manipulate the testes during indirect hernia repair |

**Which artery bleeds in bleeding duodenal ulcers?**

Gastroduodenal artery

**What is the name of the lymph nodes between the pectoralis minor and major muscles?**

Rotter's lymph nodes

**Is the left vagus nerve anterior or posterior?**

Anterior; remember the esophagus rotates during development

**What is Morrison's pouch?**

The hepatorenal recess; the most posterior cavity within the peritoneal cavity

**Give the locations of the following structures:**
    **Foregut**

Mouth to ampulla of Vater

    **Midgut**

Ampulla of Vater to distal third of transverse colon

    **Hindgut**

Distal third of transverse colon to the anus

**Where are the blood vessels on a rib?**

The vein, artery, and nerve (VAN) are underneath the rib (thus, place chest tubes and thoracentesis needles above the rib!).

**What is the order of the femoral vessels?**

The femoral vein is medial to the femoral artery (think: **NAVEL** for the order of the right femoral vessels—**N**erve, **A**rtery, **V**ein, **E**xtralymphatic tissue, **L**ymphatics).

**What is Hesselbach's triangle?**

The area bordered by:
1. Inguinal ligament
2. Epigastric vessels
3. Lateral border of the rectus sheath

**What nerve is located on top of the spermatic cord?**

Ilioinguinal nerve

**What is Calot's triangle?**

The area bordered by:
1. Cystic duct
2. Common hepatic duct
3. Cystic artery

| | |
|---|---|
| **What is Calot's node?** | Lymph node found in Calot's triangle |
| **What separates the right and left lobes of the liver?** | Cantle's line—a line drawn from the IVC to just left of the gallbladder fossa |
| **What is the gastrinoma triangle?** | A triangle where more than 90% of gastrinomas are located, bordered by:<br>1. Junction of the second and third portions of the duodenum<br>2. Cystic duct<br>3. Pancreatic neck |
| **Which artery is responsible for anterior spinal syndrome?** | Artery of Adamkiewicz |
| **Where is McBurney's point?** | One-third the distance from the anterior superior iliac spine to the umbilicus (estimate of the position of the appendix) |
| **How can you find the appendix after you find the cecum?** | Trace the taenia back as they converge on the origin of the appendix. |
| **Where is the space of Retzius?** | The preperitoneal space anterior to the bladder |
| **What are the white lines of Toldt?** | The lateral peritoneal reflections of the ascending and descending colon |
| **What is the strongest layer of the small bowel?** | Submucosa (not the serosa, think: SUbmucosa = SUperior) |
| **Which parts of the GI tract do not have a serosa?** | Esophagus<br>Middle and distal rectum |
| **What is the vein that overlies the pylorus?** | Vein of Mayo |
| **What is the pouch of Douglas?** | Pouch between the rectum and bladder or uterus |
| **What does the thoracic duct empty into?** | Left subclavian vein; left internal jugular vein junction |

| | |
|---|---|
| **What is the coronary vein?** | Left gastric vein |
| **What is the hypogastric artery?** | Internal iliac artery |
| **What is longer, the left or right renal vein?** | The left |

**What are the layers of the abdominal wall?**

1. Skin, then fat
2. Scarpa's fascia, then more fat
3. External oblique
4. Internal oblique
5. Transversus abdominis
6. Transversalis fascia
7. Preperitoneal fat
8. Peritoneum

**What are the plicae circulares?**

Plicae = folds, circulares = circular; thus, the circular folds of mucosa of the small bowel

**What is another name for the plicae circulares?**

Valvulae conniventes

**What are the major structural differences between the jejunum and ileum?**

Jejunum—long vasa rectae; large plicae circulares; thicker wall
Ileum—shorter vasa rectae; smaller plicae circulares; thinner wall (think: **I**leum = **I**nferior vasa rectae, **I**nferior plicae circulares, and **I**nferior wall)

**What are the major anatomic differences between the colon and the small bowel?**

The colon has taenia coli, haustra, and appendices epiploicae (fat appendages), whereas the small intestine is smooth.

**How far up does the diaphragm extend?**

To the nipples in men (fourth intercostal space; thus, the abdomen extends to the level of the nipples)

**What dermatome is at the umbilicus?**

T10

What are the major layers
of an artery?

Adventitia

Media

Intima

# Chapter 18

# Fluids and Electrolytes

What are the two major
body fluid compartments?

1. Intracellular
2. Extracellular

What are the two
subcompartments of
extracellular fluid?

1. Interstitial fluid (in between cells)
2. Intravascular fluid (plasma)

What percentage of body
weight is in fluid?

60%

60%

| | |
|---|---|
| **What percentage of body fluid is intracellular?** | 66% |
| **What percentage of body fluid is extracellular?** | 33% |
| **What is the composition of body fluid?** | Fluids = 60% total body weight<br>    Intracellular = 40% total body weight<br>    Extracellular = 20% total body weight<br>    (think: 60, 40, 20) |
| **How to remember the body fluid distribution by weight?** | TIE<br>**T** = **T**otal body fluid = 60% of body weight<br>**I** = **I**ntracellular = 40% of body weight<br>**E** = **E**xtracellular = 20% of body weight |
| **On average, what percentage of body weight does blood account for in adults?** | ~7% |
| **How many liters of blood are in a 70-kg man?** | 0.07 × 70 = 5 liters |
| **What are the fluid requirements every 24 hours for each of the following substances:** | |
| **Water** | ~30 to 35 mL/kg |
| **Potassium** | ~1 mEq/kg |
| **Chloride** | ~1.5 mEq/kg |
| **Sodium** | ~1–2 mEq/kg |
| **What are the levels and sources of normal daily water loss?** | Urine—1200 to 1500 mL (25–30 mL/kg)<br>Sweat—200 to 400 mL<br>Respiratory losses—500 to 700 mL<br>Feces—100 to 200 mL |
| **What are the levels and sources of normal daily electrolyte loss?** | Sodium and potassium = 100 mEq<br>Chloride = 150 mEq |

| | |
|---|---|
| **What are the levels of sodium and chloride in sweat?** | Approximately 40 mEq/L |
| **What is the major electrolyte in colonic feculent fluid?** | Potassium—65 mEq/L |
| **What is the physiologic response to hypovolemia?** | Sodium/$H_2O$ retention via renin → aldosterone, water retention via ADH, vasoconstriction via angiotensin II and sympathetics, low urine output and tachycardia (early), hypotension (late) |

## THIRD SPACING

| | |
|---|---|
| **What is it?** | Fluid accumulation in the interstitium of tissues, as in edema, e.g., loss of fluid into the interstitium and lumen of a paralytic bowel following surgery (think of the intravascular and intracellular spaces as the first two spaces) |
| **When does "third-spacing" occur postoperatively?** | Third-spaced fluid tends to mobilize back into the intravascular space around the third postoperative day; beware of fluid overload once the fluid begins to return to the intravascular space. Switch to hypotonic fluid and decrease IV rate. |
| **What are the classic signs of third spacing?** | Tachycardia<br>Decreased urine output |
| **What is the treatment?** | IV hydration with isotonic fluids |
| **What are the surgical causes of the following conditions:**<br>  **Metabolic acidosis** | Loss of bicarbonate: diarrhea, ileus, fistula, high-output ileostomy, carbonic anhydrase inhibitors<br>Increase in acids: lactic acidosis (ischemia), ketoacidosis, renal failure, necrotic tissue |
|   **Hypochloremic alkalosis** | NGT suction, loss of gastric HCl through vomiting/NGT |

| | |
|---|---|
| **Metabolic alkalosis** | Vomiting, NG suction, diuretics, alkali ingestion, mineralocorticoid excess |
| **Respiratory acidosis** | Hypoventilation (e.g., CNS depression), drugs (e.g., morphine), PTX, pleural effusion, parenchymal lung disease, acute airway obstruction |
| **Respiratory alkalosis** | Hyperventilation (e.g., anxiety, pain, fever, wrong ventilator settings) |
| **What is the "classic" acid-base finding with significant vomiting or NGT suctioning?** | Hypokalemic hypochloremic metabolic alkalosis |
| **Why hypokalemia with NGT suctioning?** | Loss in gastric fluid—loss of HCl causes alkalosis, driving $K^+$ into cells; $K^+$ loss into urine exchange for $Na^+$ |
| **What is the treatment for hypokalemic hypochloremic metabolic alkalosis?** | IVF, $Cl^-$/$K^+$ replacement |
| **What is paradoxic alkalotic aciduria?** | Seen in severe hypokalemic, hypovolemic, hypochloremic metabolic alkalosis with paradoxic metabolic alkalosis of serum and acidic urine |
| **How does paradoxic alkalotic aciduria occur?** | $H^+$ is lost in the urine in exchange for $Na^+$ in an attempt to restore volume. |
| **With paradoxic alkalotic aciduria, why is $H^+$ preferentially lost?** | $H^+$ is exchanged preferentially into the urine instead of $K^+$ because of the low concentration of $K^+$. |
| **What can be followed to assess fluid status?** | Urine output, base deficit, lactic acid, vital signs, weight changes, skin turgor, jugular venous distention (JVD), mucosal membranes, rales (crackles), central venous pressure, PCWP, chest x-ray findings |
| **With hypovolemia, what changes occur in vital signs?** | Tachycardia, tachypnea, initial rise in diastolic blood pressure because of clamping down (peripheral vasoconstriction) with subsequent decrease in both systolic and diastolic blood pressures |

| | |
|---|---|
| **What are the insensible fluid losses?** | Loss of fluid not measured:<br>Feces—100 to 200 mL/24 hours<br>Breathing—500 to 700 mL/24 hours<br>    (**Note:** increases with fever and<br>    tachypnea)<br>Skin—approximately 300 mL/24 hours,<br>    increased with fever; thus, insensible<br>    fluid loss is not directly measured |
| **What are the quantities of daily secretions:** | |
|     **Bile** | Approximately 1000 mL/24 hours |
|     **Gastric** | Approximately 2000 mL/ 24 hours |
|     **Pancreatic** | Approximately 600 mL/ 24 hours |
|     **Small intestine** | Approximately 3000 mL/day |
|     **Saliva** | Approximately 1500 mL/24 hours<br>**Note:** almost all secretions are reabsorbed. |
| **How can the estimated levels of daily secretions from bile, gastric, and small-bowel sources be remembered?** | Alphabetically and numerically: B, G, S and 1, 2, 3; or B1, G2, S3 as bile, gastric, and small bowel produce roughly 1 L, 2 L, and 3 L, respectively! |

## COMMON IV REPLACEMENT FLUIDS (ALL VALUES ARE PER LITER)

| | |
|---|---|
| **What comprises normal saline (NS)?** | 154 mEq of $Cl^-$<br>154 mEq of $Na^+$ |
| **What comprises ½ NS?** | 77 mEq of $Cl^-$<br>77 mEq of $Na^+$ |
| **What comprises ¼ NS?** | 39 mEq of $Cl^-$<br>39 mEq of $Na^+$ |
| **What comprises lactated Ringer's (LR)?** | 130 mEq $Na^+$<br>109 mEq $Cl^-$<br>28 mEq lactate<br>4 mEq $K^+$<br>3 mEq $Ca^+$ |

| | |
|---|---|
| **What comprises D5W?** | 5% dextrose (50 g) in $H_2O$ |
| **What accounts for tonicity?** | Mainly electrolytes; thus, NS and LR are both isotonic, whereas ½ NS is hypotonic to serum |
| **What happens to the lactate in LR in the body?** | Converted into bicarbonate; thus, LR cannot be used as a maintenance fluid because patients would become alkalotic |

**IVF replacement by anatomic site:**

| | |
|---|---|
| **Gastric (NGT)** | D5 1/2NS + 20 KC1 |
| **Biliary** | LR+/−sodium bicarbonate |
| **Pancreatic** | LR+/−sodium bicarbonate |
| **Small bowel (ileostomy)** | LR |
| **Colonic (diarrhea)** | LR+/−sodium bicarbonate |

## CALCULATION OF MAINTENANCE FLUIDS

| | |
|---|---|
| **What is the 100/50/20 rule?** | Maintenance IV fluids for a 24-hour period:<br>100 mL/kg for the first 10 kg<br>50 mL/kg for the next 10 kg<br>20 mL/kg for every kg over 20 (divide by 24 for hourly rate) |
| **What is the 4/2/1 rule?** | Maintenance IV fluids for hourly rate:<br>4 mL/kg for the first 10 kg<br>2 mL/kg for the next 10 kg<br>1 mL/kg for every kg over 20 |
| **What is the maintenance for a 70-kg man?** | Using 100/50/20:<br>$100 \times 10$ kg = 1000<br>$50 \times 10$ kg = 500<br>$20 \times 50$ kg = 1000<br>Total = 2500<br>Divided by 24 hours = 104 mL/hr maintenance rate |

Using 4/2/1:
    $4 \times 10$ kg = 40
    $2 \times 10$ kg = 20
    $1 \times 50$ kg = 50
    Total = 110 mL/hr maintenance rate

**What is the common adult maintenance fluid?**

D5 1/2 NS with 20 mEq KCl/L

**What is the common pediatric maintenance fluid?**

D5 1/4 NS with 20 mEq KCl/L (use 1/4 NS because of the decreased ability of children to concentrate urine)

**Why should sugar (dextrose) be added to maintenance fluid?**

To inhibit muscle breakdown

**What is the best way to assess fluid status?**

Urine output (unless the patient has cardiac or renal dysfunction, in which case central venous pressure or wedge pressure is often used)

**What is the minimal urine output for an adult on maintenance IV?**

30 mL/hr (0.5 cc/kg/hr)

**What is the minimal urine output for an adult trauma patient?**

50 mL/hr

**How many mL are in 12 oz (beer can)?**

356 mL

**How many mL are in 1 oz?**

30 mL

**How many mL are in 1 tsp?**

5 mL

**What are common isotonic fluids?**

NS, LR

**What is a bolus?**

A volume of fluid given IV in a rapid manner (e.g., 1 L over 1 hour); used for increasing intravascular volume, and isotonic fluids should be used (i.e., NS or LR)

**Why not combine bolus fluids with dextrose?**

Hyperglycemia may result.

**What is the possible consequence of hypergly-cemia in the patient with hypovolemia?**

Osmotic diuresis

**Why not combine bolus fluids with a significant amount of potassium?**

Hyperkalemia may result (the potassium in LR is very low: 4 mEq/L).

**Why should isotonic fluids be given for resuscitation (i.e., to restore intravascular volume)?**

If hypotonic fluid is given, the tonicity of the intravascular space will be decreased and $H_2O$ will freely diffuse into the interstitial and intracellular spaces. Thus, use isotonic fluids to expand the intravascular space.

**What portion of 1 L NS will stay in the intravascular space after a laparotomy?**

In 5 hours, only approximately 200 cc (or 20%) will remain in the intravascular space!

**What is the most common trauma resuscitation fluid?**

LR

**What is the most common postoperative IV fluid after a laparotomy?**

LR or D5LR for 24 to 36 hours, followed by maintenance fluid

**After a laparotomy, when should a patient's fluid be "mobilized"?**

Classically, postoperative day 3; the patient begins to "mobilize" the third-space fluid back into the intravascular space

**What IVF is used to replace duodenal or pancreatic fluid loss?**

LR (bicarbonate loss)

## ELECTROLYTE IMBALANCES

**What is a common cause of electrolyte abnormalities?**

Lab error!

**What is a major extracellular cation?**

$Na^+$

| | |
|---|---|
| **What is a major intracellular cation?** | $K^+$ |

## HYPERKALEMIA

| | |
|---|---|
| **What is the normal range for potassium level?** | 3.5–5.0 mEq/L |
| **What are the surgical causes of hyperkalemia?** | Iatrogenic overdose, blood transfusion, renal failure, diuretics, acidosis, tissue destruction (injury/hemolysis) |
| **What are the signs/symptoms?** | Decreased deep tendon reflex (DTR) or areflexia, weakness, paraesthesia, paralysis, respiratory failure |
| **What are the ECG findings?** | **Peaked T waves,** depressed ST segment, prolonged PR, wide QRS, bradycardia, ventricular fibrillation |
| **What are the critical values?** | $K^+ > 6.5$ |
| **What is the urgent treatment?** | IV calcium (cardioprotective), ECG monitoring<br>Sodium bicarbonate IV (alkalosis drives $K^+$ intracellularly)<br>Glucose and insulin<br>Albuterol<br>Sodium polystyrene sulfonate (Kayexalate) and **furosemide** (Lasix)<br>Dialysis |
| **What is the nonacute treatment?** | Furosemide (Lasix), sodium polystyrene sulfonate (Kayexalate) |
| **What is the acronym for the treatment of acute symptomatic hyperkalemia?** | "CB DIAL $K^+$":<br>**C**alcium<br>**B**icarbonate<br><br>**D**ialysis<br>**I**nsulin/dextrose<br>**A**lbuterol<br>**L**asix<br><br>**K**ayexalate |

| | |
|---|---|
| **What is "pseudohyperkalemia"?** | Spurious hyperkalemia as a result of falsely elevated $K^+$ in sample from sample hemolysis |
| **What acid-base change lowers the serum potassium?** | Alkalosis (thus, give bicarbonate for hyperkalemia) |
| **What nebulizer treatment can help lower $K^+$ level?** | Albuterol |

## HYPOKALEMIA

| | |
|---|---|
| **What are the surgical causes?** | Diuretics, certain antibiotics, steroids, alkalosis, diarrhea, intestinal fistulae, NG aspiration, vomiting, insulin, insufficient supplementation, amphotericin |
| **What are the signs/ symptoms?** | Weakness, tetany, nausea, vomiting, **ileus,** paraesthesia |
| **What are the ECG findings?** | **Flattening of T waves, U waves,** ST segment depression, PAC, PVC, atrial fibrillation |
| **What is a U wave?** |  |
| **What is the rapid treatment?** | KCl IV |
| **What is the maximum amount that can be given through a peripheral IV?** | 10 mEq/hour |
| **What is the maximum amount that can be given through a central line?** | 20 mEq/hour |
| **What is the chronic treatment?** | KCl PO |

| | |
|---|---|
| **What is the most common electrolyte-mediated ileus in the surgical patient?** | Hypokalemia |
| **What electrolyte condition exacerbates digitalis toxicity?** | Hypokalemia |
| **What electrolyte deficiency can actually cause hypokalemia?** | Low magnesium |
| **What electrolyte must you replace first before replacing $K^+$?** | Magnesium |

## HYPERNATREMIA

| | |
|---|---|
| **What is the normal range for sodium level?** | 135–145 mEq/L |
| **What are the surgical causes?** | Inadequate hydration, diabetes insipidus, diuresis, vomiting, diarrhea, diaphoresis, tachypnea, iatrogenic (e.g., TPN) |
| **What are the signs/symptoms?** | Seizures, confusion, stupor, pulmonary or peripheral edema, tremors, respiratory paralysis |
| **What is the usual treatment supplementation slowly over days?** | D5W, 1/4 NS, or 1/2 NS |
| **How fast should you lower the sodium level in hypernatremia?** | The guideline is less than 12 mEq/L per day. |
| **What is the major complication of lowering the sodium level too fast?** | Seizures (**not** central pontine myelinolysis) |

## HYPONATREMIA

| | |
|---|---|
| **What are the surgical causes of the following types:** | |
| **Hypovolemic** | Diuretic excess, hypoaldosteronism, vomiting, NG suction, burns, pancreatitis, diaphoresis |

| | |
|---|---|
| **Euvolemic** | SIADH, CNS abnormalities, drugs |
| **Hypervolemic** | Renal failure, CHF, liver failure (cirrhosis), iatrogenic fluid overload (dilutional) |
| **What are the signs/ symptoms?** | Seizures, coma, nausea, vomiting, ileus, lethargy, confusion, weakness |

**What is the treatment of the following types:**

| | |
|---|---|
| **Hypovolemic** | NS IV, correct underlying cause |
| **Euvolemic** | SIADH: furosemide and NS acutely, fluid restriction |
| **Hypervolemic** | Dilutional: fluid restriction and diuretics |
| **How fast should you lower the sodium level in hyponatremia?** | The guideline is less than 12 mEq/L per day. |
| **What may occur if you correct hyponatremia too quickly?** | Central pontine myelinolysis! |
| **What are the signs of central pontine myelinolysis?** | 1. Confusion<br>2. Spastic quadriplegia<br>3. Horizontal gaze paralysis |
| **What is the most common cause of mild postoperative hyponatremia?** | Fluid overload |
| **How do you remember the sodium level in S.I.A.D.H.?** | S.I.A.D.H. = **S**odium **I**s **A**lways **D**own **H**ere |

"PSEUDOHYPONATREMIA"

| | |
|---|---|
| **What is it?** | Spurious lab value of hyponatremia as a result of hyperglycemia, hyperlipidemia, or hyperproteinemia |

HYPERCALCEMIA

| | |
|---|---|
| **What are the causes?** | "CHIMPANZEES":<br>**C**alcium supplementation IV<br>**H**yperparathyroidism (1°/3°)<br>    hyperthyroidism |

Immobility/iatrogenic (thiazide diuretics)
Mets/Milk alkali syndrome
Paget's disease (bone)
Addison's disease/acromegaly
Neoplasm (colon, lung, breast, prostate, multiple myeloma)
Zollinger-Ellison syndrome (as part of MEN I)
Excessive vitamin D
Excessive vitamin A
Sarcoid

| | |
|---|---|
| **What are the signs/ symptoms?** | Hypercalcemia—"Stones, bones, abdominal groans, and psychiatric overtones" Polydipsia, polyuria, constipation |
| **What are the ECG findings?** | Short QT interval, prolonged PR interval |
| **What is the acute treatment of hypercalcemic crisis?** | Volume expansion with NS, diuresis with furosemide (not thiazides) |
| **What are other options for lowering Ca+ level?** | Steroids, calcitonin, bisphosphonates (pamidronate, etc.), mithramycin, dialysis (last resort) |

## HYPOCALCEMIA

| | |
|---|---|
| **How can the calcium level be determined with hypoalbuminemia?** | (4-measured albumin level) × 0.8, then add this value to the measured calcium level |
| **What are the surgical causes?** | Short bowel syndrome, intestinal bypass, vitamin D deficiency, sepsis, acute pancreatitis, osteoblastic metastasis, aminoglycosides, diuretics, renal failure, hypomagnesemia, rhabdomyolysis |
| **What is Chvostek's sign?** | Facial muscle spasm with tapping of facial nerve (think: **ch**vostek = **ch**eek) |
| **What is Trousseau's sign?** | Carpal spasm after occluding blood flow in forearm with blood pressure cuff |

| | |
|---|---|
| **What are the signs/ symptoms?** | Chvostek's and Trousseau's signs, perioral paraesthesia (early), increased deep tendon reflexes (late), confusion, abdominal cramps, laryngospasm, stridor, seizures, tetany, psychiatric abnormalities (e.g., paranoia, depression, hallucinations) |
| **What are the ECG findings?** | Prolonged QT and ST interval (peaked T-waves are also possible, as in hyperkalemia) |
| **What is the acute treatment?** | Calcium gluconate IV |
| **What is the chronic treatment?** | Calcium PO, vitamin D |
| **What is the possible complication of infused calcium if the IV infiltrates?** | **Tissue necrosis;** never administer peripherally unless absolutely necessary (calcium gluconate is less toxic than calcium chloride during an infiltration) |
| **What is the best way to check the calcium level in the ICU?** | Check ionized calcium. |

## HYPERMAGNESEMIA

| | |
|---|---|
| **What is the normal range for magnesium level?** | 1.5–2.5 mEq/L |
| **What is the surgical cause?** | TPN, renal failure, IV over supplementation |
| **What are the signs/ symptoms?** | Respiratory failure, CNS depression, decreased deep tendon reflexes |
| **What is the treatment?** | Calcium gluconate IV, insulin plus glucose, dialysis (similar to treatment of hyperkalemia), furosemide (Lasix) |

## HYPOMAGNESEMIA

| | |
|---|---|
| **What are the surgical causes?** | TPN, hypocalcemia, gastric suctioning, aminoglycosides, renal failure, diarrhea, vomiting |
| **What are the signs/ symptoms?** | Increased deep tendon reflexes, tetany, asterixis, tremor, Chvostek's sign, ventricular ectopy, vertigo, tachycardia, dysrhythmias |

| | |
|---|---|
| **What is the acute treatment?** | $MgSO_4$ IV |
| **What is the chronic treatment?** | Magnesium oxide PO (side effect: diarrhea) |
| **Hypomagnesemia may make it impossible to correct what other electrolyte abnormality?** | Hypokalemia (always fix hypomagnesemia with hypokalemia) |

## HYPERGLYCEMIA

| | |
|---|---|
| **What are the surgical causes?** | Diabetes (poor control), infection, stress, TPN, drugs, lab error, drawing over IV site, somatostatinoma, glucagonoma |
| **What are the signs/ symptoms?** | Polyuria, hypovolemia, confusion/coma, polydipsia, ileus, DKA (Kussmaul breathing), abdominal pain, hyporeflexia |
| **What is the treatment?** | Insulin |
| **What is the Weiss protocol?** | Sliding scale insulin |
| **What is the goal glucose level in the ICU?** | 80–110 mg/dL |

## HYPOGLYCEMIA

| | |
|---|---|
| **What are the surgical causes?** | Excess insulin, decreased caloric intake, insulinoma, drugs, liver failure, adrenal insufficiency, gastrojejunostomy |
| **What are the signs/ symptoms?** | Sympathetic response (diaphoresis, tachycardia, palpitations), confusion, coma, headache, diplopia, neurologic deficits, seizures |
| **What is the treatment?** | Glucose (IV or PO) |

## HYPOPHOSPHATEMIA

| | |
|---|---|
| **What is the normal range for phosphorus level?** | 2.5–4.5 mg/dL |
| **What are the signs/ symptoms of hypophosphatemia?** | Weakness, cardiomyopathy, neurologic dysfunction (e.g., ataxia), rhabdomyolysis, hemolysis, poor pressor response |

**What is a complication of severe hypophosphatemia.**

Respiratory failure

**What are the causes?**

GI losses, inadequate supplementation, medications, sepsis, alcohol abuse, renal loss

**What is the critical value?**

<1.0 mg/dL

**What is the treatment?**

Supplement with sodium phosphate or potassium phosphate IV (depending on potassium level)

## HYPERPHOSPHATEMIA

**What are the signs/ symptoms?**

Calcification (ectopic), heart block

**What are the causes?**

Renal failure, sepsis, chemotherapy, hyperthyroidism

**What is the treatment?**

Aluminum hydroxide (binds phosphate)

## MISCELLANEOUS

**This ECG pattern is consistent with which electrolyte abnormality?**

Hyperkalemia: peaked T-waves

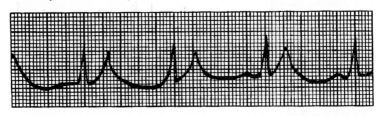

**If hyperkalemia is left untreated, what can occur?**

Ventricular tachycardia/fibrillation → death

| | |
|---|---|
| **Which electrolyte is an inotrope?** | Calcium |
| **What are the major cardiac electrolytes?** | Potassium (dysrhythmias), magnesium (dysrhythmias), calcium (dysrhythmias/inotrope) |
| **Which electrolyte must be monitored closely in patients on digitalis?** | Potassium |
| **What is the most common cause of electrolyte-mediated ileus?** | Hypokalemia |
| **What is a colloid fluid?** | Protein-containing fluid (albumin) |
| **What is the rationale for using an albumin-furosemide "sandwich"?** | The albumin will pull interstitial fluid into the intravascular space and the furosemide will then help excrete the fluid as urine. |
| **An elderly patient goes into CHF (congestive heart failure) on postoperative day 3 after a laparotomy. What is going on?** | Mobilization of the "third-space" fluid into the intravascular space, resulting in fluid overload and resultant CHF (but also must rule out MI) |
| **What fluid is used to replace NGT (gastric) aspirate?** | D5 ½NS with 20 KCl |
| **What electrolyte is associated with succinycholine?** | Hyperkalemia |

# Chapter 19

# Blood and Blood Products

**Define the following terms:**
    **PT**

**P**rothrombin **T**ime: tests extrinsic coagulation pathway

    **PTT**

**P**artial **T**hromboplastin **T**ime: tests intrinsic coagulation pathway

| | |
|---|---|
| **INR** | **I**nternational **N**ormalized **R**atio (reports PT results) |
| **Whole blood** | One unit = 450 mL ($\pm$50 mL); deficient in platelets and clotting factors V, VIII, and XI; **rarely used** |
| **Packed red blood cells (PRBCs)** | One unit ~ 300 ml ($\pm$50 mL); no platelets or clotting factors; can be mixed with NS to infuse faster |
| **Platelets** | Replace platelets with units of platelets (6–10 units from single donor or random donors) |
| **Fresh frozen plasma (FFP)** | Replaces **clotting factors;** (no RBCs/WBCs/platelets) |
| **Cryoprecipitate (cryo)** | Replaces fibrinogen, Von Willebrand factor, and some clotting factors |
| **Which electrolyte is most likely to fall with the infusion of stored blood? Why?** | Ionized calcium; the citrate preservative used for the storage of blood binds serum calcium |
| **What changes occur in the storage of PRBCs?** | $\downarrow Ca^+$, $\uparrow K^+$, $\downarrow$ 2,3-DPG, $\uparrow H^+$ ($\downarrow$ pH), $\downarrow$ PMNs |
| **What are general guidelines for blood transfusion?** | Acute blood loss, Hgb <10, and history of CAD/COPD **or** healthy symptomatic patient with Hgb <7 |
| **What is the rough formula for converting Hgb to Hct?** | Hgb $\times$ 3 = Hct |
| **One unit of PRBC increases Hct by how much?** | ~3% to 4% |
| **Which blood type is the universal donor?** | O negative |
| **What is a type and screen?** | Patient's blood type is determined and the blood is screened for antibodies; a type and cross from that sample can then be ordered if needed later. |

| | |
|---|---|
| **What is a type and cross?** | Patient's blood is sent to the blood bank and cross-matched for **specific donor units for possible blood transfusion.** |
| **Define thrombocytopenia.** | Low platelet count (<100,000) |
| **What are the common causes of thrombocytopenia in the surgical patient?** | Sepsis, $H_2$ blockers, heparin, massive transfusion, DIC, antibiotics, spurious lab value, Swann-Ganz catheter |
| **What can be given to help correct platelet dysfunction from uremia, aspirin, or bypass?** | DDAVP (desmopressin) |
| **What common medication causes platelets to irreversibly malfunction?** | Aspirin (inhibits cyclo-oxygenase) |
| **What platelet count is associated with spontaneous bleeding?** | Less than 20,000 |
| **What should the platelet count be before surgery?** | Greater than 50,000 |
| **When should "prophylactic" platelet transfusions be given?** | With platelets below 10,000 (old recommendation was 20,000) |
| **What is microcytic anemia "until proven otherwise" in a man or postmenopausal woman?** | Colon cancer |
| **Why not infuse PRBCs with lactated Ringer's?** | The calcium in LR may result in coagulation within the IV line. |
| **For how long can packed RBCs be stored?** | About 6 weeks (42 days) |
| **What is the most common cause of transfusion hemolysis?** | ABO incompatibility as a result of **clerical error** |
| **What is the risk of receiving a unit of blood infected with HIV?** | Approximately 1 in 1,000,000 |

**What are the symptoms of a transfusion reaction?**

**Fever,** chills, nausea, hypotension, lumbar pain, chest pain, abnormal bleeding

**What is the treatment for transfusion hemolysis?**

**Stop** transfusion; provide fluids; perform diuresis (Lasix) to protect kidneys; alkalinize urine (bicarbonate); give pressors as needed.

**What component of the blood transfusion can cause a fever?**

WBC

**What is the "trigger" Hct in young healthy patients?**

21%

**What is the widely stated to be "optimal" Hct in a patient with a history of heart disease or stroke?**

Approximately 30%

**When should aspirin administration be discontinued preoperatively?**

At 1 week because platelets live 7 to 10 days (must use judgment if patient is at risk for stroke or MI; it may be better to continue and use excellent surgical hemostasis in these patients)

**What can move the oxyhemoglobin dissociation curve to the right?**

Acidosis, 2,3-DPG, fever, elevated $Pco_2$ (to the right means greater ability to release the $O_2$ to the tissues)

**What is the normal life of RBCs?**

120 days

**What is the normal life of platelets?**

7 to 10 days

**What factor is deficient in hemophilia A?**

Factor VIII

**How do you remember the clotting factor for hemophilia A?**

Think: "**eight**" sounds like "**A**"

**What is the preoperative treatment of hemophilia A?**

Factor VIII infusion to $\geq 100\%$ normal preoperative levels

| | |
|---|---|
| **What coagulation study is elevated with hemophilia A?** | PTT |
| **How do you remember which coagulation study is affected by the hemophilias?** | There are two major hemophilias and two t's in PTT. |
| **What factor is deficient in hemophilia B?** | Factor IX |
| **How do you remember which factors are deficient with hemophilia A and hemophilia B?** | Alphabetically and chronologically: A before B and VIII before IX; thus, hemophilia A is factor VIII and hemophilia B is factor IX |
| **How are hemophilias A and B inherited?** | Sex-linked recessive |
| **What is Von Willebrand's disease?** | Deficiency of Von Willebrand factor (vWF) and factor VIII:C |
| **How is Von Willebrand's disease inherited?** | Autosomal dominant |
| **What is used to correct Von Willebrand's disease?** | DDAVP or cryoprecipitate |
| **What coagulation is abnormal with the following disorders:** | |
| **Hemophilia A** | PTT (elevated) |
| **Hemophilia B** | PTT (elevated) |
| **Von Willebrand's disease** | Bleeding time |
| **What is the effect on the coagulation system if the patient has a deficiency in protein C, protein S, or antithrombin III?** | A **hyper**coagulable state |

| | |
|---|---|
| **What is a "left shift" on a CBC?** | Juvenile polymorphonuclear leukocytes (bands); legend has it that the old counters for all the blood cells had the lever for bands on the LEFT of the counter |
| **What is the usual "therapeutic" PT?** | With coumadin, usually shoot for an INR of 2.0–3.0. |
| **What is the acronym basis for the word WARFARIN?** | **W**isconsin **A**lumni **R**esearch **F**oundation-**ARIN** |
| **What is the most common inherited hypercoagulable state?** | Factor V Leiden<br>Think **Le**iden = **Le**ader |
| **What is Xigris®?** | Activated protein C, which is used in severe sepsis |

# Chapter 20

# Surgical Hemostasis

| | |
|---|---|
| **What motto is associated with surgical hemostasis?** | "All bleeding stops." |
| **What is the most immediate method to obtain hemostasis?** | Pressure (finger) |
| **What is the "Bovie"?** | Electrocautery (designed by Bovie with Cushing for neurosurgery in the 1920s) |
| **What is the CUT mode on the Bovie?** | **Continuous** electrical current (20,000 Hz); cuts well with a decreased ability to coagulate |
| **What is the COAG mode on the Bovie?** | **Intermittent** electrical current (20,000 Hz); results in excellent vessel coagulation with decreased ability to cut |

**Where should a Bovie be applied to a clamp or pick-up to coagulate a vessel?**

**Anywhere** on the clamp/pick-up

**Should you ever "blindly" place a clamp in a wound to stop bleeding?**

No, you may injure surrounding tissues such as nerves.

**Define the following terms:**
   **Figure-of-eight suture**

Suture ligature placed **twice** in the tissue prior to being tied

**Vessel "tied in continuity"**  Tie, tie, cut in between

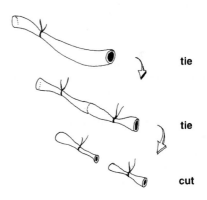

tie

tie

cut

**Surgicel®**  Cellulose sheets—act as a framework
for clotting factors/platelets to adhere to
(think: Surgi**cel** = **cell**ulose)

**Fibrin glue**  Fibrinogen and thrombin sprayed
simultaneously and mixed to produce
a fibrin "glue"

**Harmonic scalpel**  Ultrasonic scalpel that vibrates more than
50,000 times per second; seals vessels
and cuts tissue

**Clips**  Metallic clips for clipping vessels

# Chapter 21

# Common Surgical Medications

## ANTIBIOTICS

**Which antibiotics are
commonly used for
anaerobic infections?**

Metronidazole, clindamycin, cefoxitin,
cefotetan, imipenem, ticarcillin-clavulanic
acid, Unasyn®, Augmentin®

**Which antibiotics are commonly used for gram-negative infections?**
Gentamicin and other aminoglycosides, ciprofloxacin, aztreonam, third-generation cephalosporins, sulfamethoxazole-trimethoprim

**Which antibiotic, if taken with alcohol, will produce a disulfiram-like reaction?**
Metronidazole (Flagyl®) (disulfiram is Antabuse®)

**What is the drug of choice for treating amoebic infections?**
Metronidazole (Flagyl®)

**Which antibiotic is associated with cholestasis?**
Ceftriaxone (Rocephin®)

**Which antibiotic cannot be given to children or pregnant women?**
Ciprofloxacin (interferes with the growth plate)

**With which antibiotics must serum levels be determined?**
Aminoglycosides and vancomycin

**Is rash (only) in response to penicillins a contraindication to cephalosporins?**
No, but breathing problems, urticaria, and edema in response to penicillins are contraindications to the cephalosporins.

**Describe the following medications:**

**Augmentin®**
Amoxicillin and clavulanic acid

**Unasyn®**
Ampicillin and sulbactam

**Cefazolin (Ancef®)**
First-generation cephalosporin; surgical prophylaxis for **skin flora**

**Cefoxitin (Mefoxin®)**
Second-generation cephalosporin; used for mixed aerobic/anaerobic infections; effective against *Bacteroides fragilis* and anaerobic bacteria

**Ceftazidime (Ceftaz®)**
Third-generation cephalosporin; strong activity against *Pseudomonas*

**Clindamycin**
Strong activity against gram-negative **anaerobes**, such as *B. fragilis;* adequate gram-positive activity

**Gentamicin**

Aminoglycoside used to treat **gram-negative** bacteria; nephrotoxic, ototoxic; blood peak/trough levels should be monitored

**Imipenem and cilastatin (Primaxin®)**

Often used as a last resort against serious, multiresistant organisms
Usually combined with cilastin, which inhibits renal excretion of imipenem
Has a very wide spectrum

**Metronidazole (Flagyl®)**

Used for serious **anaerobic** infections (e.g., diverticulitis); also used to treat amebiasis; patient must abstain from alcohol use during therapy

**Nafcillin (Nafcil®)**

Antistaphylococcal penicillin commonly used for cellulitis

**Vancomycin**

Used to treat methicillin-resistant *Staphylococcus aureus* (**MRSA**); used orally to treat *C. difficile* pseudomembranous colitis (poorly absorbed from the gut); with IV administration, peak/trough levels should be monitored

**Percocet®**

PO narcotic pain reliever with acetaminophen and oxycodone

**Ciprofloxacin (Cipro®)**

Quinoline antibiotic with broad-spectrum activity, especially against gram-negative bacteria, including *Pseudomonas*

**Aztreonam (Azactam®)**

Monobactam with gram-negative spectrum

**Amphotericin**

IV antifungal antibiotic associated with renal toxicity, hypokalemia

**Fluconazole (Diflucan®)**

Antifungal agent (IV or PO) **not** associated with renal toxicity

**Nystatin**

PO and topical antifungal

## STEROIDS

| | |
|---|---|
| **What are the side effects?** | Adrenal suppression, immunosuppression, weight gain with central obesity, cushingoid facies, acne, hirsutism, purple striae, hyperglycemia, sodium retention/hypokalemia, hypertension, osteopenia, myopathy, ischemic bone necrosis (avascular necrosis of the hip), GI perforations |
| **What are its uses?** | Immunosuppression (transplant), autoimmune diseases, hormone replacement (Addison's disease), spinal cord trauma |
| **Can steroids be stopped abruptly?** | **No, steroids should never be stopped abruptly; always taper.** |
| **Which patients need stress-dose steroids before surgery?** | Those who are on steroids, were on steroids in the past year, have suspected hypoadrenalism, or are about to undergo adrenalectomy |
| **What is the "stress dose" for steroids?** | **100** mg of hydrocortisone IV every 8 hours and then taper (adults) |
| **Which vitamin helps counteract the deleterious effects of steroids on wound healing?** | Vitamin A |

## HEPARIN

| | |
|---|---|
| **Describe the action.** | Heparin binds with and activates antithrombin III. |
| **What are its uses?** | Prophylaxis/treatment—DVT, pulmonary embolism, stroke, atrial fibrillation, acute arterial occlusion, cardiopulmonary bypass |
| **What are the side effects?** | Bleeding complications; can cause thrombocytopenia |
| **What reverses the effects?** | **Protamine IV (1:100, 1** mg of protamine to every **100** units of heparin) |

| | |
|---|---|
| **What laboratory test should be used to follow effect?** | aPTT—activated partial thromboplastin time |
| **What is the standard lab target for therapeutic heparinization?** | 1.5–2.5 times control or measured antifactor X level |
| **Who is at risk for a protamine anaphylactic reaction?** | Patients with type 1 diabetes mellitus, s/p prostate surgery |
| **What is the half-life of heparin?** | Approximately 90 minutes (1–2 hours) |
| **How long before surgery should it be discontinued?** | From 4 to 6 hours preoperatively |
| **Does heparin dissolve clots?** | No; it stops the progression of clot formation and allows the body's own fibrinolytic systems to dissolve the clot. |
| **What is LMWH?** | **L**ow **M**olecular **W**eight **H**eparin |
| **What laboratory test do you need to follow LMWH?** | None, except in children, patients with obesity, and those with renal failure, which is the major advantage of LMWH (check factor X levels) |

## WARFARIN (COUMADIN®)

| | |
|---|---|
| **ACRONYM basis for name?** | **W**isconsin **A**lumni **R**esearch **F**oundation |
| **Describe its action.** | **Inhibits vitamin K-dependent clotting factors II, VII, IX, X,** (i.e., 2, 7, 9, **10** [think: 2 + 7 = 9 and 10]), produced in the liver |
| **What are its uses?** | Long-term anticoagulation (PO) |
| **What are its associated risks?** | Bleeding complications, teratogenic in pregnancy, skin necrosis, dermatitis |
| **What laboratory test should be used to follow its effect?** | PT (prothrombin time) as reported as INR |
| **What is INR?** | **I**nternational **N**ormalized **R**atio |

| | |
|---|---|
| **What is the classic therapeutic INR?** | INR of 2–3 |
| **What is the half-life of effect?** | 40 hours; thus, it takes about 2 days to observe a change in the PT |
| **What reverses the action?** | **Cessation,** vitamin K, fresh-frozen plasma (in emergencies) |
| **How long before surgery should it be discontinued?** | From 3 to 5 days preoperatively and IV heparin should be begun; heparin should be discontinued from 4 to 6 hours preoperatively and can be restarted postoperatively; Coumadin® can be restarted in a few days |

## MISCELLANEOUS AGENTS

**Describe the following drugs:**

| | |
|---|---|
| **Sucralfate (Carafate®)** | Treats peptic ulcers by forming an acid-resistant barrier; binds to ulcer craters; needs acid to activate and thus should not be used with $H_2$ blockers |
| **Cimetidine (Tagamet®)** | $H_2$ blocker (ulcers/gastritis) |
| **Ranitidine (Zantac®)** | $H_2$ blocker (ulcers/gastritis) |
| **Ondansetron (Zofran®)** | Anti-nausea Anti-emetic |
| **PPI** | Proton pump inhibitor: Gastric acid–secretion inhibitor; works by inhibiting the $K^+/H^+$-ATPase (e.g., omeprazole [Prilosec®]) |
| **Promethazine (Phenergan®)** | Acute antinausea agent; used postoperatively |
| **Metoclopramide (Reglan®)** | Increases gastric emptying with increase in LES pressure; **dopamine antagonist;** used in diabetic gastroparesis and to help move feeding tubes past the pylorus |
| **Haldol** | Sedative–antipsychotic (major side effect = extrapyramidal symptoms) |

| | |
|---|---|
| **Albumin** | 5% albumin—expands plasma volume<br>25% albumin—draws extravascular fluid into intravascular space by oncotic pressure |
| **Albuterol** | Inhaled beta$_2$ agonist (bronchodilator) |
| **Octreotide** | Somatostatin analog |
| **Famotidine (Pepcid®)** | H$_2$ blocker |
| **Aspirin** | Irreversibly inhibits platelets by irreversibly inhibiting cyclo-oxygenase |
| **Furosemide (Lasix®)** | Loop diuretic (watch for hypokalemia) |
| **Dantrolene (Dantrium®)** | Medication used to treat malignant hyperthermia. |
| **Misoprostol (Cytotec®)** | Prostaglandin E$_1$, analog<br>Gastroduodenal mucosal protection |
| **What is an antibiotic option for colon/appendectomy coverage if the patient is allergic to penicillin?** | 1. IV ciprofloxacin (Cipro) AND<br>2. IV clindamycin or IV Flagyl |
| **If the patient does not respond to a dose of furosemide, should the dose be repeated, increased, or decreased?** | The dose should be doubled if there is no response to the initial dose. |
| **What medication is used to treat promethazine-induced dystonia?** | Diphenhydramine hydrochloride IV (Benadryl®) |
| **Which medication is classically associated with mesenteric ischemia?** | Digitalis |
| **What type of antihypertensive medication is contraindicated in patients with renal artery stenosis?** | ACE inhibitors |
| **Does acetaminophen (Tylenol®) inhibit platelets?** | No |

| | |
|---|---|
| **What medications are used to stop seizures?** | Benzodiazepines (e.g., lorazepam [Ativan®]); phenytoin (Dilantin®) |
| **List the preop antibiotics for:**<br>    **Vascular prosthetic graft** | Ancef® (gm+ coverage) |
| **Appendectomy** | Cefoxitin, cefotetan, Unasyn® (anaerobic coverage) |
| **Colon surgery** | Cefoxitin, cefotetan, Unasyn® (anaerobic coverage) |

## NARCOTICS

| | |
|---|---|
| **What are common postoperative IV narcotics?** | Morphine (most common), meperidine (Demerol®), fentanyl, Percocet®, Dilauid® |
| **What is Demerol's claim to fame?** | It is used commonly with acute pancreatitis/biliary pathology because classically morphine may cause sphincter of Oddi spasm/constriction. |
| **What are side effects of narcotics?** | Respiratory depression, hypotension, itching, bradycardia, nausea |
| **What is the danger of prolonged use of Demerol?** | Accumulation of metabolite normeperidine (especially with renal/hepatic dysfunction), which may result in oversedation, hallucinations, and seizures! |
| **What medication reverses the effects of narcotic overdose?** | Naloxone (Narcan®), 0.4 mg IV |
| **Narcotic used to decrease postoperative shivering?** | Demerol® |

## MISCELLANEOUS

| | |
|---|---|
| **What reverses the effects of benzodiazepines?** | Flumazenil (Romazicon®), 0.2 mg IV |
| **What is Toradol®?** | Ketorolac IV NSAID |
| **What are the risks of Toradol®?** | GI bleed, renal injury, platelet dysfunction |

**Why give a patient IV Cipro when he is eating a regular diet?**

No reason—500 mg of Cipro PO gives the same serum level as 400 mg Cipro IV! And PO is much cheaper!

**What is clonidine "rebound"?**

If you stop clonidine, the patient often will have severe "rebound" hypertension.

# Chapter 22    Complications

## ATELECTASIS

**What is it?**

Collapse of the alveoli

**What is the etiology?**

Inadequate alveolar expansion (e.g., poor ventilation of lungs during surgery, inability to fully inspire secondary to pain), high levels of inspired oxygen

**What are the signs?**

Fever, decreased breath sounds with rales, tachypnea, tachycardia, and increased density on CXR

**What are the risk factors?**

Chronic obstructive pulmonary disease (COPD), smoking, abdominal or thoracic surgery, oversedation, poor pain control (**patient cannot breathe deeply secondary to pain on inspiration**)

**What is its claim to fame?**

Most common cause of fever during postoperative days 1 to 2

**What prophylactic measures can be taken?**

Preoperative smoking cessation, incentive spirometry, good pain control

**What is the treatment?**

Postoperative **incentive spirometry,** deep breathing, coughing, early ambulation, NT suctioning, and chest PT

## POSTOPERATIVE RESPIRATORY FAILURE

| | |
|---|---|
| **What is it?** | Respiratory impairment with increased respiratory rate, shortness of breath, dyspnea |
| **What is the differential diagnosis?** | Hypovolemia, pulmonary embolism, administration of supplemental $O_2$ to a patient with COPD, atelectasis, pneumonia, aspiration, pulmonary edema, abdominal compartment syndrome, pneumothorax, chylothorax, hemothorax, narcotic overdose, mucus plug |
| **What is the treatment?** | Supplemental $O_2$, chest PT; suctioning, intubation, and ventilation if necessary |
| **What is the initial workup?** | ABG, CXR, ECG, pulse oximetry, and auscultation |
| **What are the indications for intubation and ventilation?** | Cannot protect airway (unconscious), excessive work of breathing, progressive **hypoxemia** ($paO_2 < 55$ despite supplemental $O_2$), progressive **acidosis** ($pH < 7.3$ and $PCO_2 > 50$), RR > 35 |
| **What are the possible causes of postoperative pleural effusion?** | Fluid overload, pneumonia, and diaphragmatic inflammation with possible subphrenic abscess formation |
| **What is the treatment of postoperative wheezing?** | Albuterol nebulizer |
| **Why may it be dangerous to give a patient with chronic COPD supplemental oxygen?** | This patient uses relative hypoxia for respiratory drive, and supplemental $O_2$ may remove this drive! |

## PULMONARY EMBOLISM

| | |
|---|---|
| **What is a pulmonary embolism (PE)?** | DVT that embolizes to the pulmonary arterial system |

**What is DVT?**

**D**eep **V**enous **T**hrombosis—a clot forming in the pelvic or lower extremity veins

**Is DVT more common in the right or left iliac vein?**

Left is more common (4 to 1) because the aortic bifurcation crosses and possibly compresses the left iliac vein.

**What are the signs/ symptoms of DVT?**

Lower extremity pain, swelling, tenderness, Homan's sign, pulmonary embolus (PE)
Up to 50% can be asymptomatic!

**What is Homan's sign?**

Calf pain with dorsiflexion of the foot seen classically with DVT, but actually found in fewer than one-third of patients with DVT

**What test is used to evaluate for DVT?**

Duplex ultrasonography

**What is Virchow's triad?**

(1) Stasis, (2) endothelial injury, and (3) hypercoagulable state (risk factors for thrombosis)

**What are the risk factors for DVT and PE?**

Postoperative status, multiple trauma, paralysis, immobility, CHF, obesity, BCP/tamoxifen, cancer, advanced age, polycythemia, MI, HIT syndrome, hypercoagulable state (protein C/protein S deficiency)

**What are the signs/ symptoms of PE?**

Shortness of breath, tachypnea, hypotension, CP, occasionally fever, loud pulmonic component of S2, hemoptysis with pulmonary infarct

**What are the associated lab findings?**

ABG—decreased $PO_2$ and $PCO_2$ (from hyperventilation)

**Which diagnostic tests are indicated?**

CT Angiogram, V-Q scan (ventilation-perfusion scan), pulmonary A-gram is the gold standard

| | |
|---|---|
| **What are the associated CXR findings?** | 1. Westermark's sign (wedge-shaped area of decreased pulmonary vasculature resulting in hyperlucency)<br>2. Opacity with base at pleural edge from pulmonary infarction |
| **What are the associated EKG findings?** | More than 50% are abnormal; classic finding is cor pulmonale (S1Q3T3 RBBB and right-axis deviation); ECG most commonly shows flipped T waves or ST depression. |
| **What is a "saddle" embolus?** | PE that "straddles" the pulmonary artery and is in the lumen of both the right and left pulmonary arteries |
| **What is the treatment if the patient is stable?** | Anticoagulation (heparin followed by long-term [3–6 months] Coumadin®) or Greenfield filter |
| **What is a Greenfield filter?** | Metallic filter placed into IVC via jugular vein to catch emboli prior to lodging in the pulmonary artery |

| | |
|---|---|
| **Where did Dr. Greenfield get his idea for his IVC filter?** | Oil pipeline filters! |
| **When is a Greenfield filter indicated?** | If anticoagulation is contraindicated or patient has further PE on adequate anticoagulation or is high-risk (e.g., pelvic and femur fractures) |

| | |
|---|---|
| **What is the treatment if the patient's condition is unstable?** | Consider thrombolytic therapy; consult thoracic surgeon for possible Trendelenburg operation; consider catheter suction embolectomy. |
| **What is the Trendelenburg operation?** | Pulmonary artery embolectomy |
| **What is a "retrievable" IVC filter?** | An IVC filter that can be removed ("retrieved") |
| **What percentage of retrievable IVC filters are actually removed?** | Only about 20% |
| **What prophylactic measures can be taken for DVT/PE?** | LMWH (Lovenox®) 40 mg SQ QD; **or** 30 mg SQ b.i.d.; sub-Q heparin (5,000 units sub-Q every 8 hrs; must be started preoperatively), sequential compression device BOOTS beginning in OR (often used with sub-Q heparin), early ambulation |

## ASPIRATION PNEUMONIA

| | |
|---|---|
| **What is it?** | Pneumonia following aspiration of vomitus |
| **What are the risk factors?** | Intubation/extubation, impaired consciousness (e.g., drug or ETOH overdose), dysphagia (esophageal disease), nonfunctioning NGT, Trendelenburg position, OR emergent intubation with full stomach, gastric dilatation |
| **What are the signs/ symptoms?** | Respiratory failure, CP, increased sputum production, fever, cough, mental status changes, tachycardia, cyanosis, infiltrate on CXR |
| **What are the associated CXR findings?** | Early—fluffy infiltrate or normal CXR Late—pneumonia, ARDS |
| **Which lobes are commonly involved?** | Supine—RUL Sitting/semirecumbent—RLL |

| | |
|---|---|
| **Which organisms are commonly involved?** | Community acquired—gram-positive/ mixed<br>Hospital/ICU—gram-negative rods |
| **Which diagnostic tests are indicated?** | CXR, sputum, Gram stain, sputum culture, bronchoalveolar lavage |
| **What is the treatment?** | Bronchoscopy, antibiotics if pneumonia develops, intubation if respiratory failure occurs, ventilation with PEEP if ARDS develops |
| **What is Mendelson's syndrome?** | Chemical pneumonitis secondary to aspiration of stomach contents (i.e., gastric acid) |
| **Are prophylatic antibiotics indicated for aspiration pneumonitis?** | NO |

## GASTROINTESTINAL COMPLICATIONS

| | |
|---|---|
| **What are possible NGT complications?** | Aspiration-pneumonia/atelectasis<br>   (especially if NGT is clogged)<br>Sinusitis<br>Minor UGI bleeding<br>   Epistaxis<br>   Pharyngeal irritation, gastric<br>   irritation |

### GASTRIC DILATATION

| | |
|---|---|
| **What are the risk factors?** | Abdominal surgery, gastric outlet obstruction, splenectomy, narcotics |
| **What are the signs/ symptoms?** | Abdominal distension, hiccups, electrolyte abnormalities, nausea |
| **What is the treatment?** | NGT decompression |
| **What do you do if you have a patient with high NGT output?** | Check high abdominal x-ray and, if the NGT is in duodenum, pull back the NGT into the stomach. |

## POSTOPERATIVE PANCREATITIS

| | |
|---|---|
| **What is it?** | Pancreatitis resulting from manipulation of the pancreas during surgery or low blood flow during the procedure (i.e., cardiopulmonary bypass), gallstones, hypercalcemia, medications, idiopathic |
| **What lab tests are performed?** | Amylase and lipase |
| **What is the initial treatment?** | Same as that for the other causes of pancreatitis (e.g., NPO, aggressive fluid resuscitation, ± NGT PRN) |

## CONSTIPATION

| | |
|---|---|
| **What are the postoperative causes?** | Narcotics, immobility |
| **What is the treatment?** | OBR |
| **What is OBR?** | **O**rtho **B**owel **R**outine: docusate sodium (daily), dicacodyl suppository if no bowel movement occurs, Fleet® enema if suppository is ineffective |

## SHORT BOWEL SYNDROME

| | |
|---|---|
| **What is it?** | Malabsorption and diarrhea resulting from extensive bowel resection (approximately ≤120 cm of small bowel remaining) |
| **What is the initial treatment?** | TPN early, followed by many small meals chronically |

## POSTOPERATIVE SMALL BOWEL OBSTRUCTION (SBO)/ILEUS

| | |
|---|---|
| **What causes SBO?** | **Adhesions** (most of which resolve spontaneously), incarcerated hernia (internal or fascial/dehiscence) |
| **What causes ileus?** | Laparotomy, hypokalemia or narcotics, intraperitoneal infection |

| | |
|---|---|
| **What are the signs of resolving ileus/SBO?** | Flatus PR, stool PR |
| **What is the order of recovery of bowel function after abdominal surgery?** | **First**—small intestine<br>**Second**—stomach<br>**Third**—colon |
| **When can a postoperative patient be fed through a J tube?** | From 12 to 24 postoperative hours because the small intestine recovers function first in that period |

## JAUNDICE

| | |
|---|---|
| **What are the causes of the following types of postoperative jaundice:** | |
| **Prehepatic** | Hemolysis (prosthetic valve), resolving hematoma, transfusion reaction, postcardiopulmonary bypass, blood transfusions (decreased RBC compliance leading to cell rupture) |
| **Hepatic** | **Drugs,** hypotension, hypoxia, sepsis, hepatitis, "sympathetic" hepatic inflammation from adjacent right lower lobe infarction of the lung or pneumonia, preexisting cirrhosis, right-sided heart failure, hepatic abscess, pylephlebitis (thrombosis of portal vein), Gilbert syndrome, Crigler-Najjar syndrome, Dubin-Johnson syndrome, fatty infiltrate from TPN |
| **Posthepatic** | Choledocholithiasis, stricture, cholangitis, cholecystitis, biliary-duct injury, pancreatitis, sclerosing cholangitis, tumors (e.g., cholangiocarcinoma, pancreatic cancer, gallbladder cancer, metastases), biliary stasis (e.g., ceftriaxone [Rocephin®]) |
| **What blood tests would support the assumption that hemolysis was causing jaundice in a patient?** | **Decreased**—Haptoglobin, Hct<br>**Increased**—LDH, reticulocytes<br>Also, fragmented RBCs on a peripheral smear |

## BLIND LOOP SYNDROME

| | |
|---|---|
| **What is it?** | Bacterial overgrowth in the small intestine |
| **What are the causes?** | Anything that disrupts the normal flow of intestinal contents (i.e., causes stasis) |
| **What are the surgical causes of $B_{12}$ deficiency?** | Gastrectomy (decreased secretion of intrinsic factor) and excision of the terminal ileum (site of $B_{12}$ absorption) |

## POSTVAGOTOMY DIARRHEA

| | |
|---|---|
| **What is it?** | Diarrhea after a truncal vagotomy |
| **What is the cause?** | It is thought that after truncal vagotomy, a rapid transport of bile salts to the colon results in osmotic inhibition of water absorption in the colon, leading to diarrhea. |

## DUMPING SYNDROME

| | |
|---|---|
| **What is it?** | Delivery of **hyperosmotic** chyme to the small intestine causing massive fluid shifts into the bowel (normally the stomach will decrease the osmolality of the chyme prior to its emptying) |
| **With what conditions is it associated?** | Any procedure that bypasses the pylorus or compromises its function (i.e., gastroenterostomies or pyloroplasty); thus, "dumping" of chyme into small intestine |
| **What are the signs/ symptoms?** | Postprandial diaphoresis, tachycardia, abdominal pain/distention, emesis, increased flatus, dizziness, weakness |
| **How is the diagnosis made?** | History; hyperosmolar glucose load will elicit similar symptoms |
| **What is the medical treatment?** | Small, multiple, low-fat/carbohydrate meals that are high in protein content; also, **avoidance of liquids** with meals to slow gastric emptying; surgery is a last resort |

| | |
|---|---|
| **What is the surgical treatment?** | Conversion to Roux-en-Y ($\pm$ reversed jejunal interposition loop) |
| **What is a reversed jejunal interposition loop?** | A segment of jejunum is cut and then reversed to allow for a short segment of reversed peristalsis to slow intestinal transit. |

## ENDOCRINE COMPLICATIONS

### DIABETIC KETOACIDOSIS (DKA)

| | |
|---|---|
| **What is it?** | Deficiency of body insulin, resulting in hyperglycemia, formation of ketoacids, osmotic diuresis, and metabolic acidosis |
| **What are the signs of DKA?** | Polyuria, tachypnea, dehydration, confusion, abdominal pain |
| **What are the associated lab values?** | Elevated glucose, increased anion gap, hypokalemia, urine ketones, acidosis |
| **What is the treatment?** | Insulin drip, IVF rehydration, $K^+$ supplementation $\pm$ bicarbonate IV |
| **What electrolyte must be monitored closely in DKA?** | Potassium and HYPOkalemia (Remember correction of acidosis and GLC/insulin drive $K^+$ into cells and are treatment for HYPERkalemia!) |
| **What must you rule out in a diabetic with DKA?** | Infection (perirectal abscess is classically missed!) |

### ADDISONIAN CRISIS

| | |
|---|---|
| **What is it?** | Acute adrenal insufficiency in the face of a stressor (i.e., surgery, trauma, infection) |
| **How can you remember what causes addisonian crisis?** | Think: **ADD**isonian = **AD**renal **D**own |
| **What is the cause?** | Postoperatively, inadequate cortisol release usually results from steroid administration in the past year. |

| | |
|---|---|
| **What are the signs/symptoms?** | Tachycardia, nausea, vomiting, diarrhea, **abdominal pain,** ± fever, progressive lethargy, **hypotension, eventual hypovolemic shock** |
| **What is its clinical claim to infamy?** | Tachycardia and hypotension refractory to IVF and pressors! |
| **Which lab values are classic?** | Decreased $Na^+$, increased $K^+$ (secondary to decreased aldosterone) |
| **How can you remember the serum sodium level in addisonian crisis?** | Think: addisonian crisis = adre**Na**$^+$1 insufficiency = **Na**$^+$ insufficiency |
| **What is the treatment?** | IVFs (D5 NS), hydrocortisone IV, fludrocortisone PO |
| **What is fludrocortisone?** | Mineralocorticoid replacement (aldosterone) |

## SIADH

| | |
|---|---|
| **What is it?** | **S**yndrome of **I**nappropriate **A**nti**D**iuretic **H**ormone (ADH) secretion (think of **inappropriate increase** in ADH secretion) |
| **What does ADH do?** | ADH increases NaCl and $H_2O$ resorption in the kidney, increasing intravascular volume (released from posterior pituitary). |
| **What are the causes?** | **Mainly lung**/CNS: CNS trauma, oat-cell lung cancer, pancreatic cancer, duodenal cancer, pneumonia/lung abscess, increased PEEP, stroke, general anesthesia, idiopathic, postoperative, morphine |
| **What are the associated lab findings?** | Low sodium, chloride, and serum osmolality; increased urine osmolality |
| **How can you remember the serum sodium level in SIADH?** | Remember, **SIADH = S**odium **I**s **A**lways **D**own **H**ere |
| **What is the treatment?** | Treat the primary cause and restrict fluid intake. |

## DIABETES INSIPIDUS (DI)

| | |
|---|---|
| **What is it?** | Failure of ADH renal fluid conservation resulting in dilute urine in large amounts (think DI = Decreased ADH) |
| **What is the source of ADH?** | POSTERIOR pituitary |
| **What are the two major types?** | 1. Central (neurogenic) DI<br>2. Nephrogenic DI |
| **What is the mechanism of the two types?** | 1. Central DI = decreased production of ADH<br>2. Nephrogenic DI = decreased ADH effect on kidney |
| **What are the classic causes of central DI?** | **BRAIN** injury, tumor, surgery, and infection |
| **What are the classic causes of nephrogenic DI?** | Amphotericin B, hypercalcemia, and chronic kidney infection |
| **What lab values are associated with DI?** | HYPERnatremia, decreased urine sodium, decreased urine osmolality, and increased serum osmolality |
| **What is the treatment?** | Fluid replacement; follow $NA^+$ levels and urine output; central DI warrants vasopressin; nephrogenic DI may respond to thiazide diuretics |

## CARDIOVASCULAR COMPLICATIONS

| | |
|---|---|
| **What are the arterial line complications?** | Infection; thrombosis, which can lead to finger/hand necrosis; death/hemorrhage from catheter disconnection (remember to perform and document the **Allen test** before inserting an arterial line or obtaining a blood gas sample) |
| **What is an Allen test?** | Measures for adequate collateral blood flow to the hand via the ulnar artery: patient clenches fist, then both radial and ulnar arteries are occluded; patient opens the blanched hand. The ulnar artery |

is released. If the palm has an immediate strong blush, the ulnar artery should be adequate collateral flow if the radial artery thromboses.

**What are the common causes of dyspnea following central line placement?**

Pneumothorax, pericardial tamponade, carotid puncture (which can cause a hematoma that compresses the trachea), air embolism

**What is the differential diagnosis of postoperative chest pain?**

MI, atelectasis, pneumonia, pleurisy, esophageal reflux, PE, musculoskeletal pain, subphrenic abscess, aortic dissection, pneumo/chyle/hemothorax, gastritis

**What is the differential diagnosis of postoperative atrial fibrillation?**

**Fluid overload, PE, MI, pain** (excess catecholamines), atelectasis, pneumonia, digoxin toxicity, hypoxemia, thyrotoxicosis, hypercapnia, idiopathic, acidosis, electrolyte abnormalities

## MYOCARDIAL INFARCTION (MI)

**What is the most dangerous period for a postoperative MI following a previous MI?**

Six months after an MI

**What are the risk factors for postoperative MI?**

History of MI, angina, Q's on ECG, S3, JVD, CHF, aortic stenosis, advanced age, extensive surgical procedure, MI within 6 months, ECG changes

**How do postoperative MIs present?**

**Often without chest pain**
New onset **CHF,** new onset **cardiac dysrhythmia,** hypotension, chest pain, tachypnea, tachycardia, nausea/vomiting, bradycardia, neck pain, arm pain

**What ECG findings are associated with cardiac ischemia/MI?**

Flipped T waves, ST elevation, ST depression, dysrhythmias (e.g., new onset a fib, PVC, V tach)

**Which lab tests are indicated?**

Troponin I, cardiac isoenzymes (elevated CK mb fraction)

| | |
|---|---|
| **What is the treatment of postoperative MI?** | Nitrates (paste or drip), as tolerated<br>Aspirin<br>Oxygen<br>Pain control with IV morphine<br>β-blocker, as tolerated<br>Heparin (possibly; thrombolytics are contraindicated in the postoperative patient)<br>ICU monitoring |
| **How can you remember the treatment of postoperative MI?** | "BEMOAN":<br>**BE**ta-blocker (as tolerated)<br>**M**orphine<br>**O**xygen<br>**A**spirin<br>**N**itrates |
| **When do postoperative MIs occur?** | Two-thirds occur on postoperative days 2 to 5 (often silent and present with **dyspnea** or **dysrhythmia**). |

## POSTOPERATIVE CVA

| | |
|---|---|
| **What is a CVA?** | **C**erebro**V**ascular **A**ccident (stroke) |
| **What are the signs/ symptoms?** | Aphasia, motor/sensory deficits usually lateralizing |
| **What is the workup?** | Head CT; must rule out hemorrhage if anticoagulation is going to be used; carotid Doppler ultrasound study to evaluate for carotid occlusive disease |
| **What is the treatment?** | ASA, ± heparin if feasible postoperatively<br>Thrombolytic therapy is not usually postoperative option. |
| **What is the perioperative prevention?** | Avoid hypotension; continue aspirin therapy preoperatively in high-risk patients if feasible, preoperative carotid Doppler study in high-risk patients. |

## MISCELLANEOUS

### POSTOPERATIVE RENAL FAILURE

| | |
|---|---|
| **What is it?** | Increase in serum creatinine and decrease in creatinine clearance; usually associated with decreased urine output |
| **Define the following terms:** | |
|     **Anuria** | <50 cc urine output in 24 hours |
|     **Oliguria** | >50 cc and <400 cc of urine output in 24 hours |
| **What is the differential diagnosis?** | |
|     **Prerenal** | **Inadequate blood perfusing kidney:** inadequate fluids, hypotension, cardiac pump failure (CHF) |
|     **Renal** | **Kidney parenchymal dysfunction:** acute tubular necrosis, nephrotoxic contrast or drugs |
|     **Postrenal** | **Obstruction to outflow of urine from kidney:** Foley catheter obstruction/ stone, ureteral/urethral injury, BPH, bladder dysfunction (e.g., medications, spinal anesthesia) |
| **What is the work up?** | Lab tests: electrolytes, BUN, Cr, urine lytes/Cr, FENa, urinalysis, renal ultrasound |
| **What is FENa?** | **F**ractional **E**xcretion of **Na**$^+$ (sodium) |
| **What is the formula for FENa?** | "YOU NEED PEE" $(\mathbf{U}_{Na^+} \times \mathbf{P}_{cr} / P_{Na^+} \times U_{cr}) \times 100$ (U = urine, cr = creatinine, Na$^+$ = sodium, P = plasma) |

**Define the lab results with prerenal vs renal failure:**

**BUN/Cr ratio**

Prerenal: >20:1
Renal: <20:1

**Specific gravity**

Prerenal: >1.020 (as the body tries
    to hold on to fluid)
Renal: <1.020 (kidney has decreased
    ability to concentrate urine)

**FENA**

Prerenal FENa: <1
Renal: >1

**Urine Na$^+$ (sodium)**

Prerenal: >20
Renal: >40

**Urine osmolality**

Prerenal:  >500
Renal: <350 mOsm/kg

**What are the indications for dialysis?**

Fluid overload, refractory hyperkalemia,
BUN >130, acidosis, uremic
complication (encephalopathy, pericardial
effusion)

## DIC

**What is it?**

Activation of the coagulation
cascade leading to **thrombosis** and
**consumption** of clotting factors and
platelets and activation of fibrinolytic
system (fibrinolysis), resulting in
**bleeding**

**What are the causes?**

Tissue necrosis, septic shock, massive
large-vessel coagulation, shock, allergic
reactions, massive blood transfusion
reaction, cardiopulmonary bypass,
cancer, obstetric complications, snake
bites, trauma, burn injury, prosthetic
material, liver dysfunction

**What are the signs/ symptoms?**

Acrocyanosis or other signs of
thrombosis, then diffuse bleeding from
incision sites, venipuncture sites, catheter
sites, or mucous membranes

| | |
|---|---|
| **What are the associated lab findings?** | Increased fibrin-degradation products, elevated PT/PTT, decreased platelets, decreased fibrinogen (level correlates well with bleeding), presence of schistocytes (fragmented RBCs), increased D-dimer |
| **What is the treatment?** | **Removal of the cause;** otherwise supportive: IVFs, $O_2$, platelets, FFP, cryoprecipitate (fibrin), Epsilon-aminocaproic acid, as needed in predominantly thrombotic cases<br>Use of heparin is indicated in cases that are predominantly thrombotic with anti-thrombin III supplementation as needed. |

## ABDOMINAL COMPARTMENT SYNDROME

| | |
|---|---|
| **What is it?** | Increased intra-abdominal pressure usually seen after laparotomy or after massive IVF resuscitation (e.g., burn patients) |
| **What are the signs/ symptoms?** | Tight distended abdomen, decreased urine output, increased airway pressure, **increased intra-abdominal pressure** |
| **How to measure intra-abdominal pressure?** | Read intrabladder pressure (Foley catheter hooked up to manometry after instillation of 50–100 cc of water). |
| **What is normal intra-abdominal pressure?** | <15 mm Hg |
| **What intra-abdominal pressure indicates need for treatment?** | 25 mm Hg, especially if signs of compromise |
| **What is the treatment?** | Release the pressure by placing drain or by opening the abdomen and place a sheet of synthetic material to the skin to allow for more intra-abdominal volume. |

| | |
|---|---|
| **What is a "Bogata Bag"?** | A sheet of plastic (empty urology irrigation bag or IV bag) used to temporarily close the abdomen to allow for more intra-abdominal volume |

## URINARY RETENTION

| | |
|---|---|
| **What is it?** | Enlarged urinary bladder resulting from medications or spinal anesthesia |
| **How is it diagnosed?** | Physical exam (palpable bladder), bladder residual volume upon placement of a Foley catheter |
| **What is the treatment?** | Foley catheter |
| **With massive bladder distention, how much urine can you drain immediately?** | Most would clamp after 1 L and then drain the rest over time to avoid a vasovagal reaction. |

## WOUND INFECTION

| | |
|---|---|
| **What are the signs/ symptoms?** | Erythema, swelling, pain, heat, (rubor, tumor, calor, dolor) |
| **What is the treatment?** | Open wound, leave open with wet to dry dressing changes, antibiotics if cellulitis present |
| **How should one treat abdominal wound dehiscence?** | Emergently to OR for fascial reclosure |
| **What is fascial dehiscence?** | Acute separation of fascia that has been sutured closed |
| **What is the treatment?** | Bring back to the OR emergently for reclosure of the fascia. |

## WOUND HEMATOMA

| | |
|---|---|
| **What is it?** | Collection of blood (blood clot) in operative wound |
| **What is the treatment?** | Acute: remove with hemostasis<br>Subacute: observe (heat helps resorption) |

## WOUND SEROMA

| | |
|---|---|
| **What is it?** | Postoperative collection of lymph and serum in the operative wound |
| **What is the treatment?** | Needle aspiration, repeat if necessary (prevent with closed drain) |

## PSEUDOMEMBRANEOUS COLITIS

| | |
|---|---|
| **What is it also called?** | Antibiotic-associated diarrhea |
| **What are the signs/symptoms?** | **Diarrhea,** fever, hypotension/tachycardia |
| **What *classic* antibiotic causes C. diff ?** | Clindamycin (but almost all antibiotics can cause it) |
| **How is it diagnosed?** | *C. difficile* toxin in stool, fecal WBC, flex sig (see a mucus pseudomembrane in lumen of colon = hence the name) |
| **What is the treatment?** | 1. Flagyl (PO or IV)<br>2. PO Vancomycin if refractory to Flagyl |

# Chapter 23

# Common Causes of Ward Emergencies

| | |
|---|---|
| **What can cause hypotension?** | Hypovolemia (iatrogenic, hemorrhage), sepsis, MI, cardiac dysrhythmia, hypoxia, false reading (e.g., wrong cuff/arterial line twist or clot), pneumothorax, PE, cardiac tamponade, medications (e.g., morphine) |
| **How do you act?** | A, B, C's, examine, recheck BP, IV access, IV bolus, labs (e.g., HCT), ECG, pulse ox/vital signs monitoring, CXR, supplemental oxygen, check medications/history, give IV antibiotics "stat" if sepsis likely |

**What are the common causes of postoperative hypertension?**

**Pain** (from catecholamine release), anxiety, hypercapnia, hypoxia (which may also cause hypotension), preexisting condition, bladder distention

**What can cause hypoxia/ shortness of breath?**

Atelectasis, pneumonia, mucous plug, pneumothorax, PE, MI/dysrhythmia, venous blood in ABG syringe, SAT% machine malfunction/probe malposition, iatrogenic (wrong ventilator settings), severe anemia/hypovolemia, low cardiac output, CHF, ARDS, fluid overload

**How do you act?**

A, B, C's, physical exam, vital signs/pulse oximetry monitoring, supplemental oxygen, IV access, ABG, ECG, CXR

**What can cause mental status change?**

**Hypoxia** until ruled out, hypotension (e.g., cardiogenic shock), hypovolemia, iatrogenic (narcotics/benzodiazepines), drug reaction, alcohol withdrawal, drug withdrawal, seizure, ICU psychosis, CVA, sepsis, metabolic derangements, intracranial bleeding, **urinary retention in the elderly**

**What are the signs of alcohol withdrawal?**

**Confusion,** tachycardia/autonomic instability, seizure, hallucinations

**What are the causes of tachycardia?**

Hypovolemia/third-spacing, pain, alcohol withdrawal, anxiety/agitation, urinary retention, cardiac dysrhythmia (e.g., sinoventricular tachycardia, atrial fibrillation with rapid rate), MI, PE, β-blocker withdrawal

**What are the causes of decreased urine output?**

Hypovolemia, urinary retention, Foley catheter malfunction, cardiac failure, MI, acute tubular necrosis (ATN), ureteral/ urethral injury, abdominal compartment syndrome, sepsis

**How do you act initially in a case of decreased urine output?**

A, B, C's, examine, vital signs, check or place Foley catheter, irrigate Foley catheter, IV fluid bolus

# Chapter 24

# Surgical Respiratory Care

**What is the most common cause of fever in the first 48 hours postop?**

Atelectasis

**What is absorption atelectasis?**

Elevated inhaled oxygen replaces the nitrogen in the alveoli resulting in collapse of the air sac (atelectasis). Nitrogen keeps alveoli open by "stenting" it.

**What is incentive spirometry?**

The patient can document tidal volume and will have an "incentive" to increase it.

**What is oxygen-induced hypoventilation?**

Some patients with COPD have low oxygen as the main stimulus for the respiratory drive. If given supplemental oxygen, they will have a decreased respiratory drive and hypoventilation.

**Why give supplemental oxygen to a patient with a pneumothorax?**

Pneumothorax is almost completely nitrogen—thus increasing the oxygen in the alveoli increases the nitrogen gradient and results in faster absorption of the pneumothorax!

**What is a Venturi mask?**
The holes on the side of the mask allow for mixing of oxygen and air.

**What is a nonrebreather mask?**
100% oxygen with a reservoir bag

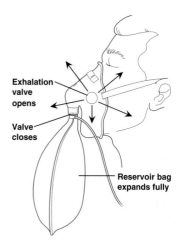

**Why do nonrebreather masks have a "reservoir" bag?**
Inhalation flow will exceed the delivery rate of the tubing and the bag allows for extra oxygen.

**What is the maximum oxygen FiO₂ delivered by a nonrebreather mask?**
Approximately 80%–90%

**How do you figure out the PaO$_2$ from an O$_2$ sat?**

PaO$_2$ of 40, 50, 60 roughly equals 70, 80, 90 in sats

**What is an oxygen nasal cannula?**

Oxygen delivered via tubing with prongs into nares

**How much do you increase the FiO$_2$ by each liter added to the nasal cannula?**

Approximately 3%

**What is the max effective flow for a nasal cannula?**

6 liters

# Chapter 25          Surgical Nutrition

**What is the motto of surgical nutrition?**

If the gut works, use it.

**What are the normal daily dietary requirements for adults of the following:**
    **Protein**

1 g/kg/day

    **Calories**

30 kcal/kg/day

| | |
|---|---|
| **By how much is basal energy expenditure (BEE) increased or decreased in the following cases:** | |
| Severe head injury | Increased $\approx 1.7 \times$ |
| Severe burns | Increased $\approx 2-3 \times$ |
| **What are the calorie contents of the following substances:** | |
| Fat | 9 kcal/g |
| Protein | 4 kcal/g |
| Carbohydrate | 4 kcal/g |
| **What is the formula for converting nitrogen requirement/loss to protein requirement/loss?** | Nitrogen $\times$ 6.25 = protein |
| **What is RQ?** | **R**espiratory **Q**uotient: the ratio of $CO_2$ produced to $O_2$ consumed |
| **What is the normal RQ?** | 0.8 |
| **What can be done to decrease the RQ?** | More fat, less carbohydrates |
| **What dietary change can be made to decrease $CO_2$ production in a patient in whom $CO_2$ retention is a concern?** | Decrease carbohydrate calories and increase calories from fat |
| **What lab tests are used to monitor nutritional status?** | Blood levels of:<br>**Prealbumin** (T 1/2 $\approx$ 2–3 days)—acute change determination<br>Transferrin (T 1/2 $\approx$ 8–9 days)<br>Albumin (T 1/2 $\approx$ 14–20 days)—more chronic determination |

Total lymphocyte count
Anergy
Retinol-binding protein (T $1/2 \approx$
12 hours)

**Where is iron absorbed?**　　　　　Duodenum (some in proximal jejunum)

**Where is vitamin $B_{12}$**　　　　　Terminal ileum
**absorbed?**

**What are the surgical causes**　　　Gastrectomy, excision of terminal ileum,
**of vitamin $B_{12}$ deficiency?**　　　blind loop syndrome

**Where are bile salts**　　　　　　　Terminal ileum
**absorbed?**

**Where are fat-soluble**　　　　　　　Terminal ileum
**vitamins absorbed?**

**Which vitamins are fat**　　　　　　K, A, D, E ("KADE")
**soluble?**

**What are the signs of the**
**following disorders:**
　**Vitamin A deficiency**　　　　　　Poor wound healing

　**Vitamin $B_{12}$/folate**　　　　　　Megaloblastic anemia
　**deficiency**

　**Vitamin C deficiency**　　　　　　Poor wound healing, bleeding gums

　**Vitamin K deficiency**　　　　　　$\downarrow$ in the vitamin K-dependent clotting
　　　　　　　　　　　　　　　　　factors (II, VII, IX, and X); bleeding;
　　　　　　　　　　　　　　　　　elevated PT

　**Chromium deficiency**　　　　　　Diabetic state

　**Zinc deficiency**　　　　　　　　Poor wound healing, alopecia, dermatitis,
　　　　　　　　　　　　　　　　　taste disorder

　**Fatty acid deficiency**　　　　　　Dry, flaky skin; alopecia

**What vitamin increases the**　　　　PO vitamin C (ascorbic acid)
**PO absorption of iron?**

**What vitamin lessens the deleterious effects of steroids on wound healing?**

Vitamin A

**What are the common indications for total parenteral nutrition (TPN)?**

NPO more than 7 days
Enterocutaneous fistulas
Short bowel syndrome
Prolonged ileus

**What is TPN?**

**T**otal **P**arenteral **N**utrition = IV nutrition

**What is in TPN?**

Protein
Carbohydrates
Lipids
($H_2O$, electrolytes, minerals/vitamins,
  ± insulin, ± $H_2$ blocker)

**How much of each in TPN:**

**Lipids**

20% to 30% of calories (lipid from soybeans, etc.)

**Protein**

1.7 g/kg/day (10–20% of calories) as amino acids

**Carbohydrates**

50% to 60% of calories as dextrose

**What are the possible complications of TPN?**

Line infection, fatty infiltration of the liver, electrolyte/glucose problems, pneumothorax during placement of central line, loss of gut barrier, acalculus cholecystitis, refeeding syndrome, hyperosmolality

**What are the advantages of enteral feeding?**

Keeps gut barrier healthy, thought to lessen translocation of bacteria, not associated with complications of line placement, associated with fewer electrolyte/glucose problems

**What is the major nutrient of the gut (small bowel)?**

Glutamine

**What is "refeeding syndrome"?**

Decreased serum **potassium, magnesium,** and **phosphate** after refeeding (via TPN or enterally) a starving patient

**What are the vitamin K-dependent clotting factors?**

2, 7, 9, 10 (think: 2 + 7 = 9, and then 10)

**What is an elemental tube feed?**

Very low residue tube feed in which almost all the tube feed is absorbed

**Where is calcium absorbed?**

Duodenum (actively)
Jejunum (passively)

**What is the major nutrient of the colon?**

**Butyrate** (and other short-chain fatty acids)

**What must bind $B_{12}$ for absorption?**

Intrinsic factor from the gastric parietal cells

**What sedative medication has caloric value?**

Propofol delivers 1 kcal/cc in the form of lipid!

**Why may all the insulin placed in a TPN bag not get to the patient?**

Insulin will bind to the IV tubing.

**What is the best way to determine the caloric requirements of a patient on the ventilator?**

Metabolic chart

**How can serum bicarbonate be increased in patients on TPN?**

Increase acetate (which is metabolized into bicarbonate)

**What are "trophic" tube feeds?**

Very low rate of tube feeds (i.e., approximately 10 cc/hr), which are thought to keep mucosa alive and healthy

**When should PO feedings be started after a laparotomy?**

Classically after flatus or stool PR (usually postoperative days 3–5)

**What is the best parameter to check adequacy of nutritional status?**

Prealbumin

# Chapter 26

# Shock

| | |
|---|---|
| **What is the definition of shock?** | Inadequate tissue perfusion |
| **What are the different types (5)?** | Hypovolemic<br>Septic<br>Cardiogenic<br>Neurogenic<br>Anaphylactic |
| **What are the signs of shock?** | Pale, diaphoretic, cool skin<br>Hypotension, tachycardia, tachypnea<br>↓ mental status and pulse pressure<br>Poor capillary refill<br>Poor urine output |
| **What are the best indicators of tissue perfusion?** | Urine output, mental status |
| **What lab tests help assess tissue perfusion?** | Lactic acid (elevated with inadequate tissue perfusion), base deficit, pH from ABG (acidosis associated with inadequate tissue perfusion) |

## HYPOVOLEMIC SHOCK

| | |
|---|---|
| **What is the definition?** | Decreased intravascular volume |
| **What are the common causes?** | Hemorrhage<br>Burns<br>Bowel obstruction<br>Crush injury<br>Pancreatitis |
| **What are the signs?** | **Early**—Orthostatic hypotension, mild tachycardia, anxiety, diaphoresis, vaso-constriction (decreased pulse pressure with increased diastolic pressure)<br>**Late**—Changed mental status, decreased BP, marked tachycardia |

**What are the signs/ symptoms with:**

**Class I hemorrhage (<15% or 750 cc blood loss)?**

Mild anxiety, normal vital signs

**Class II hemorrhage (15–30% or 750–1500 cc blood loss)?**

Normal systolic BP with decreased pulse pressure, tachycardia, tachypnea, anxiety

**Class III hemorrhage (30–40% or 1500–2000 cc blood loss)?**

Tachycardia (heart rate >120), tachypnea (respiratory rate >30), **decreased systolic BP,** decreased pulse pressure, confusion

**Class IV hemorrhage (>40% or >2000 cc blood loss)?**

Decreased systolic BP, tachycardia (heart rate >140), tachypnea (respiratory rate >35), decreased pulse pressure, confused and lethargic, no urine output

**What is the treatment?**

1. **Stop the bleeding**
2. **Volume:** IVF (isotonic LR) then blood as needed

**How is the effectiveness of treatment evaluated:**

**Bedside indicator?**

Urine output, BP, heart rate, mental status, extremity warmth, capillary refill, body temperature

**Labs?**

pH, base deficit, and lactate level

**What usually causes failure of resuscitation?**

Persistent massive hemorrhage, requiring emergent surgical procedure

**Why does decreased pulse pressure occur with early hypovolemic shock?**

Pulse pressure (systolic–diastolic BP) decreases because of vasoconstriction, resulting in an elevated diastolic BP.

**What is the most common vital sign change associated with early hypovolemic shock?**

Tachycardia

| | |
|---|---|
| **What type of patient does not mount a normal tachycardiac response to hypovolemic shock?** | Patients on β-blockers, spinal shock (loss of sympathetic tone), endurance athletes |
| **Should vasopressors be used to treat hypovolemic shock?** | No |
| **Should patients with hypovolemic shock be put into the Trendelenburg position?** | No |

## SEPTIC SHOCK

| | |
|---|---|
| **What is the definition?** | Documented infection and hypotension |
| **What is the specific etiology?** | Most common—gram-negative septicemia<br>Less common—gram-positive septicemia, fungus |
| **What factors increase the susceptibility to septic shock?** | Any mechanism that increases susceptibility to infection (e.g., trauma, immunosuppression, corticosteroids, hematologic disease, diabetes) |
| **What complications are major risks in septic shock?** | Multiple organ failure, DIC, **death** |
| **What are the signs/symptoms?** | Initial—vasodilation, resulting in warm skin and full pulses; normal urine output<br>Delayed—vasoconstriction and poor urine output; mental status changes; hypotension |
| **What percentage of blood cultures are positive in patients with bacterial septic shock?** | Only about 50%! |
| **What are the associated findings?** | Fever, hyperventilation, tachycardia |

**Which are the associated lab findings?**

Early—hyperglycemia/glycosuria, respiratory alkalosis, hemoconcentration, leukopenia

Late—leukocytosis, acidosis, elevated lactic acid

**Note:** Identifying organism is important to direct treatment/antibiotics.

**What is the treatment?**

1. Volume (IVF)
2. Antibiotics (empiric)
3. Drainage of infection
4. Pressors PRN
5. Zygris® PRN

**What is Zygris®?**

Activated protein C, shown to decrease mortality in septic shock and multiple organ failure

## CARDIOGENIC SHOCK

**What is the definition?**

Cardiac insufficiency; left ventricular failure (usually), resulting in inadequate tissue perfusion

**What are the causes?**

MI, papillary muscle dysfunction, massive cardiac contusion, cardiac tamponade, tension pneumothorax, cardiac valve failure

**What are the signs/ symptoms on exam?**

Dyspnea
Rales
Pulsus alternans (increased pulse with greater filling following a weak pulse)
Loud pulmonic component of $S_2$
Gallop rhythm

**What are the associated vital signs/parameters?**

Hypotension, decreased cardiac output, elevated CVP/wedge pressure, decreased urine output (low renal blood flow), tachycardia (possibly)

**What are the signs on CXR?**

Pulmonary edema

| | |
|---|---|
| **What is the treatment?** | Based on diagnosis/mechanism:<br>1. CHF: diuretics and afterload reduction (e.g., ACE inhibitors), with or without pressors<br>2. Left ventricular failure (MI): pressors, afterload reduction |
| **What are the last resort support mechanisms?** | Intra-aortic balloon pump (IABP), ventricular assist device (VAD) |

## NEUROGENIC SHOCK

| | |
|---|---|
| **What is the definition?** | Inadequate tissue perfusion from loss of sympathetic vasoconstrictive tone |
| **What are the common causes?** | Spinal cord injury<br>   Complete transection of spinal cord<br>   Partial cord injury with spinal shock<br>   Spinal anesthesia |
| **What are the signs/ symptoms?** | **Hypotension** and **bradycardia,** neurologic deficit |
| **Why are heart rate and BP decreased?** | Loss of sympathetic tone (but hypovolemia [e.g., hemoperitoneum] must be ruled out) |
| **What are the associated findings?** | Neurologic deficits suggesting cord injury |
| **What MUST you rule out in a trauma patient who has what you think is spinal shock?** | Hemorrhagic shock! |
| **What is the treatment?** | **IV fluids** (vasopressors reserved for hypotension refractory to fluid resuscitation) |
| **What percentage of patients with hypotension and spinal neurologic deficits have hypotension of purely neurogenic origin?** | About two thirds (67%) of patients |
| **What is spinal shock?** | Complete flaccid paralysis immediately following spinal cord injury; may or may not be associated with circulatory shock |

| | |
|---|---|
| **What is the lowest reflex available to the examiner?** | Bulbocavernous reflex: checking for contraction of the anal sphincter upon compression of the glans penis or clitoris |
| **What is the lowest level voluntary muscle?** | External anal sphincter |
| **What are the classic findings associated with spinal cord shock?** | Hypotension<br>Bradycardia or lack of compensatory tachycardia |

## MISCELLANEOUS

| | |
|---|---|
| **What is the acronym for treatment options for anaphylactic shock?** | "BASE":<br>**B**enadryl<br>**A**minophylline<br>**S**teroids<br>**E**pinephrine |

# Chapter 27          **Surgical Infection**

| | |
|---|---|
| **What are the classic signs/symptoms of inflammation/infection?** | Tumor (mass = swelling/edema)<br>Calor (heat)<br>Dolor (pain)<br>Rubor (redness = erythema) |
| **Define:** | |
| **Bacteremia** | Bacteria in the blood |
| **SIRS** | **S**ystemic **I**nflammatory **R**esponse **S**yndrome (fever, tachycardia, tachypnea, leukocytosis) |
| **Sepsis** | Documented infection and SIRS |
| **Septic shock** | Sepsis and hypotension refractory to fluid resuscitation |
| **Cellulitis** | **Blanching erythema** from superficial dermal/epidermal infection (usually strep > staph) |

| | |
|---|---|
| **Abscess** | Collection of pus within a cavity |
| **Superinfection** | A new infection arising while a patient is receiving antibiotics for the original infection at a different site (e.g., *C. difficile* colitis) |
| **Nosocomial infection** | Infection originating in the hospital |
| **Empiric** | Use of antibiotic based on previous sensitivity information or previous experience awaiting culture results in an established infection |
| **Prophylactic** | Antibiotics used to prevent an infection |
| **What is the most common nosocomial infection?** | Urinary tract infection (UTI) |
| **What is the most common nosocomial infection causing death?** | Respiratory tract infection (pneumonia) |

## URINARY TRACT INFECTIONS (UTIs)

| | |
|---|---|
| **What diagnostic tests are used?** | Urinalysis, culture, urine microscopy for WBC |
| **What constitutes a POSITIVE urine analysis?** | Positive nitrite (from bacteria)<br>Positive leukocyte esterase (from WBC)<br>More than 10 WBC/HPF<br>Presence of bacteria (supportive) |
| **What number of colony-forming units (CFU) confirms the diagnosis of UTI?** | On urine culture, classically 100,000 or $10^5$ CFU |
| **What are the common organisms?** | *Escherichia coli, Klebsiella, Proteus* (*Enterococcus, Staphylococcus aureus*) |
| **What is the treatment?** | Antibiotics with gram-negative spectrum (e.g., sulfamethoxazole/trimethoprim [Bactrim™], gentamicin, ciprofloxacin, aztreonam); check culture and sensitivity |

| What is the treatment of bladder candidiasis? | 1. Remove or change Foley catheter.<br>2. Administer systemic fluconazole or amphotericin bladder washings. |

## CENTRAL LINE INFECTIONS

| What are the signs of a central line infection? | **Unexplained hyperglycemia,** fever, mental status change, hypotension, tachycardia → **shock,** pus, and erythema at central line site |
| What is the most common cause of "catheter-related bloodstream infections"? | Coagulase-negative staphylococcus (37%), followed by enterococci, *Staphylococcus aureus,* gram-negative rods |
| When should you change central lines? | When they are infected; there is NO advantage to changing them every 7 days |
| What central line infusion increases the risk of infection? | Hyperal (TPN) |
| What is the treatment for central line infection? | 1. Remove central line (send for culture) +/− IV antibiotics.<br>2. Place NEW central line in a different site. |
| When should you change peripheral IV short angiocatheters? | Every 72 to 96 hours |

## WOUND INFECTION

| What is it? | Infection in an operative wound |
| When do these infections arise? | Classically, postoperative days 5 to 7 |
| What are the signs/ symptoms? | **Pain** at incision site, erythema, drainage, induration, warm skin, fever |
| What is the treatment? | Remove skin sutures/staples, perform digital examination to rule out fascial dehiscence, pack wound open, send wound culture, administer antibiotics |

| | |
|---|---|
| **What are the most common bacteria found in postoperative wound infections?** | *Staphylococcus aureus* (20%)<br>*Escherichia coli* (10%)<br>Enterococcus (10%) |
| | Other causes: *Staphylococcus epidermidis, Pseudomonas,* anaerobes, other gram-negative organisms, *Streptococcus* |
| **Which bacteria cause fever and wound infection in the first 24 hours after surgery?** | 1. *Streptococcus*<br>2. *Clostridium* (bronze-brown weeping tender wound) |

## CLASSIFICATION OF OPERATIVE WOUNDS

| | |
|---|---|
| **What is a "clean" wound?** | Elective, nontraumatic wound without acute inflammation; usually closed primarily without the use of drains |
| **What is the infection rate of a clean wound?** | Less than 1.5% |
| **What is a clean-contaminated wound?** | Operation on the GI or respiratory tract without unusual contamination or entry into the biliary or urinary tract |
| **Without infection present, what is the infection rate of a clean-contaminated wound?** | Less than 3% |
| **What is a contaminated wound?** | Acute inflammation, traumatic wound, GI tract spillage, or a major break in sterile technique |
| **What is the infection rate of a contaminated wound?** | Approximately 5% |
| **What is a dirty wound?** | Pus present, perforated viscus, or dirty traumatic wound |
| **What is the infection rate of a dirty wound?** | Approximately 33% |

**What are the possible complications of wound infections?**

Fistula, sinus tracts, sepsis, abscess, suppressed wound healing, superinfection (i.e., a new infection that develops during antibiotic treatment for the original infection), hernia

**What factors influence the development of infections?**

A foreign body (e.g., suture, drains, grafts)
Decreased blood flow (poor delivery of PMNs and antibiotics)
Strangulation of tissues with excessively tight sutures
Necrotic tissue or excessive local tissue destruction (e.g., too much Bovie)
Long operations (>2 hrs)
Hypothermia
Hematomas or seromas
Dead space that prevents the delivery of phagocytic cells to bacterial foci
Poor approximation of tissues

**What patient factors influence the development of infections?**

Uremia
Hypovolemic shock
Vascular occlusive states
Advanced age
Distant area of infection

**What are examples of an immunosuppressed state?**

Immunosuppressant treatment
Chemotherapy
Systemic malignancy
Trauma or burn injury
Diabetes mellitus
Obesity
Malnutrition
AIDS
Uremia

**Which lab tests are indicated?**

CBC: leukocytosis or leukopenia (as an abscess may act as a WBC sink), blood cultures, imaging studies (e.g., CT to locate an abscess)

**What is the treatment?**

Incision and drainage—an abscess must be drained (**Note:** fluctuation is a sign of a *subcutaneous* abscess. Most abdominal abscesses are drained percutaneously.)
Antibiotics for deep abscesses

| | |
|---|---|
| **What are the indications for antibiotics after drainage of a subcutaneous abscess?** | Diabetes mellitus, surrounding cellulitis, prosthetic heart valve, or an immuno-compromised state |

## PERITONEAL ABSCESS

| | |
|---|---|
| **What is a peritoneal abscess?** | Abscess within the peritoneal cavity |
| **What are the causes?** | Postoperative status after a laparotomy, ruptured appendix, peritonitis, any inflammatory intraperitoneal process, anastomotic leak |
| **What are the sites of occurrence?** | Pelvis, Morison's pouch, subphrenic, paracolic gutters, periappendiceal, lesser sac |
| **What are the signs/ symptoms?** | Fever (classically spiking), abdominal pain, mass |
| **How is the diagnosis made?** | Abdominal CT (or ultrasound) |
| **When should an abdominal CT be obtained looking for a postoperative abscess?** | After postoperative day 7 (otherwise, abscess will not be "organized" and will look like a normal postoperative fluid collection) |
| **What CT findings are associated with abscess?** | Fluid collection with fibrous rind, **gas** in fluid collection |
| **What is the treatment?** | Percutaneous CT-guided drainage |
| **What is an option for drainage of pelvic abscess?** | Transrectal drainage (or transvaginal) |
| **All abscesses must be drained except which type?** | Amebiasis! |
| **What is a "stitch" abscess?** | Subcutaneous abscess centered around a subcutaneous stitch, which is a "foreign body"; treat with drainage and stitch removal |

## NECROTIZING FASCIITIS

| | |
|---|---|
| **What is it?** | Bacterial infection of underlying fascia (spreads rapidly along fascial planes) |
| **What are the causative agents?** | Classically, group A *Streptococcus pyogenes,* but most often polymicrobial with anaerobes/gram-negative organisms |
| **What are the signs/symptoms?** | Fever, pain, crepitus, cellulitis, skin discoloration, blood blisters (hemorrhagic bullae), weeping skin, increased WBCs, subcutaneous air on x-ray, septic shock |
| **What is the treatment?** | IVF, IV antibiotics and aggressive early extensive surgical debridement, cultures, tetanus prophylaxis |
| **Is necrotizing fasciitis an emergency?** | YES, patients must be taken to the OR immediately! |

## CLOSTRIDIAL MYOSITIS

| | |
|---|---|
| **What is it?** | Clostridial muscle infection |
| **What is another name for this condition?** | Gas gangrene |
| **What is the most common causative organism?** | *Clostridium perfringens* |
| **What are the signs/symptoms?** | Pain, fever, shock, crepitus, foul-smelling brown fluid, subcutaneous air on x-ray |
| **What is the treatment?** | IV antibiotics, aggressive surgical debridement of involved muscle, tetanus prophylaxis |

## SUPPURATIVE HIDRADENITIS

| | |
|---|---|
| **What is it?** | Infection/abscess formation in **apocrine** sweat glands |
| **In what three locations does it occur?** | Perineum/buttocks, inguinal area, axilla (site of apocrine glands) |

| | |
|---|---|
| **What is the most common causative organism?** | *Staphylococcus aureus* |
| **What is the treatment?** | Antibiotics<br>Incision and drainage (excision of skin with glands for chronic infections) |

## PSEUDOMEMBRANOUS COLITIS

| | |
|---|---|
| **What is it?** | Antibiotic-induced colonic overgrowth of *C. difficile,* secondary to loss of competitive nonpathogenic bacteria that comprise the normal colonic flora<br>**Note:** it can be caused by any antibiotic, but especially penicillins, cephalosporins, and clindamycin. |
| **What are the signs/ symptoms?** | **Diarrhea,** ± fever, ± increased WBCs, ± abdominal cramps, ± abdominal distention |
| **What causes the diarrhea?** | Exotoxin released by *C. difficile* |
| **How is the diagnosis made?** | Assay stool for exotoxin titer; fecal leukocytes may or may not be present; on colonoscopy, there is an exudate that looks like a membrane (hence, "pseudomembranous") |
| **What is the treatment?** | PO vancomycin (97% sensitive) or PO metronidazole (Flagyl®; 93% sensitive); discontinuation of causative agent<br>**Never** give antiperistaltics |

## PROPHYLACTIC ANTIBIOTICS

| | |
|---|---|
| **What are the indications for prophylactic IV antibiotics?** | Accidental wounds with heavy contamination and tissue damage<br>Accidental wounds requiring surgical therapy that has had to be delayed<br>Prosthetic heart valve or valve disease<br>Penetrating injuries of hollow intra-abdominal organs<br>Large bowel resections and anastomosis |

Cardiovascular surgery with the use of a
prosthesis/vascular procedures
Patients with open fractures (start in ER)
Traumatic wounds occurring more than
8 hours prior to medical attention

**What must a prophylactic antibiotic cover for procedures on the large bowel/abdominal trauma/appendicitis?**

Anaerobes

**What commonly used antibiotics offer anaerobic coverage?**

Cefoxitin (Mefoxin®), clindamycin, metronidazole (Flagyl®), cefotetan, ampicillin-sulbactam (Unasyn®), Zosyn™, Timentin®, Imipenem®

**What antibiotic is used prophylactically for vascular surgery?**

Ancef (if patient is significantly allergic to PCN—hives/swelling/shortness of breath—then erythromycin or clindamycin)

**When is the appropriate time to administer prophylactic antibiotics?**

Must be in adequate levels in the blood stream **prior to surgical incision!**

## PAROTITIS

**What is it?**

Infection of the parotid gland

**What is the most common causative organism?**

*Staphylococcus*

**What are the associated risk factors?**

Age older than 65 years, malnutrition, poor oral hygiene, presence of NG tube, NPO, dehydration

**What is the most common time of occurrence?**

Usually 2 weeks postoperative

**What are the signs?**

Hot, red, tender parotid gland and increased WBCs

**What is the treatment?**

Antibiotics, operative drainage as necessary

## MISCELLANEOUS

| | |
|---|---|
| **Which bacteria can be found in the stool (colon)?** | Anaerobic—*Bacteroides fragilis*<br>Aerobic—*Escherichia coli* |
| **Which bacteria are found in infections from human bites?** | *Streptococcus viridans, S. aureus,*<br>    *Peptococcus,* **Eikenella** |
| **What is the most common ICU pneumonia bacteria?** | Gram-negative organisms |
| **What is Fournier's gangrene?** | Perineal infection starting classically in the scrotum in patients with diabetes; treat with triple antibiotics and wide debridement; a surgical emergency! |
| **Does adding antibiotics to peritoneal lavage solution lower the risk of abscess formation?** | No ("Dilution is the solution to pollution.") |
| **What is the classic finding associated with a *Pseudomonas* infection?** | Green exudate and "fruity" smell |
| **What are the classic antibiotics for "triple" antibiotics?** | Ampicillin, gentamycin, and metronidazole (Flagyl®) |
| **Which antibiotic is used to treat ameba infection?** | Metronidazole (Flagyl®) |
| **Which bacteria commonly infect prosthetic material and central lines?** | *Staphylococcus* **epidermis** |
| **What is the antibiotic of choice for *Actinomyces*?** | Penicillin G (exquisitely sensitive) |
| **What is a furuncle?** | A staphylococcal abscess that forms in a hair follicle (think: **f**ollicle = **f**uruncle) |

**What is a carbuncle?**

A subcutaneous staphylococcal abscess (usually an extension of a furuncle), most commonly seen in patients with diabetes (i.e., rule out diabetes)

**What is a felon?**

Infection of the finger pad (think: **f**elon = **f**inger printing)

**What microscopic finding is associated with *Actinomyces*?**

Sulfur granules

**What organism causes tetanus?**

*Clostridium tetani*

**What are the signs of tetanus?**

Lockjaw, muscle spasm, laryngospasm, convulsions, respiratory failure

**What are the appropriate prophylactic steps in tetanus-prone (dirty) injury in the following patients:**

    **Three previous immunizations?**

None (tetanus toxoid only if >5 years since last toxoid)

    **Two previous immunizations?**

Tetanus toxoid

    **One previous immunization?**

Tetanus immunoglobulin IM and tetanus toxoid IM (at different sites!)

    **No previous immunizations?**

Tetanus immunoglobulin IM and tetanus toxoid IM (at different sites!)

**What is Fitz-Hugh-Curtis syndrome?**

Right upper quadrant pain from gonococcal perihepatitis in women

**What is bacterial translocation?**

Bacteria gain access to lymphatics and blood stream from the colon via compromised mucosal barrier.

# Chapter 28     **Fever**

| | |
|---|---|
| **Define postoperative fever.** | Temperature >38.5° C or 101.5° F |
| **What are the classic W's of postoperative fever? (5)** | **W**ind—atelectasis<br>**W**ater—urinary tract infection (UTI)<br>**W**ound—wound infection<br>**W**alking—DVT/thrombophlebitis<br>**W**onder drugs—drug fever |
| **Give the classic postoperative timing for the following causes of postoperative fever:** | |
|     **Atelectasis (Wind)** | First 24 to 48 hours |
|     **UTI (Water)** | Anytime after postoperative day 3 |
|     **Wound infection (Wound)** | Usually after postoperative day 5 (but it can be anytime!) |
|     **DVT/PE/thrombophlebitis (Walking)** | Postoperative days 7 to 10 |
|     **Drug fever (Wonder drugs)** | Anytime |
| **What is the most common cause of fever on postoperative days 1 to 2?** | Atelectasis |
| **What is a "complete" fever work up?** | Physical exam (look at wound, etc.), CXR, urinalysis, blood cultures, CBC |
| **What causes fever before 24 postoperative hours?** | Atelectasis, β-hemolytic streptococcal or clostridial wound infections, anastomotic leak |
| **What causes fever from postoperative days 3 to 5?** | UTI, pneumonia, IV site infection, wound infection |
| **What is an anesthetic cause of fever INTRAoperatively?** | Malignant hyperthermia—treat with **dantrolene** |

**What causes fever from postoperative days 5 to 10?**

Wound infection, pneumonia, abscess, infected hematoma, *C. difficile* colitis, anastomotic leak
**DVT, peritoneal abscess, drug fever**
Pulmonary embolism, abscess, parotitis

**What causes wound infection on postoperative days 1 to 2?**

*Streptococcus*
Clostridia (painful bronze-brown weeping wound)

**What can cause fever at any time?**

1. IV site infection
2. Central line infection

**What is the classic preoperative "bowel prep"?**

1. Bowel prep: lower bacterial count in colon by catharsis (GoLYTELY or Fleets)
2. PO antibiotics (neomycin, erythromycin) preoperatively
3. Preoperative IV antibiotic with spectrum versus anaerobes (e.g., Cefoxitin)

**What treatment provides protection from OPSS after splenectomy?**

Immunization against *H. influenza, Streptococcus, Meningococcus*, and penicillin when illness/fever occurs

**What treatment provides protection from endocarditis with faulty heart valve or prosthetic heart valve?**

Antibiotics prior to dental procedure or any surgery

**What treatment provides protection from tetanus infection?**

Tetanus toxoid (and tetanus immune globulin, if one or no previous toxoid with dirty wound)

**What treatment provides protection from ETOH withdrawal?**

Chlordiazepoxide (Librium®), also give Rally pack

**What treatment provides protection from Wernicke's encephalopathy?**

**Rally pack** (A.K.A. banana bag since the IV is yellow with the vitamins in it); pack includes thiamine, folate, and magnesium

**What is Wernicke's encephalopathy?**

Condition resulting from thiamine deficiency in patients with alcoholism, causing a **triad** of symptoms:
1. Confusion
2. Ataxia
3. Ophthalmoplegia

**What treatment decreases the risk of perioperative adrenal crisis in a patient on chronic steroids?**

"Stress-dose" steroids: 100 mg hydrocortisone administered preoperatively, continued postoperatively Q 8 hours, and then tapered off

---

# Chapter 29

# Surgical Prophylaxis

**What medications provide protection from postoperative GI bleeding?**

$H_2$ blockers, PPI (proton pump inhibitor), sucralfate (binds ulcer craters)

**What measures provide protection from postoperative atelectasis/ pneumonia?**

Incentive spirometry, coughing, **smoking cessation,** ambulation

**What treatments provide protection from postoperative DVT?**

Low-molecular-weight heparin (LMWH), subcutaneous low-dose unfractionated heparin, sequential compression device (SCD) for lower extremities, or both; early ambulation

**What measures provide protection from wound infection?**

Shower the night before surgery with chlorhexidine scrub.
**Never use a razor** for hair removal (electric shavers only).
Ensure adequate skin prep in OR.
Do not close the skin in a contaminated case.
Ensure preoperative antibiotics in the bloodstream **before incision.**
Ensure no excess Bovie (necrotic tissue).

| | |
|---|---|
| **Why not use a razor to remove hair?** | The micro cuts are a nidus for bacteria and subsequent wound infection. |
| **How long should you give "prophylactic antibiotics"?** | <24 hrs |
| **What treatment provides protection from oral/ esophageal fungal infection during IV antibiotic treatment?** | PO nystatin |
| **What measures prevent ventilator-associated pneumonia (VAP)?** | Head of bed >30°, handwashing, patient oral hygiene, avoidance of gastric over-distention |

# Chapter 30 — Surgical Radiology

## CHEST

| | |
|---|---|
| **What defines a technically adequate CXR?** | The film must be "RIPE":<br>**R**otation: Clavicular heads are equidistant from the thoracic spinous processes.<br>**I**nspiration: Diaphragm is at or below ribs 8–10 posteriorly and ribs 5–6 anteriorly.<br>**P**enetration: Disk spaces are visible but there is no bony detail of the spine; bronchovascular structures are seen through the heart.<br>**E**xposure: Make sure all of the lung fields are visible. |
| **How should a CXR be read?** | Check the following:<br>**Tubes and lines:** Check placement<br>**Patient data:** Name, date, history number<br>**Orientation:** Up/down, left-right<br>**Technique:** AP or PA, supine or erect, decubitus |

**Trachea:** Midline or deviated, caliber
**Lungs:** CHF, mass
**Pulmonary vessels:** Artery or vein enlargement
**Mediastinum:** Aortic knob, nodes
**Hila:** Masses, lymphadenopathy
**Heart:** Transverse diameter should be ≤half the transthoracic diameter
**Pleura:** Effusion, thickening, pneumothorax
**Bones:** Fractures, lesions
**Soft tissues:** Periphery and below the diaphragm

**What CXR is better: P-A or A-P?**

P-A, less magnification of the heart (heart is closer to the x-ray plate)

**Classically, how much pleural fluid can the diaphragm hide on upright CXR?**

It is said that the diaphragm can overshadow up to 500 cc.

**How can CXR confirm that the last hole on a chest tube is in the pleural cavity?**

The last hole is through the radiopaque line on the chest tube; thus, look for the break in the radiopaque line to be in the rib cage.

**How can a loculated pleural effusion be distinguished from a free-flowing pleural effusion?**

Ipsilateral decubitus CXR; if fluid is not loculated (or contained) it will layer out

**How do you recognize a pneumothorax on CXR?**

Air without lung markings is seen outside the white pleural line—best seen in the apices on an upright CXR.

**What x-ray should be obtained before feeding via a nasogastric or nasoduodenal tube?**

Low CXR to ensure the tube is in the GI tract and not in the lung

**What C-spine views are used to rule out bony injury?**

A-P, lateral, **open mouth odontoid** views

**What plain x-rays are used to look for ligamentous C-spine injury?**

Lateral flex and extension C-spine films

**What CXR findings may provide evidence of traumatic aortic injury?**

Widened mediastinum >8 cm (most common)
Apical pleural capping
Loss of aortic knob
Inferior displacement of left main bronchus; NG tube displaced to the right, tracheal deviation, hemothorax

**How do you read a CT scan?**

Cross section with the patient in supine position looking at the feet

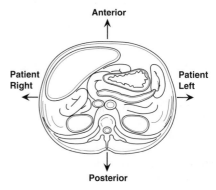

## ABDOMEN

**How should an abdominal x-ray (AXR) be read?**

Check the following:
**Patient data**: Name, date, history number
**Orientation**: up/down, left-right
**Technique**: A-P or P-A, supine or erect, decubitus
**Air:** free air under diaphragm, air-fluid levels
**Gas dilatation** (3, 6, 9 rule)
**Borders**: psoas shadow, preperitoneal fat stripe
**Mass**: look for organomegaly, kidney shadow
**Stones/calcification**: urinary, biliary, fecalith
**Stool**
**Tubes**
**Bones**
**Foreign bodies**

**How can you tell the difference between a small bowel obstruction (SBO) and an ileus?**

In SBO there is a transition point (cut-off sign) between the distended proximal bowel and the distal bowel of normal caliber. The distal bowel may be gasless. The bowel in ileus is *diffusely* distended.

**What is the significance of an air-fluid level?**

Seen in obstruction or ileus on an upright x-ray; intraluminal bowel diameter increases, allowing for separation of fluid and gas

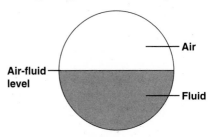

**What are the normal calibers of the small bowel, transverse colon, and cecum?**

Use the "**3, 6, 9 rule.**"
Small bowel <3 cm
Transverse colon <6 cm
Cecum <9 cm

**What is the "rule of 3s" for the small bowel?**

The bowel wall should be less than 3 mm thick.
The bowel folds should be less than 3 mm thick.
The bowel diameter should be less than 3 cm wide.

**How can the small and large bowel be distinguished on AXR?**

By the intraluminal folds; the small bowel plicae circulares are complete, whereas the plicae semilunares of the large bowel are only partially around the inner circumference of the lumen

**Where does peritoneal fluid accumulate in the supine position?**

Morison's pouch (hepatorenal recess), the space between the anterior surface of the right kidney and the posterior surface of the right lobe of the liver

**What percentage of kidney stones are radiopaque?**

Approximately 90%

**What percentage of gallstones are radiopaque?**

Approximately 10%

**What percentage of patients with acute appendicitis have a radiopaque fecalith?**

Approximately 5%

**What are the radiographic signs of appendicitis?**

Fecalith; sentinel loops; scoliosis away from the right because of pain; mass effect (abscess); loss of psoas shadow; loss of preperitoneal fat stripe; and, very rarely, a small amount of free air, if perforated

**What does KUB stand for?**

**K**idneys, **U**reters, and **B**ladder—commonly used term for a plain film AXR (abdominal flat plate)

**What is the "parrot's beak" or "bird's beak" sign?**

Evidence of sigmoid volvulus on barium enema; evidence of achalasia on barium swallow

**What is a "cut-off sign"?**

Seen in obstruction, bowel distention, and distended bowel that is "cut-off" from normal bowel

**What are "sentinel loops"?**

Distention or air-fluid levels (or both) near a site of abdominal inflammation (e.g., seen in RLQ with appendicitis)

**What is loss of the psoas shadow?**

Loss of the clearly defined borders of the psoas muscle on AXR; loss signifies inflammation or ascites

**What is loss of the peritoneal fat stripe (A.K.A. preperitoneal fat stripe)?**

Loss of the lateral peritoneal/preperitoneal fat interface; implies inflammation

**What is "thumbprinting"?**

Nonspecific colonic mucosal edema resembling thumb indentations on AXR

**What is pneumatosis intestinalis?**

Gas within the intestinal wall (usually means **dead gut**) that can be seen in patients with congenital variant or chronic steroids

**What is free air?**

Air free within the peritoneal cavity (air or gas should be seen only within the bowel or stomach); results from bowel or stomach perforation; arrows show air under the right diaphragm.

**What is the best position for the detection of FREE AIR (free intraperitoneal air)?**

**Upright CXR**—air below the right diaphragm

**If you cannot get an upright CXR, what is the second best plain x-ray for free air?**

Left lateral decubitus, because it prevents confusion with gastric air bubble; with free air **both** sides of the bowel wall can be seen; can detect as little as 1 cc of air

**How long after a laparotomy can there be free air on AXR?**

Usually 7 days or less

**What is Chilaiditi's sign?**

Transverse colon over the liver simulating free air on x-ray

**When should a postoperative abdominal/pelvic CT looking for a peritoneal abscess be performed?**

Postoperative day 7 or later, to give time for the abscess to form

**What is the best test to evaluate the biliary system and gallbladder?**

Ultrasound (U/S)

**What is the normal diameter of the common bile duct with gallbladder present?**

<4 mm until age 40, then add 1 mm per decade (e.g., 7 mm at age 70)

**What is the normal common bile duct diameter after removal of the gallbladder?**

8 to 10 mm

**What U/S findings are associated with acute cholecystitis?**

Gallstones, thickened gallbladder wall (>3 mm), distended gallbladder (>4 cm A-P), impacted stone in gallbladder neck, pericholecystic fluid

**What type of kidney stone is not seen on AXR?**

Uric acid (think: **u**ric acid = **u**nseen)

**What medication should be given prophylactically to a patient with a true history of contrast allergy?**

Methylprednisolone or dexamethasone; the patient should also receive nonionic contrast (associated with one-fifth as many reactions as ionic contrast, the less expensive standard)

**What is a C-C mammogram?**

A cranio-caudal mammogram, in which the breast is compressed top to bottom

**What is an MLO mammogram?**

Medio-lateral oblique mammogram, in which the breast is compressed in a 45° angle from the axilla to the lower sternum

**What are the best studies to evaluate for a pulmonary embolus?**

Spiral thoracic CT scan, V-Q ventilation-perfusion scan, pulmonary angiogram (gold standard)

# Chapter 31    Anesthesia

**Define the following terms:**

**Anesthesia**

Loss of sensation/pain

**Local anesthesia**

Anesthesia of a small confined area of the body (e.g., lidocaine for an elbow laceration)

**Epidural anesthesia**

Anesthetic drugs/narcotics infused into epidural space

**Spinal anesthesia**

Anesthetic agents injected into the thecal sac

**Regional anesthesia**

Blocking of the sensory afferent nerve fibers from a **region** of the body (e.g., radial nerve block)

| | |
|---|---|
| **General anesthesia** | Unconsciousness/amnesia (e.g., inhalational anesthetics) |
| **GET or GETA** | **G**eneral **E**ndotracheal **A**nesthesia |

**Give examples of the following terms:**

| | |
|---|---|
| **Local anesthetic** | Lidocaine, bupivacaine (Marcaine®) |
| **Regional anesthetic** | Lidocaine, bupivacaine (Marcaine®) |
| **General anesthesia** | Isoflurane, enflurane, sevoflurane, desflurane, nitrous oxide, halothane |
| **Dissociative agent** | Ketamine (children/burn patients) |
| **What is cricoid pressure?** | Manual pressure on cricoid cartilage occluding the esophagus and thus decreasing the chance of aspiration of gastric contents during intubation (A.K.A. Sellick's maneuver) |

**What is "rapid-sequence" anesthesia induction?**

1. Oxygenation and short-acting induction agent
2. Muscle relaxant
3. Cricoid pressure
4. Intubation
5. Inhalation anesthetic (rapid: boom, boom, boom → to lower the risk of aspiration during intubation)

| | |
|---|---|
| **Give examples of induction agents.** | Propofol, midazolam, sodium thiopental |
| **What are contraindications of the depolarizing agent succinylcholine?** | Patients with burns, neuromuscular diseases/paraplegia, eye trauma, or increased ICP |
| **Why is succinylcholine contraindicated in these patients?** | Depolarization can result in life-threatening **hyperkalemia; succinylcholine also increases intraocular pressure.** |
| **Why doesn't lidocaine work in an abscess?** | Lidocaine does not work in an **acidic** environment. |

| | |
|---|---|
| **Why does lidocaine burn on injection and what can be done to decrease the burning sensation?** | Lidocaine is acidic, which causes the burning; add sodium bicarbonate to decrease the burning sensation. |
| **Why does some lidocaine come with epinephrine?** | Epinephrine is meant to vasoconstrict the small vessels and thus decrease bleeding and blood flow, therefore washing out the lidocaine from the area, prolonging its effect. |
| **In what locations is lidocaine with epinephrine contraindicated?** | Fingers, toes, penis, etc., because of the possibility of ischemic injury/necrosis resulting from vasoconstriction |
| **What are the contraindications to nitrous oxide?** | Nitrous oxide is poorly soluble in serum and thus expands into any air-filled body pockets; avoid in patients with middle ear occlusions, **pneumothorax, small bowel obstruction,** etc. |
| **What is the feared side effect of bupivacaine (Marcaine®)?** | Cardiac dysrhythmia after intravascular injection leading to fatal refractory dysrhythmia |
| **What are the side effects of morphine?** | Constipation, respiratory failure, hypotension (from histamine release), spasm of sphincter of Oddi (use Demerol® in pancreatitis and biliary surgery), decreased cough reflex |
| **What are the side effects of meperidine?** | Similar to those of morphine but causes less sphincteric spasm and can cause tachycardia and seizures |
| **Limit to the duration of Demerol® postoperatively?** | Build up of the metabolites (normeperidine) |
| **What medication is a contraindication to Demerol®?** | Monoamine oxidase inhibitor |
| **What metabolite of Demerol® breakdown causes side effects (e.g., seizures)?** | Normeperidine |

| | |
|---|---|
| What is the treatment of life-threatening respiratory depression with morphine or Demerol®? | **Narcan®** IV (naloxone) |
| What are the side effects of epidural analgesia? | **Orthostatic hypotension,** decreased motor function, urinary retention |
| What is the advantage of epidural analgesia? | Analgesia without decreased cough reflex |
| What must be taken out only after removal of the epidural catheter? | The Foley catheter should be removed after the epidural is removed; otherwise, patient is likely to suffer from urinary retention. |
| What are the side effects of spinal anesthesia? | **Urinary retention** Hypotension (neurogenic shock) |
| What is the side effect of inhalational (volatile) anesthesia? | Halothane—**hypotension** (cardiac depression, decreased baroreceptor response to hypotension, and peripheral vasodilation), malignant hyperthermia |

## MALIGNANT HYPERTHERMIA

| | |
|---|---|
| What is it? | Inherited predisposition to an anesthetic reaction, causing uncoupling of the excitation–contraction system in skeletal muscle, which in turn causes **malignant hyperthermia;** hypermetabolism is fatal if untreated |
| What is the incidence? | Very rare |
| What are the causative agents? | General anesthesia, succinylcholine |
| What are the signs/ symptoms? | **Increased body temperature;** hypoxia; acidosis; tachycardia, $\uparrow$ $PCO_2$ ($\uparrow$ end tidal $CO_2$) |
| What is the treatment? | **IV dantrolene,** body cooling, discontinuation of anesthesia |

## MISCELLANEOUS

| | |
|---|---|
| **What are some of the nonde-polarizing muscle blockers?** | Vecuronium<br>Pancuronium |
| **What are the antidotes to the nondepolarizing neuro muscular blocking agents?** | Edrophonium<br>Neostigmine<br>Pyridostigmine |
| **How do these agents work?** | They inhibit anticholinesterase. |
| **Which muscle blocker is depolarizing?** | Succinylcholine |
| **What is the duration of action of succinylcholine?** | Less than 6 minutes |
| **What is the antidote to reverse succinylcholine?** | Time; endogenous blood pseudocholines-terase (patients deficient in this enzyme may be paralyzed for hours!) |
| **What is the maximum dose of lidocaine:**<br>    **With epinephrine?**<br>    **Without epinephrine?** | <br>7 mg/kg<br>4 mg/kg |
| **What is the duration of lidocaine local anesthesia?** | 30 to 60 minutes (up to 4 hours with epinephrine) |
| **What are the early signs of lidocaine toxicity?** | Tinnitus, perioral/tongue numbness, metallic taste, blurred vision, muscle twitches, drowsiness |
| **What are the signs of lidocaine toxicity with large overdose (>10 mcg/mL)?** | Seizures, coma, respiratory arrest<br>Loss of consciousness<br>Apnea |
| **When should the Foley catheter be removed in a patient with an epidural catheter?** | Several hours **after** the epidural catheter is removed (to prevent urinary retention) |
| **What is a PCA pump?** | **P**atient-**C**ontrolled **A**nalgesia; a pump delivers a set amount of pain reliever when the patient pushes a button (e.g., 1 mg of morphine every 6 minutes) |

| | |
|---|---|
| **What are the advantages of a PCA pump?** | Better pain control<br>Patients actually use less pain medication with a PCA!<br>If given a moderate dose without a basal rate, patients should not be able to overdose (they will fall asleep and not be able to push the button!) |
| **What is a "basal rate" on the PCA?** | A steady continuous infusion rate of the narcotic (e.g., 1–2 mg of morphine) continuously infused per hour; patient can supplement with additional doses as needed |
| **What is used to reverse narcotics?** | Naloxone (Narcan®) |
| **What is used to reverse benzodiazepines?** | Flumazenil |
| **What is fentanyl?** | Very potent narcotic (number one drug of abuse by anesthesiologists) |
| **Name an IV NSAID.** | Ketorolac (has classic side effects of NSAIDs: PUD, renal insufficiency) |
| **What is a feared but very rare complication of halothane anesthetic?** | Halothane hepatitis |

# Chapter 32     Surgical Ulcers

| | |
|---|---|
| **Define the following terms:**<br>   **Peptic ulcer** | General term for gastric/duodenal ulcer disease |
|    **Gastric ulcer** | Ulcer in the stomach |

**Curling's ulcer**

Gastric ulcer after burn injury (think: Curling's — curling iron burn — burn)

**Cushing's ulcer**

Peptic ulcer after neurologic insult (think: Cushing — famous neurosurgeon)

**Dieulafoy's ulcer**

Pinpoint gastric mucosal defect bleeding from underlying arterial vessel malformation

**Marjolin's ulcer**

Squamous cell carcinoma ulceration overlying chronic osteomyelitis or burn scar

**Aphthous ulcer**

GI tract ulcer seen in Crohn's disease

**Marginal ulcer**

Mucosal ulcer seen at a site of GI tract anastomosis

**Decubitus ulcer**

Skin/subcutaneous ulceration from pressure necrosis, classically on the buttocks/sacrum

**Venous stasis ulcer**

Skin ulceration on **medial malleolus** caused by venous stasis of a lower extremity

**LE arterial insufficiency ulcer**

Skin ulcers usually located on the toes/feet

# Chapter 33

# Surgical Oncology

**Define:**

| | |
|---|---|
| **Surgical oncology** | Surgical treatment of tumors |
| **XRT** | Radiation therapy |
| **In situ** | Not invading basement membrane |
| **Benign** | Nonmalignant tumor—does not invade or metastasize |
| **Malignant** | Tumors with anaplasia that invade and metastasize |
| **Adjuvant RX** | Treatment that aids or assists surgical treatment = Chemo or XRT |
| **Neoadjuvant RX** | Chemo, XRT, or both BEFORE surgical resection |
| **Brachytherapy** | XRT applied directly or very close to the target tissue (e.g., implantable radioactive seeds) |
| **Metachronous tumors** | Tumors occurring at different times |
| **Synchronous tumors** | Tumors occurring at the same time |
| **What do the T, M, and N stand for in TMN staging?** | **T**-**T**umor size<br>**M**-**M**ets (distant)<br>**N**-**N**odes |
| **What tumor marker is associated with colon cancer?** | CEA |
| **What tumor marker is associated with hepatoma?** | Alpha-fetoprotein |

| | |
|---|---|
| **What is a paraneoplastic syndrome?** | Syndromes of dysfunction not directly associated with tumor mass or mets (autoimmune or released substance) |
| **What are the most common cancers in women?** | 1. Lung<br>2. Breast<br>3. Colorectal |
| **What are the most common cancers in men?** | 1. Prostate<br>2. Lung<br>3. Colorectal |
| **What is the most common cancer causing death in both men and women?** | Lung! |

General Surgery

# Chapter 34

**GI Hormones
and Physiology**

## OVERVIEW

| | |
|---|---|
| **Define the products of the following stomach cells:** | |
|     **Gastric parietal cells** | HCl<br>Intrinsic factor |
|     **Chief cells** | Pepsinogen (think: "a peppy chief") |
|     **G cells** | Gastrin, G cells are found in the antrum<br>(think: G = Gastrin) |
|     **Mucous neck cells** | Bicarbonate mucus |
| **What is pepsin?** | A proteolytic enzyme that hydrolyzes peptide bonds |
| **What is intrinsic factor?** | A protein secreted by the parietal cells that combines with vitamin $B_{12}$ and enables absorption in the terminal ileum |
| **Name three receptors on the parietal cell that stimulate HCl release.** | 1. Histamine<br>2. Acetylcholine<br>3. Gastrin |
| **What is the enterohepatic circulation?** | Circulation of bile acids from the liver to the gut and back to the liver via the portal vein |
| **Where are most of the bile acids absorbed?** | The terminal ileum |
| **How many times is the entire bile acid pool circulated during a typical meal?** | Two times |

| | |
|---|---|
| **What are the stimulators of gallbladder emptying?** | Cholecystokinin, vagal input |
| **What are the inhibitors of gallbladder emptying?** | Somatostatin, sympathetics (it is impossible to flee and digest food at the same time), VIP |

## CHOLECYSTOKININ

| | |
|---|---|
| **What is its source?** | Duodenal mucosal cells |
| **What stimulates its release?** | Fat, protein, amino acids, HCl |
| **What inhibits its release?** | Trypsin and chymotrypsin |
| **What are its actions?** | Empties gallbladder<br>Opens ampulla of Vater<br>Slows gastric emptying<br>Stimulates pancreatic acinar cell growth and release of exocrine products |

## SECRETIN

| | |
|---|---|
| **What is its source?** | Duodenal cells (specifically the argyrophil S cells) |
| **What stimulates its release?** | pH less than 4.5 (acid), fat in the duodenum |
| **What inhibits its release?** | High pH in the duodenum |
| **What are its actions?** | Releases pancreatic bicarbonate/enzymes/$H_2O$, releases bile/bicarbonate, decreases LES tone, decreases release of gastric acid |

## GASTRIN

| | |
|---|---|
| **What is its source?** | Gastric antrum G cells |
| **What stimulates its release?** | Stomach peptides/amino acids<br>Vagal input<br>Calcium |

| | |
|---|---|
| **What inhibits its release?** | pH less than 3.0 |
| | Somatostatin |
| **What are its actions?** | Release of HCl from parietal cells |
| | Trophic effect on mucosa of the stomach and small intestine |

## SOMATOSTATIN

| | |
|---|---|
| **What is its source?** | Pancreatic D cells |
| **What stimulates its release?** | Food |
| **What are its actions?** | Globally inhibits GI function |

## MISCELLANEOUS

| | |
|---|---|
| **What is the purpose of the colon?** | Reabsorption of $H_2O$ and storage of stool |
| **What is the main small bowel nutritional source?** | Glutamine |
| **What is the main nutritional source of the colon?** | Butyrate (short-chain fatty acid) |
| **Where is calcium absorbed?** | Duodenum actively, jejunum passively |
| **Where is iron absorbed?** | Duodenum |
| **Where is vitamin $B_{12}$ absorbed?** | Terminal ileum |
| **Which hormone primarily controls gallbladder contraction?** | CCK |
| **What supplement does a patient need after removal of the terminal ileum or stomach?** | Vitamin $B_{12}$ |
| **Name the main constituents of bile.** | Water, phospholipids (lecithins), bile acids, cholesterol, and bilirubin |

**What are most gallstones made of?**

Cholesterol

**How do opiates affect the bowel?**

Opiates stimulate sodium absorption and inhibit secretion in the ileum, as well as decreasing GI motility by incoordinated peristalsis. Therefore, place patients on stool softeners when dispensing pain medication.

**Which type of muscle fibers, smooth or striated, does the esophagus contain?**

Both
Upper third—striated muscle control of motor nerves
Middle third—mixed
Lower third—smooth muscle, primarily under control of vagal motor fibers

**Which electrolytes does the colon actively absorb?**

$Na^+$, $Cl^-$

**Which electrolytes does the colon actively secrete?**

$HCO_3$ (plays a role in diarrhea causing the patient to have a normal anion gap acidosis)

**Which electrolytes does the colon passively secrete?**

$K^+$

**What is the gastrocolic reflex?**

Increased secretory and motor functions of the stomach result in increased colonic motility

**What is the blood supply to the liver?**

Seventy-five percent from the portal vein, rich in products of digestion
Twenty-five percent from the hepatic artery, rich in $O_2$ (but each provide for 50% of oxygen)

**What are Peyer patches?**

Nodules of lymphoid tissue with B and T lymphocytes in the small intestine that selectively sample lumenal antigens found in the terminal ileum

# Chapter 35

# **Acute Abdomen and Referred Pain**

| | |
|---|---|
| **What is an "acute abdomen"?** | Acute abdominal pain so severe that the patient seeks medical attention (not the same as a "surgical abdomen," because most cases of acute abdominal pain do not require surgical treatment) |
| **What are peritoneal signs?** | Signs of peritoneal irritation: extreme tenderness, percussion tenderness, rebound tenderness, voluntary guarding, motion pain, **involuntary** guarding/ rigidity (late) |

**Define the following terms:**

| | |
|---|---|
| **Rebound tenderness** | Pain upon releasing the palpating hand pushing on the abdomen |
| **Motion pain** | Abdominal pain upon moving, pelvic rocking, moving of stretcher, or heel strike |
| **Voluntary guarding** | Abdominal muscle contraction with palpation of the abdomen |
| **Involuntary guarding** | Rigid abdomen as the muscles "guard" involuntarily |
| **Colic** | Intermittent severe pain (usually because of intermittent contraction of a hollow viscus against an obstruction) |
| **What conditions can mask abdominal pain?** | Steroids, diabetes, paraplegia |
| **What is the most common cause of acute abdominal surgery in the United States?** | Acute appendicitis (7% of the population will develop it sometime during their lives) |

**What important questions should be asked when obtaining the history of a patient with an acute abdomen?**

"Have you had this pain before?"
"On a scale from 1 to 10, what would you rank this pain?"
"Fevers/chills?"
"Duration?" (comes and goes vs. constant)
"Quality?" (sharp vs. dull)
"Does anything make the pain better or worse?"
"Migration?"
"Point of maximal pain?"
"Urinary symptoms?"
"Nausea, vomiting, or diarrhea?"
"Anorexia?"
"Constipation?"
"Last bowel movement?"
"Any change in bowel habits?"
"Any relation to eating?"
"Last menses?"
"Last meal?"
"Vaginal discharge?"
"Melena?"
"Hematochezia?"
"Hematemesis?"
"Medications?"
"Allergies?"
"Past medical history?"
"Past surgical history?"
"Family history?"
"Tobacco/ETOH/Drugs?"

**What should the acute abdomen physical exam include?**

**Inspection** (e.g., surgical scars, distention)
**Auscultation** (e.g., bowel sounds, bruits)
**Palpation** (e.g., tenderness, R/O hernia, CVAT, rectal, pelvic exam, rebound, voluntary guard, motion tenderness)
**Percussion** (e.g., liver size, spleen size)

**What is the best way to have a patient localize abdominal pain?**

"Point with **one** finger where the pain is worse."

**What is the classic position of a patient with peritonitis?**

Motionless (often with knees flexed)

**What is the classic position of a patient with a kidney stone?**

Cannot stay still, restless, writhing in pain

**What is the best way to examine a scared child or histrionic adult's abdomen?**

Use stethoscope to palpate abdomen

**What lab tests are used to evaluate the patient with an acute abdomen?**

CBC with **differential,** chem-10, amylase, type and screen, urinalysis, LFTs

**What is a "left shift" on CBC differential?**

Sign of inflammatory response: Immature neutrophils (bands) (today many call more than 80% of WBCs as neutrophils a left shift)

**What lab test should every woman of childbearing age with an acute abdomen receive?**

Human chorionic gonadotropin ($\beta$-hCG) to rule out pregnancy/ectopic pregnancy

**Which x-rays are used to evaluate the patient with an acute abdomen?**

Upright chest x-ray, upright abdominal film, supine abdominal x-ray (if patient cannot stand, left lateral decubitus abdominal film)

**How is free air ruled out if the patient cannot stand?**

Left lateral decubitus—free air collects over the liver and does not get confused with the gastric bubble

**What diagnosis must be considered in every patient with an acute abdomen?**

**Appendicitis!**

**What are the differential diagnoses by quadrant?**
    **RUQ**

Cholecystitis, hepatitis, PUD, perforated ulcer, pancreatitis, liver tumors, gastritis, hepatic abscess, choledocholithiasis, cholangitis, pyelonephritis, nephrolithiasis, appendicitis (**especially during pregnancy**); thoracic causes (e.g., pleurisy/pneumonia), PE, pericarditis, MI (especially inferior MI)

| | |
|---|---|
| **LUQ** | PUD, perforated ulcer, gastritis, splenic injury, abscess, reflux, dissecting aortic aneurysm, thoracic causes, pyelonephritis, nephrolithiasis, hiatal hernia (strangulated paraesophageal hernia), Boerhaave's syndrome, Mallory-Weiss tear, splenic artery aneurysm, colon disease |
| **LLQ** | Diverticulitis, sigmoid volvulus, perforated colon, colon cancer, urinary tract infection, small bowel obstruction, inflammatory bowel disease, nephrolithiasis, pyelonephritis, fluid accumulation from aneurysm or perforation, referred hip pain; gynecologic causes (e.g., ectopic pregnancy), PID, mittelschmerz, ovarian cyst, fibroid degeneration, endometriosis, gynecologic tumor, torsion of cyst or fallopian tube |
| **RLQ** | Same as LLQ, especially **appendicitis,** also mesenteric lymphadenitis, cecal diverticulitis, Meckel's diverticulum, intussusception |
| **What is the differential diagnosis of epigastric pain?** | PUD, gastritis, MI, pancreatitis, biliary colic, gastric volvulus, Mallory-Weiss |
| **What is the differential diagnosis of gynecologic pain?** | Ovarian cyst, ovarian torsion, PID, tubo-ovarian abscess, fibroid, necrotic fibroid, pregnancy, ectopic pregnancy, endometritis, cancer of the cervix/uterus/ovary, endometrioma |
| **What is the differential diagnosis of thoracic causes of abdominal pain?** | MI (especially inferior), pneumonia, dissecting aorta, aortic aneurysm, empyema, esophageal rupture/tear, PTX, esophageal foreign body |
| **What is the differential diagnosis of scrotal causes of lower abdominal pain?** | Testicular torsion, epididymitis, orchitis, inguinal hernia, referred pain from nephrolithiasis or appendicitis |
| **What are nonsurgical causes of abdominal pain?** | Gastroenteritis, DKA, sickle cell crisis, rectus sheath hematoma, |

acute porphyria, PID, kidney stone, pyelonephritis, hepatitis, pancreatitis, pneumonia, MI, *C. difficile* colitis

**What are unique differential diagnoses for the patient with AIDS and abdominal pain?**

In addition to all common abdominal conditions:
**C**MV (most **c**ommon)
Kaposi's sarcoma
Lymphoma
TB
MAI (*Mycobacterium avium intracellulare*)

**What are the possible causes of suprapubic pain?**

Cystitis, colonic pain, gynecologic causes (and of course appendicitis)

**What causes pain limited to specific dermatomes?**

Early zoster before vesicles erupt

**What is referred pain?**

Pain felt at a site distant from a disease process; caused by the convergence of multiple pain afferents in the posterior horn of the spinal cord

**What is gastroenteritis?**

Viral or bacterial infection of the GI tract, usually with vomiting and diarrhea, pain (usually **after** vomiting), nonsurgical

**What is classically stated to be the "great imitator"?**

Constipation

**Name the classic locations of referred pain:**
  **Cholecystitis**

Right subscapular pain (also epigastric)

  **Appendicitis**

Early: periumbilical
Rarely: testicular pain

  **Diaphragmatic irritation (from spleen, perforated ulcer, or abscess)**

Shoulder pain (on the left a + Kehr's sign)

  **Pancreatitis/cancer**

Back pain

  **Rectal disease**

Pain in the small of the back

| | |
|---|---|
| **Nephrolithiasis** | Testicular pain/flank pain |
| **Rectal pain** | Midline small of back pain |
| **Small bowel** | Periumbilical |
| **Uterine pain** | Midline small of back pain |

**Give the classic diagnosis for the following cases:**

| | |
|---|---|
| "Abdominal pain out of proportion to exam" | Rule out mesenteric ischemia |
| **Hypotension and pulsatile abdominal mass** | Ruptured AAA; go to the OR |
| **Fever, LLQ pain, and change in bowel habits** | Diverticulitis |

**Give the test of choice for the following conditions:**

| | |
|---|---|
| **Cholelithiasis** | Ultrasound (U/S) |
| **Bile duct obstruction** | U/S |
| **Mesenteric ischemia** | Mesenteric A-gram |
| **Ruptured abdominal aortic aneurysm** | Emergent laparotomy |
| **AAA** | Abdominal CT or U/S |
| **Abdominal abscess** | Abdominal CT |
| **Severe diverticulitis** | Abdominal CT |

| | |
|---|---|
| **What is the most common cause of RUQ pain?** | Cholelithiasis |
| **What is the most common cause of surgical RLQ pain?** | Acute appendicitis |
| **What is the most common cause of GI tract LLQ pain?** | Diverticulitis |

| | |
|---|---|
| **Classically, what endocrine problems can cause abdominal pain?** | 1. Addisonian crisis<br>2. DKA (**D**iabetic **K**eto**A**cidosis) |

---

# Chapter 36     Hernias

| | |
|---|---|
| **What is a hernia?** | (**L. rupture**) The protrusion of a peritoneal sac through a musculoaponeurotic barrier (e.g., abdominal wall); a fascial defect |
| **What is the incidence?** | Between 5% and 10% lifetime; 50% are indirect inguinal, 25% are direct inguinal, and approximately 5% are femoral |
| **What are the precipitating factors?** | Increased intra-abdominal pressure: straining at defecation or urination (rectal cancer, colon cancer, prostatic enlargement, constipation), obesity, pregnancy, ascites, valsavagenic (coughing) COPD; an abnormal congenital anatomic route (i.e., patent processus vaginalis) |
| **Why should hernias be repaired?** | To avoid complications of incarceration/ strangulation, bowel necrosis, SBO, pain |
| **What is more dangerous: a small or large hernia defect?** | A small defect is more dangerous because a tight defect is more likely to strangulate if incarcerated. |
| **Define the following descriptive terms:**<br>    **Reducible** | The ability to return the displaced organ or tissue/hernia contents to their usual anatomic site |
|     **Incarcerated** | Swollen or fixed within the hernia sac (incarcerated = imprisoned); may cause intestinal obstruction (i.e., an irreducible hernia) |

| | |
|---|---|
| **Strangulated** | Incarcerated hernia with resulting ischemia; will result in signs and symptoms of ischemia and intestinal obstruction or bowel necrosis (think: strangulated = choked) |
| **Complete** | Hernia sac and its contents protrude all the way through the defect |
| **Incomplete** | Defect present without sac or contents protruding completely through it |

**Define the following types of hernias:**

| | |
|---|---|
| **Sliding hernia** | Hernia sac partially formed by the wall of a viscus (i.e., bladder/cecum) |
| **Littre's hernia** | Hernia involving a Meckel's diverticulum (think alphabetically: **L**ittre's **M**eckel's = L.M.) |
| **Spigelian hernia** | Hernia through the linea semilunaris (or spigelian fascia); also known as spontaneous lateral ventral hernia (think: **S**pigelian = **S**emilunaris) |
| **Internal hernia** | Hernia into or involving intra-abdominal structure |
| **Obturator hernia** | Hernia through obturator canal (females ≥ males) |
| **Lumbar hernia** | Petit's hernia or Grynfeltt's hernia |
| **Petit's hernia** | (Rare) hernia through Petit's triangle (A.K.A. inferior lumbar triangle) (think: petit = small = inferior) |
| **Grynfeltt's hernia** | Hernia through Grynfeltt-Lesshaft triangle (superior lumbar triangle) |
| **Pantaloon hernia** | Hernia sac exists as **both a direct and indirect** hernia straddling the inferior epigastric vessels and protruding through the floor of the canal as well as the internal ring (two sacs separated by |

the inferior epigastric vessels [the pant crotch] like a pair of pantaloon pants)

**Incisional hernia**

Hernia through an incisional site; most common cause is a wound infection

**Ventral hernia**

Incisional hernia in the ventral abdominal wall

**Parastomal hernia**

Hernia adjacent to an ostomy (e.g., colostomy)

**Sciatic hernia**

Hernia through the sciatic foramen

**Richter's hernia**

Incarcerated or strangulated hernia involving only **one sidewall of the bowel,** which can spontaneously reduce, resulting in gangrenous bowel and perforation within the abdomen without signs of obstruction

**Epigastric hernia**
Hernia through the linea alba above the umbilicus

**Umbilical hernia**
Hernia through the umbilical ring, in adults associated with ascites, pregnancy, and obesity

**Intraparietal hernia**
Hernia in which abdominal contents migrate between the layers of the abdominal wall

**Femoral hernia**
Hernia medial to femoral vessels (under inguinal ligament)

**Hesselbach's hernia**
Hernia under inguinal ligament **lateral** to femoral vessels

**Bochdalek's hernia**
Hernia through the posterior diaphragm, usually on the left (think: Boch de lek = "back to the left" on the diaphragm)

**Morgagni's hernia**
Anterior parasternal diaphragmatic hernia

**Properitoneal hernia**
Intraparietal hernia between the peritoneum and transversalis fascia

**Cooper's hernia**
Hernia through the femoral canal and tracking into the scrotum or labia majus

**Indirect inguinal**
Inguinal hernia lateral to Hesselbach's triangle

**Direct inguinal**
Inguinal hernia within Hesselbach's triangle

**Hiatal hernia**
Hernia through esophageal hiatus

**Amyand's hernia**
Hernia sac containing a ruptured appendix (think: **A**myand's = **A**ppendix)

**What are the boundaries of Hesselbach's triangle?**

1. Inferior epigastric vessels
2. Inguinal ligament (Poupart's)
3. Lateral border of the rectus sheath

Floor consists of internal oblique and the transversus abdominis muscle.

**What are the layers of the abdominal wall?**

Skin
Subcutaneous fat
Scarpa's fascia
External oblique
Internal oblique
Transversus abdominus
Transversalis fascia
Preperitoneal fat
Peritoneum
**Note:** all three muscle layer aponeuroses form the anterior rectus sheath, with the posterior rectus sheath being deficient below the arcuate line.

## GROIN HERNIAS

**What are the differential diagnoses of a groin mass?**

Lymphadenopathy, hematoma, seroma, abscess, hydrocele, femoral artery aneurysm, EIC, undescended testicle, sarcoma, hernias, testicle torsion

### DIRECT INGUINAL HERNIA

**What is it?**

A hernia within the floor of Hesselbach's triangle, i.e., the hernia sac does not traverse the internal ring (think of **directly** through the abdominal wall)

**What is the cause?**

Acquired defect from mechanical breakdown over the years

**What is the incidence?**

Approximately 1% of all men; frequency increases with advanced age

**What nerve runs with the spermatic cord in the inguinal canal?**

Ilioinguinal nerve

## INDIRECT INGUINAL HERNIA

**What is it?**

Hernia through the internal ring of the inguinal canal, traveling down toward the external ring; it may enter the scrotum upon exiting the external ring (i.e., if complete); think of the hernia sac traveling **indirectly** through the abdominal wall from the internal ring to the external ring

**What is the cause?**

Patent processus vaginalis (i.e., congenital)

**What is the incidence?**

Approximately 5% of all men; most common hernia in both men **and** women

**How is an inguinal hernia diagnosed?**

Relies mainly on history and physical exam with index finger invaginated into the external ring and palpation of hernia; examine the patient standing up if diagnosis is not obvious
**Note:** if swelling occurs below the inguinal ligament, it is possibly a femoral hernia.

**What is the differential diagnosis of an inguinal hernia?**

Lymphadenopathy, psoas abscess, ectopic testis, hydrocele of the cord, saphenous varix, lipoma, varicocele, testicular torsion, femoral artery aneurysm, abscess

| | |
|---|---|
| **What is the risk of strangulation?** | Higher with indirect than direct inguinal hernia, but highest in femoral hernias |
| **What is the treatment?** | Emergent herniorrhaphy is indicated if strangulation is suspected or acute incarceration is present; otherwise, elective herniorrhaphy is indicated to prevent the chance of incarceration/strangulation. |

## INGUINAL HERNIA REPAIRS

**Define the following procedures:**

| | |
|---|---|
| **Bassini** | **Sutures** approximate reflection of inguinal ligament (Poupart's) to the transversus abdominis aponeurosis/conjoint tendon |
| **McVay** | **Cooper's** ligament sutured to transversus abdominis aponeurosis/conjoint tendon |
| **Lichtenstein** | "Tension-free repair" using mesh |
| **Shouldice** | Imbrication of the floor of the inguinal canal (A.K.A. "Canadian repair") |
| **Plug and patch** | Placing a plug of mesh in hernia defect and then overlaying a patch of mesh over inguinal floor (requires few if any sutures in mesh!) |
| **High ligation** | Ligation and transection of indirect hernia sac without repair of inguinal floor (used only in **children**) |
| **TAPP procedure** | **T**rans**A**bdominal **P**re**P**eritoneal inguinal hernia repair |
| **TEPA procedure** | **T**otally **E**xtra**P**eritoneal **A**pproach |

| | |
|---|---|
| **What are the indications for laparoscopic inguinal hernia repair?** | 1. Bilateral inguinal hernias<br>2. Recurring hernia<br>3. Need to resume full activity as soon as possible |

## CLASSIC INTRAOPERATIVE INGUINAL HERNIA QUESTIONS

| | |
|---|---|
| **What is the first identifiable subcutaneous named layer?** | Scarpa's fascia (thin in adults) |
| **What is the name of the subcutaneous vein that is ligated?** | Superficial epigastric vein |
| **What happens if you cut the ilioinguinal nerve?** | Numbness of inner thigh or lateral scrotum; usually goes away in 6 months |
| **From what abdominal muscle layer is the cremaster muscle derived?** | Internal oblique muscle |
| **From what abdominal muscle layer is the inguinal ligament (A.K.A. Poupart's ligament) derived?** | External oblique muscle aponeurosis |
| **To what does the inguinal (Poupart's) ligament attach?** | Anterior superior iliac spine to the pubic tubercle |
| **Which nerve travels on the spermatic cord?** | Ilioinguinal nerve |
| **Why do some surgeons deliberately cut the ilioinguinal nerve?** | First they obtain preoperative consent and cut so as to remove the risk of entrapment and postoperative pain. |
| **What is in the spermatic cord (6)?** | 1. Cremasteric muscle fibers<br>2. Vas deferens<br>3. Testicular artery<br>4. Testicular pampiniform venous plexus<br>5. ± hernia sac<br>6. Genital branch of the genitofemoral nerve |
| **What is the hernia sac made of?** | Peritoneum (direct) or a patent processus vaginalis (indirect) |
| **What attaches the testicle to the scrotum?** | The gubernaculum |

**What is the most common organ in an inguinal hernia sac in men?**

Small intestine

**What is the most common organ in an inguinal hernia sac in women?**

Ovary/fallopian tube

**What lies in the inguinal canal in the female instead of the VAS?**

Round ligament

**Where in the inguinal canal does the hernia sac lie in relation to the other structures?**

Anteromedially

**What is a "cord lipoma"?**

Preperitoneal fat on the cord structures (pushed in by the hernia sac); not a real lipoma; remove surgically, if feasible

**What is a small outpouching of testicular tissue off of the testicle?**

Testicular appendage (A.K.A. the appendix testes); remove with electrocautery

**What action should be taken if a suture is placed through the femoral artery or vein during an inguinal herniorrhaphy?**

Remove the suture as soon as possible and apply pressure (i.e., do not tie the suture down!)

**What nerve is found on top of the spermatic cord?**

Ilioinguinal nerve

**What nerve travels within the spermatic cord?**

The genital branch of the genitofemoral nerve

**What are the borders of Hesselbach's triangle?**

1. Epigastric vessels
2. Inguinal ligament
3. Lateral border of the rectus sheath

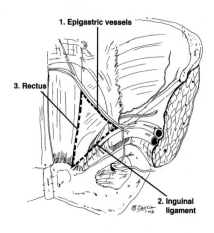

1. Epigastric vessels

3. Rectus

2. Inguinal ligament

**What type of hernia goes through Hesselbach's triangle?**

A direct hernia due to a weak abdominal floor

**What is a "relaxing incision"?**

Incision(s) in the rectus sheath to relax the conjoint tendon so that it can be approximated to the reflection of the inguinal ligament without tension

**What is the conjoint tendon?**

The aponeurotic attachments of the "conjoining" of the internal oblique and transversus abdominis to the pubic tubercle

**Define inguinal anatomy.**

1. Inguinal ligament (Poupart's ligament)
2. Transversus aponeurosis
3. Conjoint tendon

**How tight should the new internal inguinal ring be?**

Should allow entrance of the tip of a Kelly clamp but not a finger (the new external inguinal ring should not be tight and should allow entrance of a finger)

**What percentage of the strength of an inguinal floor repair does the external oblique aponeurosis represent?**

ZERO

## FEMORAL HERNIA

**What is it?**

Hernia traveling beneath the inguinal ligament down the femoral canal medial to the femoral vessels (think: FM, or **F**emoral hernia = **M**edial)

**What are the boundaries of the femoral canal?**

1. Cooper's ligament posteriorly
2. Inguinal ligament anteriorly
3. Femoral vein laterally
4. Lacunar ligament medially

**What factors are femoral hernias associated with?**

Women, pregnancy, and exertion

**What percentage of all hernias are femoral hernias?**

5%

**What percentage of patients with a femoral hernia are female?**

85%!

**What are the complications?**

Approximately one-third incarcerate (due to narrow, unforgiving neck)

**What is the most common hernia in women?**

Indirect inguinal hernia

**What is the repair of a femoral hernia?**

McVay (Cooper's ligament repair), mesh plug repair

## HERNIA REVIEW QUESTIONS

| | |
|---|---|
| **Should elective TURP or elective herniorrhaphy be performed first?** | TURP |
| **Which type of esophageal hiatal hernia is associated with GE reflux?** | Sliding esophageal hiatal hernia |
| **Classically, how can an incarcerated hernia be reduced in the ER?** | 1. Apply ice to incarcerated hernia.<br>2. Sedate.<br>3. Use the Trendelenburg position for inguinal hernias.<br>4. Apply steady gentle manual pressure.<br>5. Admit and observe for signs of necrotic bowel after reduction.<br>6. Perform surgical herniorrhaphy ASAP. |
| **What is appropriate if you cannot reduce an incarcerated hernia with steady, gentle compression?** | Go directly to OR for repair. |
| **What is the major difference in repairing a pediatric indirect inguinal hernia and an adult inguinal hernia?** | In babies and children it is rarely necessary to repair the inguinal floor; repair with "high ligation" of the hernia sac. |
| **What is the Howship-Romberg sign?** | Pain along the medial aspect of the proximal thigh from nerve compression caused by an obturator hernia |
| **What is the "silk glove" sign?** | The inguinal hernia sac in an infant/toddler feels like a finger of a silk glove when rolled under the examining finger. |
| **What must you do before leaving the OR after an inguinal hernia repair?** | Pull the testicle back down to the scrotum. |

## ESOPHAGEAL HIATAL HERNIAS

| | |
|---|---|
| **What is a type I and a type II hiatal hernia?** | 1. Type I = sliding<br>2. Type II = paraesophageal |

## SLIDING ESOPHAGEAL HIATAL HERNIA

**What is it?**

Both the stomach and GE junction herniate into the thorax via the esophageal hiatus; also known as type I hiatal hernia.

**What is the incidence?**

More than 90% of all hiatal hernias

**What are the symptoms?**

Most patients are asymptomatic, but the condition can cause **reflux,** dysphagia (from inflammatory edema), esophagitis, and pulmonary problems secondary to aspiration.

**How is it diagnosed?**

UGI series, manometry, EGD with biopsy for esophagitis

**What are the complications?**

Reflux → esophagitis → Barrett's esophagus → cancer and stricture formation; aspiration pneumonia; it can also result in UGI bleeding from esophageal ulcerations

**What is the treatment?**

85% of cases treated medically with antacids, $H_2$ blockers/PPIs, head elevation after meals, small meals, and no food prior to sleeping; 15% of cases require surgery for persistent symptoms despite adequate medical treatment

**What is the surgical treatment?**

Laparoscopic Nissen fundoplication (LAP NISSEN) involves wrapping the fundus around the LES and suturing it in place

## PARAESOPHAGEAL HIATAL HERNIA

**What is it?**

Herniation of all or part of the stomach through the esophageal hiatus into the thorax without displacement of the gastroesophageal junction; also known as type II hiatal hernia

**What is the incidence?**

Less than 5% of all hiatal hernias (rare)

**What are the symptoms?**

Derived from mechanical obstruction; dysphagia, stasis gastric ulcer, and strangulation; many cases are asymptomatic and not associated with reflux because of a relatively normal position of the GE junction

**What are the complications?**

Hemorrhage, incarceration, obstruction, and strangulation

**What is the treatment?**

Surgical, because of frequency and severity of potential complications

# Chapter 37

# Laparoscopy

**What is laparoscopy?**

Minimally invasive surgical technique using gas to insufflate the peritoneum and instruments manipulated through ports introduced through small incisions with video camera guidance

**What gas is used and why?**

$CO_2$ because of better solubility in blood and, thus, less risk of gas embolism, noncombustible

**Which operations are performed with the laparoscope?**

**Frequently**—cholecystectomy; appendectomy; inguinal hernia repair; ventral hernia repair, Nissen fundoplication

**Infrequently**—bowel resection, colostomy, surgery for PUD (PGV, perforation), colectomy, splenectomy, adrenalectomy

**What are the contraindications?**

**Absolute**—hypovolemic shock, severe cardiac decompensation

**Relative**—extensive intraperitoneal adhesions, diaphragmatic hernia, COPD

**What are the associated complications?**

Pneumothorax, bleeding, perforating injuries, infection, intestinal injuries, solid organ injury, major vascular injury, **$CO_2$ embolus,** bladder injury, hernia at larger trocar sites, DVT

**What prophylactic measure should every patient get when they are going to have a laparoscopic procedure?**

SCD boots—**S**equential **C**ompression **D**evice (and most add an OGT to decompress the stomach; Foley catheter is usually used for pelvic procedures)

**What are the cardiovascular effects of a pneumoperitoneum?**

**Increased afterload** and **decreased preload** (but the CVP and PCWP are deceivingly elevated!)

**What is the effect of $CO_2$ insufflation on end tidal $CO_2$ levels?**

Increased as a result of absorption of $CO_2$ into the bloodstream; the body compensates with increased ventilation and blows the extra $CO_2$ off and thus there is no acidosis

**What are the advantages over laparotomy?**

Shorter hospitalization, less pain and scarring, lower cost, decreased ileus

**What is the Veress needle?**

Needle with spring-loaded, retractable, blunt inner-protective tube that protrudes from the needle end when it enters peritoneal cavity; used for blind entrance and then insufflation of $CO_2$ through the Veress needle

**How can it be verified that the Veress needle is in the peritoneum?**

Syringe of saline; saline should flow freely without pressure through the needle "drop test"

**If the Veress needle is not in the peritoneal cavity, what happens to the $CO_2$ flow/ pressure?**

Flow decreases and pressure is high

**What is the Hasson technique?**

No Veress needle—cut down and place trocar under **direct visualization**

**What is the cause of post-laparoscopic shoulder pain?**

Referred pain from $CO_2$ on diaphragm and diaphragm stretch

**What is a laparoscopic-assisted procedure?**

Laparoscopic dissection; then, part of the procedure is performed through an open incision

**What is FRED®?**

**F**og **R**eduction **E**limination **D**evice; sponge with antifog solution used to coat the camera lens

**Give some tips for "driving" the camera during laparoscopy.**

1. Keep the camera centered on the action.
2. Watch all trocars as they enter the peritoneal cavity (and the tissues beyond, so they can be avoided!).

3. Watch all instruments as they come through the trocars (unless directed otherwise).
4. Ask if you want to come out and clean and re-FRED the lens.
5. Look outside the body at the trocars and instrument angles to reorient yourself.
6. Keep the camera oriented at all times (i.e., up and down); usually the camera cord is on the bottom of the camera—orient yourself to the camera before entering the abdomen.
7. You may clean the camera lens at times by lightly touching the lens to the liver or peritoneum.
8. Never let the camera lens come into contact with the bowel because the camera may get very hot and you can burn a hole in the bowel or burn the drapes!
9. Put your helmet on (i.e., expect to get yelled at!).
10. Never act agitated when the surgeons are a little abrupt (e.g., "Center—center the camera!").
11. Always watch the trocars as they are removed from the abdominal wall for bleeding from the site and view the layers of the abdominal wall, looking for bleeding as you pull the camera trocar out at the end of the case.

**At what length must you close trocar sites?**

≥ 7 mm should be closed.

**How do you get the spleen out after a laparoscopic splenectomy?**

Crush it in a bag—then pull the bag out of a trocar site.

**What is an IOC?**

**I**ntra**O**perative **C**holangiogram (done during a lap chole to evaluate the common bile duct anatomy and to look for any retained duct stone)

# Chapter 38        Trauma

| | |
|---|---|
| **What widely accepted protocol does trauma care in the United States follow?** | The Advanced Trauma Life Support (ATLS) precepts of the American College of Surgeons |
| **What are the three main elements of the ATLS protocol?** | 1. Primary survey/resuscitation<br>2. Secondary survey<br>3. Definitive care |
| **How and when should the patient history be obtained?** | It should be obtained while completing the primary survey; often the rescue squad, witnesses, and family members must be relied upon. |

## PRIMARY SURVEY

| | |
|---|---|
| **What are the five steps of the primary survey?** | Think: "ABCDEs":<br>**A**irway (and C-spine stabilization)<br>**B**reathing<br>**C**irculation<br>**D**isability<br>**E**xposure and **E**nvironment |
| **What principles are followed in completing the primary survey?** | Life-threatening problems discovered during the primary survey are **always** addressed **before** proceeding to the next step. |

### AIRWAY

| | |
|---|---|
| **What are the goals during assessment of the airway?** | Securing the airway and protecting the spinal cord |
| **In addition to the airway, what MUST be considered during the airway step?** | Spinal immobilization |
| **What comprises spinal immobilization?** | Use of a full backboard and rigid cervical collar |

**In an alert patient, what is the quickest test for an adequate airway?**

Ask a question; if the patient can speak, the airway is intact.

**What is the first maneuver used to establish an airway?**

Chin lift, jaw thrust, or both; if successful, often an oral or nasal airway can be used to temporarily maintain the airway

**If these methods are unsuccessful, what is the next maneuver used to establish an airway?**

Endotracheal intubation, either nasal or oral (oral if the patient is not breathing with inline C-spine traction)

**When is nasotracheal intubation contraindicated?**

In patients with maxillofacial fracture or apnea

**If all other methods are unsuccessful, what is the definitive airway?**

Cricothyroidotomy, A.K.A. "surgical airway": incise the cricothyroid membrane between the cricoid cartilage inferiorly and the thyroid cartilage superiorly and place an endotracheal or tracheostomy tube into the trachea

**What must always be kept in mind during difficult attempts at establishing an airway?**

Spinal immobilization and adequate oxygenation; if at all possible, patients must be adequately ventilated with 100% oxygen using a bag and mask before any attempt at establishing an airway

## BREATHING

| | |
|---|---|
| **What are the goals in assessing breathing?** | Securing oxygenation and ventilation<br>Treating life-threatening thoracic injuries |
| **What comprises adequate assessment of breathing?** | Inspection—for air movement, respiratory rate, cyanosis, tracheal shift, jugular venous distention, asymmetric chest expansion, use of accessory muscles of respiration, open chest wounds<br>Auscultation—for breath sounds<br>Percussion—for hyperresonance or dullness over either lung field<br>Palpation—for presence of subcutaneous emphysema, flail segments |
| **What are the life-threatening conditions that MUST be diagnosed and treated during the breathing step?** | Tension pneumothorax, open pneumothorax, massive hemothorax |

### Pneumothorax

| | |
|---|---|
| **What is it?** | Injury to the lung, resulting in release of air into the pleural space between the normally apposed parietal and visceral pleura |
| **How is it diagnosed?** | **Tension pneumothorax is a clinical diagnosis:** dyspnea, jugular venous distention, tachypnea, anxiety, pleuritic chest pain, unilateral decreased or absent breath sounds, tracheal shift away from the affected side, hyperresonance on the affected side |
| **What is the treatment of a tension pneumothorax?** | **Immediate** decompression by **needle thoracostomy** in the second intercostal space midclavicular line, followed by **tube thoracostomy** placed in the anterior/midaxillary line in the fourth intercostal space (level of the nipple in men) |
| **What is the medical term for a "sucking chest wound"?** | Open pneumothorax |

**How is an open pneumothorax diagnosed and treated?**

**Diagnosis:** usually obvious, with air movement through a chest wall defect and pneumothorax on CXR

**Treatment in the ER:** +/− intubation with positive-pressure ventilation, tube thoracostomy (chest tube), occlusive dressing over chest wall defect

**What does a pneumothorax look like on chest X-ray?**

Loss of lung markings. Figure shows a right-sided pneumothorax. Arrows point out edge of lung-air interface.

## *Flail Chest*

**What is it?**

Two separate fractures in three or more consecutive ribs

**How is it diagnosed?**

A flail segment of chest wall that moves **paradoxically** (sucks in with inspiration and pushes out with expiration opposite the rest of the chest wall)

**What is the major cause of respiratory compromise with flail chest?**

Underlying pulmonary contusion!

**What is the treatment?**

**Intubation** with positive pressure ventilation and PEEP PRN (let ribs heal on their own)

### Cardiac Tamponade

**What is it?**

Bleeding into the pericardial sac, resulting in constriction of heart, decreasing inflow and resulting in decreased cardiac output (the pericardium does not stretch!)

**What are the signs and symptoms?**

Tachycardia/shock with **Beck's triad,** pulsus paradoxus, Kussmaul's sign

**Define the following:**
    **Beck's triad**

1. Hypotension
2. Muffled heart sounds
3. JVD

    **Kussmaul's sign**

JVD with inspiration

**How is cardiac tamponade definitely diagnosed?**

Ultrasound (echocardiogram)

**What is the treatment?**

Immediate IV fluid bolus; with pericardiocentesis, subsequent surgical exploration is mandatory (pericardiocentesis is a temporizing option; rare)

### Massive Hemothorax

**How is it diagnosed?**

Hypotension; unilaterally decreased or absent breath sounds; dullness to percussion; CXR, CT scan, chest tube output

| | |
|---|---|
| **What is the treatment?** | Volume replacement |
| | **Tube thoracostomy** (chest tube) |
| | Use of cell saver, if available |
| | Removal of the blood (which will allow apposition of the parietal and visceral pleura, sealing the defect and slowing the bleeding) |
| **What are indications for emergent thoracotomy for hemothorax?** | Massive hemothorax = |
| | 1. >1500 cc of blood on initial placement of chest tube |
| | 2. Persistent >200 cc of bleeding via chest tube per hour × 4 hours |

## CIRCULATION

| | |
|---|---|
| **What are the goals in assessing circulation?** | Securing adequate tissue perfusion; treatment of external bleeding |
| **What is the initial test for adequate circulation?** | Palpation of pulses: as a rough guide, if a radial pulse is palpable, then systolic pressure is at least 80 mm Hg; if a femoral or carotid pulse is palpable, then systolic pressure is at least 60 mm Hg. |
| **What comprises adequate assessment of circulation?** | Heart rate, blood pressure, peripheral perfusion, urinary output, mental status, capillary refill (normal <2 seconds), exam of skin: cold, clammy = hypovolemia |
| **Who can be hypovolemic with normal blood pressure?** | The young; autonomic tone can maintain blood pressure until cardiovascular collapse is imminent |
| **Which patients may not mount a tachycardic response to hypovolemic shock?** | Those with concomitant spinal cord injuries |
| | Those on β-blockers |
| | Well-conditioned athletes |
| **How are sites of external bleeding treated?** | By direct pressure; +/− tourniquets |

**What is the best and preferred intravenous (IV) access in the trauma patient?**

"Two large-bore IV's" (14–16 gauge), IV catheters in the upper extremities (peripheral IV access)

**What are alternate sites of IV access?**

Percutaneous and cutdown catheters in the lower leg saphenous; central access into femoral, jugular, subclavian veins

**For a femoral vein catheter, how can the anatomy of the right groin be remembered?**

Lateral to medial "NAVEL":
**N**erve
**A**rtery
**V**ein
**E**xtralymphatic material
**L**ymphatics
Thus, the vein is medial to the femoral artery pulse (or think: "venous close to penis").

**What is the trauma resuscitation fluid of choice?**

Lactated Ringer's (LR) solution (isotonic, and the lactate helps buffer the hypovolemia-induced metabolic acidosis)

**What types of decompression do trauma patients receive?**

Gastric decompression with an NG tube and Foley catheter bladder decompression after **normal rectal exam**

**What are the contraindications to placement of a Foley?**

Signs of urethral injury:
Severe pelvic fracture in men
Blood at the urethral meatus (penile opening)
"High-riding" "ballotable" prostate (loss of urethral tethering)
Scrotal/perineal injury/ecchymosis

**What test should be obtained prior to placing a Foley catheter if urethral injury is feared?**

A retrograde urethrogram (RUG; dye in penis retrograde to the bladder and x-ray looking for extravasation of dye)

**How is gastric decompression achieved with a maxillofacial fracture?**

**Not** with an NG tube because the tube may perforate through the cribriform plate into the brain; place an **oral**-gastric tube (OGT), not an NG tube

## DISABILITY

| | |
|---|---|
| **What are the goals in assessing disability?** | Determination of neurologic injury (think: neurologic disability) |
| **What comprises adequate assessment of disability?** | Mental status—Glasgow Coma Scale (GCS)<br><br>Pupils—a blown pupil suggests ipsilateral brain mass (blood) as herniation of the brain compresses CN III<br><br>Motor/sensory—screening exam for lateralizing extremity movement, sensory deficits |
| **Describe the GCS scoring system.** | **Eye opening (E)**<br>4—Opens spontaneously<br>3—Opens to voice (command)<br>2—Opens to painful stimulus<br>1—Does not open eyes<br>(think: eyes = "four eyes")<br>**Motor response (M)**<br>6—Obeys commands<br>5—Localizes painful stimulus<br>4—Withdraws from pain<br>3—Decorticate posture<br>2—Decerebrate posture<br>1—No movement<br>(think: motor = "6-cylinder motor")<br>**Verbal response (V)**<br>5—Appropriate and oriented<br>4—Confused<br>3—Inappropriate words<br>2—Incomprehensible sounds<br>1—No sounds<br>(think: verbal = "Jackson 5") |
| **What is the GCS score for a dead man?** | GCS 3 |
| **What is the GCS score for a patient in a "coma"?** | GCS ≤8 |
| **How does scoring differ if the patient is intubated?** | The verbal evaluation is omitted and replaced with a "T"; thus, the highest score for an intubated patient is 11 T. |

## EXPOSURE AND ENVIRONMENT

| | |
|---|---|
| **What are the goals in obtaining adequate exposure?** | Complete disrobing to allow a thorough visual inspection and digital palpation of the patient during the secondary survey |
| **What is the "environment" of the E?** | Keep a warm **E**nvironment (i.e., keep the patient warm; a hypothermic patient can become coagulopathic). |

## SECONDARY SURVEY

| | |
|---|---|
| **What principle is followed in completing the secondary survey?** | Complete physical exam, including all orifices: ears, nose, mouth, vagina, rectum |
| **Why look in the ears?** | Hemotympanum is a sign of basilar skull fracture; otorrhea is a sign of basilar skull fracture. |
| **Examination of what part of the trauma patient's body is often forgotten?** | The patient's back (logroll the patient and examine!) |
| **What are typical signs of basilar skull fracture?** | Raccoon eyes, Battle's sign, clear otorrhea or rhinorrhea, hemotympanum |
| **What diagnosis in the anterior chamber must not be missed on the eye exam?** | Traumatic hyphema = blood in the anterior chamber of the eye |
| **What potentially destructive lesion must not be missed on the nasal exam?** | Nasal septal hematoma; the hematoma must be evacuated; if not, it can result in pressure necrosis of the septum! |
| **What is the best indication of a mandibular fracture?** | Dental malocclusion; tell the patient to "bite down" and ask: "Does that feel normal to you?" |
| **What signs of thoracic trauma are often found on the neck exam?** | Crepitus or subcutaneous emphysema from tracheobronchial disruption/PTX; tracheal deviation from tension pneumothorax; jugular venous distention from cardiac tamponade; carotid bruit heard with seatbelt neck injury resulting in carotid artery injury |

**What is the best physical exam for broken ribs or sternum?**

Lateral and anterior-posterior compression of the thorax to elicit pain/instability

**What physical signs are diagnostic for thoracic great vessel injury?**

None; diagnosis of great vessel injury requires a high index of suspicion based on the mechanism of injury, associated injuries, and CXR/radiographic findings (e.g., widened mediastinum)

**What must be considered in every penetrating injury of the thorax at or below the level of the nipple?**

Concomitant injury to the abdomen; remember, the diaphragm extends to the level of the nipples in the male on full expiration

**What is the significance of subcutaneous air?**

Indicates PTX, until proven otherwise

**What is the proper technique for examining the thoracic and lumbar spine?**

Logrolling the patient to allow complete visualization of the back and palpation of the spine to elicit pain over fractures, step off (spine deformity)

**What conditions must exist to pronounce an abdominal physical exam negative?**

An alert patient without any evidence of head/spinal cord injury or drug/ETOH intoxication (even then, the abdominal exam is not 100% accurate)

**What physical signs may indicate intra-abdominal injury?**

Tenderness; guarding, peritoneal signs; progressive distention (always use a gastric tube for decompression of air); seatbelt sign

**What is the seatbelt sign?**

Ecchymosis on lower abdomen from wearing a seatbelt (approximately 10% of patients with this sign have a small bowel perforation!)

**What must be documented from the rectal exam?**

Sphincter tone (as an indication of spinal cord injury); presence of blood (as an indication of colon or rectal injury); prostate position (as an indication of urethral injury)

**What is the best physical exam technique to test for pelvic fractures?**

Lateral compression of the iliac crests and greater trochanters and anterior-posterior compression of the symphysis pubis to elicit pain/instability

**What is the "halo" sign?**

Cerebrospinal fluid from nose/ear will form a clear "halo" around the blood on a cloth.

**What physical signs indicate possible urethral injury, thus contraindicating placement of a Foley catheter?**

**High-riding ballotable prostate** on rectal exam; presence of blood at the meatus; scrotal or perineal ecchymosis

**What must be documented from the extremity exam?**

Any fractures or joint injuries; any open wounds; motor and sensory exam, particularly distal to any fractures; distal pulses; peripheral perfusion

**What complication after prolonged ischemia to the lower extremity must be treated immediately?**

Compartment syndrome

**What is the treatment for this condition?**

Fasciotomy (four-compartment below the knee)

**What injuries must be suspected in a trauma patient with a progressive decline in mental status?**

Epidural hematoma, subdural hematoma, brain swelling with rising intracranial pressure
But **hypoxia/hypotension must be ruled out!**

## TRAUMA STUDIES

**What are the classic blunt trauma ER x-rays?**

1. AP (anterior-to-posterior) chest film
2. AP pelvis film

**What are the common trauma labs?**

Blood for complete blood count, chemistries, amylase, liver function tests, lactic acid, coagulation studies, and **type and crossmatch;** urine for urinalysis

**Will the hematocrit be low after an acute massive hemorrhage?**

No (no time to equilibrate)

**How can a C-spine be evaluated?**

1. Clinically by physical exam
2. Radiographically

**What patients can have their C-spines cleared by a physical exam?**

No neck pain on palpation with full range of motion (FROM) with no neurologic injury (GCS 15), no ETOH/drugs, no distracting injury, no pain meds

**How do you rule out a C-spine bony fracture?**

With a CT scan of the C-spine

**What do you do if no bony C-spine fracture is apparent on CT scan and you cannot obtain an MRI in a COMATOSE patient?**

This is controversial; the easiest answer is to leave the patient in a cervical collar.

**Which x-rays are used for evaluation of cervical spine LIGAMENTOUS injury?**

MRI, lateral flexion and extension C-spine films

**What findings on chest film are suggestive of thoracic aortic injury?**

**Widened mediastinum (most common finding),** apical pleural capping, loss of aortic contour/KNOB/AP window, depression of left main stem bronchus, nasogastric tube/tracheal deviation, pleural fluid, elevation of right mainstem bronchus, clinical suspicion, high-speed mechanism

**What study is used to rule out thoracic aortic injury?**

Spiral CT of mediastinum looking for mediastinal hematoma with CTA
Thoracic arch aortogram (gold standard)

**What percentage of thoracic aortograms will reveal an aortic injury?**

Only about 10% of studies are positive

**What is the most common site of thoracic aortic traumatic tear?**

Just distal to the take off of the left subclavian artery

**What studies are available to evaluate for intra-abdominal injury?**

FAST, CT, DPL

**What is a FAST exam?**

Ultrasound: **F**ocused **A**ssessment with **S**onography for **T**rauma = FAST

**What does the FAST exam look for?**

Blood in the peritoneal cavity looking at Morison's pouch, bladder, spleen, and pericardial sac

**What does DPL stand for?**

**D**iagnostic **P**eritoneal **L**avage

**What diagnostic test is the test of choice for evaluation of the unstable patient with blunt abdominal trauma?**

FAST

**What is the indication for abdominal CT in blunt trauma?**

Normal vital signs with abdominal pain/ tenderness

**What is the indication for DPL or FAST in blunt trauma?**

Unstable vital signs (hypotension)

**How is a DPL performed?**

Place a catheter below the umbilicus (in patients without a pelvic fracture) into the peritoneal cavity.
Aspirate for blood and if less than 10 cc are aspirated, infuse 1 L of saline or LR.
Drain the fluid (by gravity) and analyze.

**What is a "grossly positive" DPL?**

≥10 cc blood aspirated

**Where should the DPL catheter be placed in a patient with a pelvic fracture?**

Above the umbilicus
A common error—if you go below the umbilicus, you may get into a pelvic hematoma tracking between the fascia layers and thus obtain a false-positive DPL.

**What constitutes a positive peritoneal tap?**

Prior to starting a peritoneal lavage, the DPL catheter should be aspirated. If more than 10 mL of blood or enteric contents are aspirated, then this constitutes a positive tap and requires laparotomy.

**What are the indicators of a positive peritoneal lavage in blunt trauma?**

Classic: inability to read newsprint through lavaged fluid
RBC ≥100,000/mm$^3$
WBC ≥500/mm$^3$ (Note: mm$^3$, not mm$^2$)
Lavage fluid (LR/NS) drained from chest tube, Foley, NG tube
Less common:
  Bile present
  Bacteria present
  Feces present
  Vegetable matter present
  Elevated amylase level

**What must be in place before a DPL is performed?**

NG tube and Foley catheter (to remove the stomach and bladder from the firing line!)

**What injuries does CT miss?**

Small bowel injuries and diaphragm injuries

**What injuries does DPL miss?**

Retroperitoneal injuries

**What study is used to evaluate the urethra in cases of possible disruption due to blunt trauma?**

Retrograde urethrogram (RUG)

**What are the most emergent orthopaedic injuries?**

1. Hip dislocation—must be reduced immediately
2. Exsanguinating pelvic fracture (binder or external fixator)

**What findings would require a celiotomy in a blunt trauma victim?**

Peritoneal signs, free air on CXR/CT, unstable patient with positive FAST exam or positive DPL results

**What is the treatment of a gunshot wound to the belly?**

Exploratory laparotomy

**What is the evaluation of a stab wound to the belly?**

If there are peritoneal signs, heavy bleeding, shock, unstable vital signs, perform exploratory laparotomy. Otherwise, many surgeons either observe the asymptomatic stab wound patient closely, use local wound exploration to rule out fascial penetration, or use DPL.

## PENETRATING NECK INJURIES

**What depth of neck injury must be further evaluated?**

Penetrating injury through the platysma

**Define the anatomy of the neck by trauma zones:**
  **Zone III**

Angle of the mandible and up

  **Zone II**

Angle of the mandible to the cricoid cartilage

  **Zone I**

Below the cricoid cartilage
Note: the zones are in the same anatomic order as the LeFort facial fractures (III, II, I) (or I, II, III following carotid blood flow).

**How do most surgeons treat penetrating neck injuries (those that penetrate the platysma) by neck zone:**

**Zone III**

Selective exploration

**Zone II**

Surgical exploration vs. selective exploration

**Zone I**

Selective exploration

**What is selective exploration?**

Selective exploration is based on diagnostic studies that include A-gram or CT A-gram, bronchoscopy, esophagoscopy

**What are the indications for surgical exploration in all penetrating neck wounds (Zones I, II, III)?**

"**Hard** signs" of significant neck damage: **shock,** exsanguinating hemorrhage, expanding hematoma, pulsatile hematoma, neurologic injury, SUBQ emphysema

## MISCELLANEOUS TRAUMA FACTS

**What is the "3-for-1" rule?**

The trauma patient in hypovolemic shock acutely requires 3 L of crystalloid (LR) for every 1 L of blood loss.

**What is the minimal urine output for an adult trauma patient?**

50 mL/hr

| | |
|---|---|
| **How much blood can be lost into the thigh with a closed femur fracture?** | Up to 1.5 L of blood |
| **Can an adult lose enough blood in the "closed" skull from a brain injury to cause hypovolemic shock?** | Absolutely not! But infants can lose enough blood from a brain injury to cause shock. |
| **Can a patient be hypotensive after an isolated head injury** | Yes, but rule out hemorrhagic shock! |
| **What is the brief ATLS history?** | An "AMPLE" history:<br>**A**llergies<br>**M**edications<br>**P**MH<br>**L**ast meal (when)<br>**E**vents (of injury, etc.) |
| **In what population is a surgical cricothyroidotomy not recommended?** | Any patient younger than 12 years; instead perform needle cricothyroidotomy |
| **What are the signs of a laryngeal fracture?** | Subcutaneous emphysema in neck<br>Altered voice<br>Palpable laryngeal fracture |
| **What is the treatment of rectal penetrating injury?** | **Diverting proximal colostomy;** closure of perforation (if easy, and definitely if intraperitoneal); and **presacral drainage** |
| **What is the treatment of extraperitoneal minor bladder rupture?** | "Bladder catheter" (Foley) drainage and observation; intraperitoneal or large bladder rupture requires operative closure. |
| **What intra-abdominal injury is associated with seatbelt use?** | Small bowel injuries (L2 fracture, pancreatic injury) |
| **What is the treatment of a pelvic fracture?** | +/− Pelvic binder until the external fixator is placed; IVF/blood; +/− A-gram to embolize bleeding pelvic vessels |

**Bleeding from pelvic fractures is most commonly caused by arterial or venous bleeding?**

Venous (approximately 90%)

**If a patient has a laceration through an eyebrow, should you shave the eyebrow prior to suturing it closed?**

No—20% of the time, the eyebrow will not grow back if shaved!

**What is the treatment of extensive irreparable biliary, duodenal, and pancreatic head injury?**

Trauma Whipple

**What is the most common intra-abdominal organ injured with penetrating trauma?**

Small bowel

**How high up do the diaphragms go?**

To the nipples (intercostal space # 4); thus, intra-abdominal injury with penetrating injury below the nipples must be ruled out

**Classic trauma question: "If you have only one vial of blood from a trauma victim to send to the lab, what test should be ordered?"**

Type and cross (for blood transfusion)

**What is the treatment of penetrating injury to the colon?**

If the patient is in shock, resection and colostomy.
If the patient is stable, the trend is primary anastomosis/repair.

**What is the treatment of small bowel injury?**

Primary closure or resection and primary anastomosis

**What is the treatment of minor pancreatic injury?**

Drainage (e.g., JP drains)

**What is the most commonly injured abdominal organ with blunt trauma?**

Liver (in recent studies)

**What is the treatment for significant duodenal injury?**

Pyloric exclusion:
1. Close duodenal injury
2. Staple off pylorus
3. Gastrojejunostomy

**What is the treatment for massive tail of pancreas injury?**

Distal pancreatectomy (usually perform splenectomy also)

**What is "damage control" surgery?**

Stop major hemorrhage and GI soilage. Pack and get out of the OR ASAP to bring the patient to the ICU to warm, correct coags, and resuscitate. Return patient to OR when stable, warm and not acidotic.

**What is the "lethal triad"?**

ACHe
1. Acidosis
2. Coagulopathy
3. Hypothermia
(think: **ACHe** = **A**cidosis, **C**oagulopathy, **H**ypothermia)

**What comprises the workup/ treatment of a stable parasternal chest gunshot/ stab wound?**

1. CXR
2. FAST, chest tube, +/− OR for sub xiphoid window; if blood returns, then sternotomy to assess for cardiac injury

**What is the diagnosis with NGT in chest on CXR?**

Ruptured diaphragm with stomach in pleural cavity

**What films are typically obtained to evaluate extremity fractures?**

Complete views of the involved extremity, including the joints above and below the fracture

**Outline basic work up for a victim of severe blunt trauma :**

In E.R.: Airway, physical exam. IV X 2, 2 L LR, labs, spun HCT,
type and cross, OGT/NGT, Foley, chest tube PRN
X-rays: CXR, Pelvis, Femur
(if femur fracture is suspected)

[Note: +/− = if indicated. A-gram = aortogram. AP = anteroposterior.
Ext = extremity. ICU = Intensive Care Unit. OGT = orogastric tube.
FAST = Focused Assessment Sonogram for Trauma. lat = lateral.
C = cervical. T = thoracic. L = lumbar. PRN = as needed.]

| | |
|---|---|
| **What lab tests are used to look for intra-abdominal injury in children?** | Liver function tests (LFTs) = ↑AST and/or ↑ALT |
| **What is the only real indication for MAST trousers?** | Prehospitalization, pelvic fracture |
| **What is the treatment for human and dog bites?** | Leave wound open, irrigation, antibiotics |

---

# Chapter 39    Burns

| | |
|---|---|
| **Define:** | |
| **TBSA** | **T**otal **B**ody **S**urface **A**rea |
| **STSG** | **S**plit **T**hickness **S**kin **G**raft |
| **Are acid or alkali chemical burns more serious?** | In general, **ALKALI** burns are more serious because the body cannot buffer the alkali, thus allowing them to burn for much longer. |
| **Why are electrical burns so dangerous?** | Most of the destruction from electrical burns is internal because the route of least electrical resistance follows nerves, blood vessels, and fascia. Injury is usually worse than external burns at entrance and exit sites would indicate. **Cardiac dysrhythmias,** myoglobinuria, acidosis, and renal failure are common. |
| **How is myoglobinuria treated?** | To avoid renal injury, think "HAM": **H**ydration with IV fluids **A**lkalization of urine with IV bicarbonate **M**annitol diuresis |
| **Define level of burn injury: First degree burns** | Epidermis only |

**Second degree burns**  Epidermis and varying levels of dermis

**Third degree burns**  A.K.A. "full thickness"; all layers of the skin including the entire dermis (think: "getting the third degree")

**Fourth degree burns**  Burn injury into bone or muscle

**How do first degree burns present?**  Painful, dry, red areas that do not form blisters (think of sunburn)

**How do second degree burns present?**  Painful, hypersensitive, swollen, mottled areas with **blisters** and open weeping surfaces

**How do third degree burns present?**  Painless, insensate, swollen, dry, mottled white, and charred areas; often described as dried leather

**What is the major clinical difference between second and third degree burns?**  Third degree burns are painless, and second degree burns are painful (laudable pain).

**By which measure is burn severity determined?**  Depth of burn and total body surface area (TBSA) affected by second and third degree burns

TBSA is calculated by the "rule of nines" in adults and by a modified rule in children to account for the disproportionate size of the head and trunk

**What is the "rule of nines"?**  In an adult, the total body surface area that is burned can be estimated by the following:
Each upper limb = 9%
Each lower limb = 18%
Anterior and posterior trunk = 18% each
Head and neck = 9%
Perineum and genitalia = 1%

| | |
|---|---|
| **What is the "rule of the palm"?** | The surface area of the patient's palm is approximately 1% of the TBSA used for estimating size of small burns |
| **What is the burn center referral criteria for the following?** | |
| **Second degree burns** | >20% TBSA |
| **Third degree burns** | >5% TBSA<br>Second degree >10% TBSA in children and the elderly<br>Any burns involving the face, hands, feet, or perineum<br>Any burns with inhalation injury<br>Any burns with associated trauma<br>Any electrical burns |
| **What is the treatment of first degree burns?** | Keep clean, ± Neosporin®, pain meds |

**What is the treatment of second degree burns?**

Remove blisters; apply antibiotic ointment (usually Silvadene®) and dressing; pain meds. Most second degree burns do not require skin grafting (epidermis grows from hair follicles and from margins).

**What are some newer options for treating a second degree burn?**

1. Biobrane® (silicone artificial epidermis—temporary)
2. Silverlon® (silver ion dressings)

**What is the treatment of third degree burns?**

Early excision of eschar (within first week postburn) and split-thickness skin grafting (STSG)

**How can you decrease bleeding during excision?**

Tourniquets as possible, topical epinephrine, topical thrombin

**What is an autograft STSG?**

STSG from the patient's own skin

**What is an allograft STSG?**

STSG from a cadaver (temporary coverage)

**What thickness is the STSG?**

10/1000 to 15/1000 of an inch (down to the dermal layer)

**What prophylaxis should the burn patient get in the ED?**

Tetanus

**What is used to evaluate the eyes after a third degree burn?**

Fluorescein

**What principles guide the initial assessment and resuscitation of the burn patient?**

Airway, breathing, circulation, disability, and exposure. Check for eschar and compartment syndromes.

**What are the signs of smoke inhalation?**

Smoke and soot in sputum/mouth/nose; nasal/facial hair burns, carboxyhemoglobin, throat/mouth erythema, history of loss of consciousness/explosion/fire in small enclosed area, dyspnea, low $O_2$ saturation, confusion, headache, coma

**What lab value assesses smoke inhalation?**

**Carboxyhemoglobin** level (a carboxyhemoglobin level of more than 60% is associated with a 50% mortality); treat with 100% $O_2$ and time

**How should the airway be managed in the burn patient with an inhalational injury?**

With a low threshold for **intubation;** oropharyngeal swelling may occlude the airway so that intubation is impossible; 100% oxygen should be administered immediately and continued until significant carboxyhemoglobin is ruled out

**What is "burn shock"?**

**Burn shock** describes the loss of fluid from the intravascular space as a result of burn injury, which causes "leaking capillaries" that require crystalloid infusion.

**What is the "Parkland formula"?**

V = Total Body Surface Area Burn (%) × Weight (kg) × 4

Formula widely used to estimate the volume (V) of crystalloid necessary for the initial resuscitation of the burn patient; half of the calculated volume is given in the **first 8 hours,** the rest in the next 16 hours

**What burns qualify for the Parkland formula?**

>10% TBSA second and third-degree burns only

**How is the crystalloid given?**

Through two large-bore peripheral venous catheters

**Can you place an IV or central line through burned skin?**

YES

**Why is glucose-containing IVF contraindicated in burn patients in the first 24 hours postburn?**

The patient's serum glucose will be elevated on its own because of the stress response

**What fluid is used after the first 24 hrs postburn?**

Colloid; use D5W **and** 5% albumin at 0.5 cc/kg/% burn surface area

**Why should D5W IV be administered after 24 hours postburn?**

Because of the massive sodium load in the first 24 hrs of LR infusion and because of the massive evaporation of $H_2O$ from the burn injury, the patient will need free water; after 24 hours, the capillaries begin to work and then the patient can usually benefit from **albumin** and D5W.

**What is the minimal urine output for burn patients?**

Adults >0.5 cc/kg/hr; children 1–2 cc/kg/hr

**How is volume status monitored in the burn patient?**

**Urine output**, blood pressure, heart rate, peripheral perfusion, and mental status; Foley catheter is mandatory and may be supplemented by central venous pressure and pulmonary capillary wedge pressure monitoring

**Why do most severely burned patients require nasogastric decompression?**

Patients with greater than 20% TBSA burns usually develop a paralytic ileus → vomiting → aspiration risk → pneumonia

**What stress prophylaxis must be given to the burn patient?**

$H_2$ blocker to prevent burn stress ulcer (Curling's ulcer)

**What are the signs of burn wound infection?**

Increased WBC with left shift, **discoloration of burn eschar** (most common sign), green pigment, necrotic skin lesion in unburned skin, edema, ecchymosis tissue below eschar, second degree burns that turn into third degree burns, hypotension

**Is fever a good sign of infection in burn patients?**

NO

**What are the common organisms found in burn wound infections?**

*Staphylococcus aureus, Pseudomonas, Streptococcus, Candida albicans*

**How is a burn wound infection diagnosed?**

Send burned tissue in question to the laboratory for quantitative burn wound bacterial count. If the count is more than $10^5$/gram, infection is present and IV antibiotics should be administered.

**How are minor burns dressed?**

Gentle cleaning with nonionic detergent and debridement of loose skin and broken blisters; the burn is dressed with a topical antibacterial (e.g., neomycin) and covered with a sterile dressing

**How are major burns dressed?**

Cleansing and application of topical antibacterial agent

**Why are systemic IV antibiotics contraindicated in fresh burns?**

The bacteria live in the eschar, which is avascular (the systemic antibiotic will not be delivered to the eschar); thus, apply topical antimicrobial agents.

**Note some advantages and disadvantages of the following topical antibiotic agents:**

    **Silver sulfadiazine (Silvadene®)**

Painless, but little eschar penetration, misses *Pseudomonas*, and has idiosyncratic **neutropenia**; sulfa allergy is contraindication

    **Mafenide acetate (Sulfamylon®)**

Penetrates eschars, broad spectrum (but misses *Staphylococcus*), causes pain on application; triggers allergic reaction in 7% of patients; may cause **acid-base imbalances** (think: **M**afenide **AC**etate = **M**etabolic **AC**idosis); agent of choice in already-contaminated burn wounds

    **Polysporin®**

Polymyxin B sulfate; painless, clear, used for facial burns; does not have a wide antimicrobial spectrum

**Are prophylactic systemic antibiotics administered to burn patients?**

No. Prophylactic antibiotics have not been shown to reduce the incidence of sepsis, but rather have been shown to select for resistant organisms. IV antibiotics are reserved for established wound infections, pneumonia, urinary tract infections, etc.

**Are prophylactic antibiotics administered for inhalational injury?**

No

**Circumferential, full-thickness burns to the extremities are at risk for what complication?**

Distal neurovascular impairment, similar to compartment syndrome

**How is it treated?**

Escharotomy: full-thickness longitudinal incision through the eschar with scalpel or electrocautery; incision must extend into healthy fat

**What is the major infection complication (other than wound infection) in burn patients?**

Pneumonia, central line infection (change central lines prophylactically every 3 to 4 days)

**Is tetanus prophylaxis required in the burn patient?**

Yes, it is mandatory in all patients except those actively immunized within the past 12 months (with complete immunization: toxoid ×3).

**From which burns is water evaporation highest?**

Third degree

**Can infection convert a partial-thickness injury into a full-thickness injury?**

Yes!

**How is carbon monoxide inhalation overdose treated?**

100% $O_2$ (± hyperbaric $O_2$)

**Which electrolyte must be closely followed acutely after a burn?**

$Na^+$ (sodium)

**When should central lines be changed in the burn patient?**

Most burn centers change them every 3 to 4 days.

**What is the name of the gastric/duodenal ulcer associated with burn injury?**

Curling's ulcer (think: curling iron burn = Curling's burn ulcer)

**How are STSGs nourished in the first 24 hours?**

IMBIBITION (fed from wound bed exudate)

# Chapter 40     **Upper GI Bleeding**

**What is it?**

Bleeding into the lumen of the proximal GI tract, proximal to the ligament of Treitz

**What are the signs/symptoms?**

Hematemesis, melena, syncope, shock, fatigue, coffee-ground emesis, hematochezia, epigastric discomfort, epigastric tenderness, signs of hypovolemia, guaiac-positive stools

**Why is it possible to have hematochezia?**

Blood is a cathartic and hematochezia usually indicates a vigorous rate of bleeding from the UGI source.

**Are stools melenic or melanotic?**

Melenic (melanotic is incorrect)

**How much blood do you need to have melena?**

>50 cc of blood

**What are the risk factors?**

Alcohol, cigarettes, liver disease, burn/trauma, aspirin/NSAIDs, vomiting, sepsis, steroids, previous UGI bleeding, history of peptic ulcer disease (PUD), esophageal varices, portal hypertension, splenic vein thrombosis, abdominal aortic aneurysm repair (aortoenteric fistula), burn injury, trauma

**What is the most common cause of significant UGI bleeding?**

PUD—duodenal and gastric ulcers (50%)

**What are the *common* differential diagnoses of UGI bleeding?**

1. **Acute gastritis**
2. **Duodenal ulcer**
3. Esophageal varices
4. Gastric ulcer
5. Esophageal
6. Mallory-Weiss tear

**What are the *uncommon* differential diagnoses of UGI bleeding?**

Gastric cancer, hemobilia, duodenal diverticula, gastric volvulus, Boerhaave's syndrome, aortoenteric fistula, paraesophageal hiatal hernia, epistaxis, NGT irritation, Dieulafoy's ulcer, angiodysplasia

**Which diagnostic tests are useful?**

History, NGT aspirate, abdominal x-ray, endoscopy (EGD)

**What is the diagnostic test of choice with UGI bleeding?**

EGD (>95% diagnosis rate)

**What are the treatment options with the endoscope during an EGD?**

Coagulation, injection of epinephrine (for vasoconstriction), injection of sclerosing agents (varices), variceal ligation (banding)

**Which lab tests should be performed?**

Chem-7, bilirubin, LFTs, CBC, **type & cross,** PT/PTT, amylase

**Why is BUN elevated?**

Because of absorption of blood by the GI tract

**What is the initial treatment?**

1. **IVFs** (16 G or larger peripheral IVS × 2), **Foley** catheter (monitor fluid status)
2. **NGT** suction (determine rate and amount of blood)
3. Water lavage (use warm $H_2O$—will remove clots)
4. **EGD:** Endoscopy (determine etiology/ location of bleeding and possible treatment—coagulate bleeders)

**Why irrigate in an upper GI bleed?**

To remove the blood clot that has fibrino- lytic and factor so you can see the mucosa

**What test may help identify the site of MASSIVE UGI bleeding when EGD fails to diagnose cause and blood continues per NGT?**

Selective mesenteric angiography

**What are the indications for surgical intervention in UGI bleeding?**

Refractory or recurrent bleeding and site known, >3 u PRBCS to stabilize or >6 u PRBCs overall

| | |
|---|---|
| **What percentage of patients require surgery?** | Approximately 10% |
| **What percentage of patients spontaneously stop bleeding?** | Approximately 80% to 85% |
| **What is the mortality of acute UGI bleeding?** | Overall 10%, 60–80 years of age 15%, older than 80 years of age 25% |
| **What are the risk factors for death following UGI bleed?** | Age older than 60 years<br>Shock<br>More than 5 units of PRBC transfusion<br>Concomitant health problems |

## PEPTIC ULCER DISEASE (PUD)

| | |
|---|---|
| **What is it?** | Gastric and duodenal ulcers |
| **What is the incidence in the United States?** | Approximately 10% of the population will suffer from PUD during their lifetime! |
| **What are the possible consequences of PUD?** | Pain, hemorrhage, perforation, obstruction |
| **What percentage of patients with PUD develop bleeding from the ulcer?** | Approximately 20% |
| **Which bacteria are associated with PUD?** | *Helicobacter pylori* |
| **What is the treatment?** | Treat *H. pylori* with MOC or ACO two-week antibiotic regimens:<br>**MOC: M**etronidazole, **O**meprazole, **C**larithromycin (think: "**MOCK**")<br>or<br>**ACO: A**mpicillin, **C**larithromycin, **O**meprazole |
| **What is the name of the sign with RLQ pain/peritonitis as a result of succus collecting from a perforated peptic ulcer?** | Valentino's sign |

## DUODENAL ULCERS

| | |
|---|---|
| **In which age group are these ulcers most common?** | Between 40 and 65 years of age (younger than patients with gastric ulcer) |
| **What is the ratio of male to female patients?** | Men > women (3 to 1) |
| **What is the most common location?** | Most are within 2 cm of the pylorus in the duodenal bulb. |
| **What is the classic pain response to food intake?** | Food classically relieves duodenal ulcer pain (think: **D**uodenum = **D**ecreased with food). |
| **What is the cause?** | Increased production of gastric acid |
| **What syndrome must you always think of with a duodenal ulcer?** | Z-E syndrome (Zollinger-Ellison) |
| **What are the associated risk factors?** | Male gender, smoking, aspirin and other NSAIDs, uremia, Z-E syndrome, *H. pylori*, trauma, burn injury |
| **What are the symptoms?** | Epigastric pain—burning or aching, usually several hours after a meal (food, milk, or antacids initially relieve pain)<br>Bleeding<br>Back pain<br>Nausea, vomiting, and anorexia<br>↓ appetite |
| **What are the signs?** | Tenderness in epigastric area (possibly), guaiac-positive stool, melena, hematochezia, hematemesis |
| **What is the differential diagnosis?** | Acute abdomen, pancreatitis, cholecystitis, **all causes of UGI bleeding,** Z-E syndrome, gastritis, MI, gastric ulcer, reflux |
| **How is the diagnosis made?** | History, PE, EGD, UGI series (**if patient is not actively bleeding**) |

**When is surgery indicated with a bleeding duodenal ulcer?**

Most surgeons use: >6 u PRBC transfusions, >3 u PRBCs needed to stabilize, or significant rebleed

**What EGD finding is associated with rebleeding?**

Visible vessel in the ulcer crater, recent clot, active oozing

**What is the medical treatment?**

PPIs (proton pump inhibitors) or $H_2$ receptor antagonists—heal ulcers in 4 to 6 weeks in most cases
Treatment for *H. pylori*

**When is surgery indicated?**

The acronym "I HOP":
**I**ntractability
**H**emorrhage (massive or relentless)
**O**bstruction (gastric outlet obstruction)
**P**erforation

**How is a bleeding duodenal ulcer surgically corrected?**

Opening of the duodenum through the pylorus
Oversewing of the bleeding vessel

**What artery is involved with bleeding duodenal ulcers?**

Gastroduodenal artery

**What are the common surgical options for the following conditions:**
    **Truncal vagotomy?**

Pyloroplasty

    **Duodenal perforation?**

Graham patch (poor candidates, shock, prolonged perforation)
Truncal vagotomy and pyloroplasty incorporating ulcer
Graham patch and highly selective vagotomy
Truncal vagotomy and antrectomy (higher mortality rate, but lowest recurrence rate)

    **Duodenal obstruction resulting from duodenal ulcer scarring (gastric outlet obstruction)?**

Truncal vagotomy, antrectomy, and gastroduodenostomy (BI or BII)
Truncal vagotomy and drainage procedure (gastrojejunostomy)

| | |
|---|---|
| **Duodenal ulcer intractability?** | PGV (highly selective vagotomy) |
| | Vagotomy and pyloroplasty |
| | Vagotomy and antrectomy BI or BII (especially if there is a coexistent pyloric/prepyloric ulcer) but associated with a higher mortality |
| **Which ulcer operation has the highest ulcer recurrence rate and the lowest dumping syndrome rate?** | PGV (proximal gastric vagotomy) |
| **Which ulcer operation has the lowest ulcer recurrence rate and the highest dumping syndrome rate?** | Vagotomy and antrectomy |
| **Why must you perform a drainage procedure (pyloroplasty, antrectomy) after a truncal vagotomy?** | Pylorus will not open after a truncal vagotomy. |
| **Which duodenal ulcer operation has the lowest mortality rate?** | PGV (1/200 mortality), truncal vagotomy and pyloroplasty (1–2/200), vagotomy and antrectomy (1%–2% mortality) |
| | Thus, PGV is the operation of choice for intractable duodenal ulcers with the cost of increased risk of ulcer recurrence. |
| **What is a "kissing" ulcer?** | Two ulcers are each on opposite sides of the lumen so that they can "kiss." |
| **Why may a duodenal rupture be initially painless?** | Fluid can be sterile, with a nonirritating pH of 7.0 initially. |
| **Why may a perforated duodenal ulcer present as lower quadrant abdominal pain?** | Fluid from stomach/bile drains down paracolic gutters to lower quadrants and causes localized irritation. |

## GASTRIC ULCERS

| | |
|---|---|
| **In which age group are these ulcers most common?** | Between 40 and 70 years old (older than the duodenal ulcer population) |
| | Rare in patients younger than 40 years |

**How does the incidence in men compare with that of women?**

Men > women

**Which is more common overall: gastric or duodenal ulcers?**

Duodenal ulcers are more than twice as common as gastric ulcers; (think **D**uodenal = **D**ouble rate).

**What is the classic pain response to food?**

Food classically increases gastric ulcer pain.

**What is the cause?**

**Decreased cytoprotection** or gastric protection (i.e., decreased bicarbonate/mucous production)

**Is gastric acid production high or low?**

Gastric acid production is normal or low!

**Which gastric ulcers are associated with increased gastric acid?**

Prepyloric
Pyloric
Coexist with duodenal ulcers

**What are the associated risk factors?**

Smoking, alcohol, burns, trauma, CNS tumor/trauma, NSAIDs, steroids, shock, severe illness, male gender, advanced age

**What are the symptoms?**

Epigastric pain
+/− vomiting, anorexia, and nausea

**How is the diagnosis made?**

History, PE, EGD with multiple biopsy (looking for gastric cancer)

**What is the most common location?**

Approximately 70% are on the lesser curvature; 5% are on the greater curvature.

**When and why should biopsy be performed?**

With all gastric ulcers, to rule out gastric cancer
If the ulcer does not heal in 6 weeks after medical treatment, **rebiopsy** (always biopsy in OR also) must be performed.

**What is the medical treatment?**

Similar to that of duodenal ulcer—PPIs or $H_2$ blockers, *Helicobacter pylori* treatment

**When do patients with gastric ulcers need to have an EGD?**

1. For diagnosis with biopsies
2. 6 weeks postdiagnosis to confirm healing and rule out gastric cancer!

**What are the indications for surgery?**

The acronym "I CHOP":
**I**ntractability
**C**ancer (rule out)
**H**emorrhage (massive or relentless)
**O**bstruction (gastric outlet obstruction)
**P**erforation
(Surgery is indicated if gastric cancer cannot be ruled out.)

**What is the common operation for hemorrhage, obstruction, and perforation?**

Distal gastrectomy with excision of the ulcer **without** vagotomy unless there is duodenal disease (i.e., BI or BII)

**What are the options for concomitant duodenal and gastric ulcers?**

Resect (BI, BII) and **truncal vagotomy**

**What is a common option for surgical treatment of a pyloric gastric ulcer?**

Truncal vagotomy and antrectomy (i.e., BI or BII)

**What is a common option for a poor operative candidate with a perforated gastric ulcer?**

Graham patch

**What must be performed in every operation for gastric ulcers?**

Biopsy looking for gastric cancer

**Define the following terms:**
  **Cushing's ulcer**

PUD/gastritis associated with neurologic trauma or tumor (think: Dr. **C**ushing = **n**eurosurgeon)

  **Curling's ulcer**

PUD/gastritis associated with major burn injury (think: curling iron burn)

  **Marginal ulcer**

Ulcer at the margin of a GI anastomosis

  **Dieulafoy's ulcer**

Pinpoint gastric mucosal defect bleeding from an underlying vascular malformation

## PERFORATED PEPTIC ULCER

| | |
|---|---|
| **What are the symptoms?** | **Acute** onset of upper abdominal pain |
| **What causes pain in the lower quadrants?** | Passage of perforated fluid along colic gutters |
| **What are the signs?** | Decreased bowel sounds, tympanic sound over the liver (air), peritoneal signs, tender abdomen |
| **What are the signs of posterior duodenal erosion/perforation?** | Bleeding from gastroduodenal artery (and possibly acute pancreatitis) |
| **What sign indicates anterior duodenal perforation?** | Free air (anterior perforation is more common than posterior) |
| **What is the differential diagnosis?** | Acute pancreatitis, acute cholecystitis, perforated acute appendicitis, colonic diverticulitis, MI, any perforated viscus |
| **Which diagnostic tests are indicated?** | X-ray: free air under diaphragm or in lesser sac in an upright CXR (if upright CXR is not possible, then left lateral decubitus can be performed because air can be seen over the liver and not confused with the gastric bubble) |
| **What are the associated lab findings?** | Leukocytosis, high amylase serum (secondary to absorption into the blood stream from the peritoneum) |
| **What is the initial treatment?** | NPO: NGT ($\downarrow$ contamination of the peritoneal cavity)<br>IVF/Foley catheter<br>Antibiotics/PPIs<br>Surgery |
| **What is a Graham patch?** | A piece of omentum incorporated into the suture closure of perforation |
| **What are the surgical options for treatment of a duodenal perforation?** | Graham patch<br>Truncal vagotomy and pyloroplasty incorporating ulcer |

Graham patch and highly selective vagotomy

**What are the surgical options for perforated gastric ulcer?**

Antrectomy incorporating perforated ulcer, Graham patch or wedge resection in unstable/poor operative candidates

**What is the significance of hemorrhage and perforation with duodenal ulcer?**

May indicate two ulcers (kissing); posterior is bleeding and anterior is perforated with free air

**What type of perforated ulcer may present just like acute pancreatitis?**

Posterior perforated duodenal ulcer into the pancreas (i.e., epigastric pain radiating to the back; high serum amylase)

**What is the classic difference between duodenal and gastric ulcer symptoms as related to food ingestion?**

Duodenal = decreased pain
Gastric = increased pain
(think: **D**uodenal = **D**ecreased pain)

## TYPES OF SURGERIES

**Define the following terms:**
**Graham patch**

For treatment of duodenal perforation in poor operative candidates/unstable patients
Place viable omentum over perforation and tack into place with sutures

**Truncal vagotomy**

Resection of a 1- to 2-cm segment of each vagal **trunk** as it enters the abdomen on the distal esophagus, decreasing gastric acid secretion

**What other procedure must be performed along with a truncal vagotomy?**

A "drainage procedure" (pyloroplasty, antrectomy, or gastrojejunostomy), because vagal fibers provide relaxation of the pylorus and if you cut them, the pylorus will not open

**Define the following terms:**
**Vagotomy and pyloroplasty**

Pyloroplasty performed with vagotomy to compensate for decreased gastric emptying

**Vagotomy and antrectomy**

Remove antrum and pylorus in addition to vagotomy; reconstruct as a Billroth I or II

**What is the goal of duodenal ulcer surgery?**

Decrease gastric acid secretion (and fix IHOP)

**What is the advantage of proximal gastric vagotomy (highly selective vagotomy)?**

No drainage procedure is needed; vagal fibers to the pylorus are preserved; rate of dumping syndrome is low.

**What is a Billroth I (BI)?**

Truncal vagotomy, antrectomy, and gastroduodenostomy (think: BI = one limb off of the stomach remnant)

**What are the contraindications for a Billroth I?**

Gastric cancer or suspicion of gastric cancer

**What is a Billroth II (BII)?**

Truncal vagotomy, antrectomy, and gastrojejunostomy (think: BII = two limbs off of the stomach remnant)

**What is the Kocher maneuver?**

Dissect the left lateral peritoneal attachments to the duodenum to allow visualization of posterior duodenum.

## STRESS GASTRITIS

**What is it?**

**Superficial** mucosal erosions in the stressed patient

| | |
|---|---|
| **What are the risk factors?** | Sepsis, intubation, trauma, shock, burn, brain injury |
| **What is the prophylactic treatment?** | $H_2$ blockers, antacids, sucralfate |
| **What are the signs/ symptoms?** | NGT blood (usually), painless (usually) |
| **How is it diagnosed?** | EGD, if bleeding is significant |
| **What is the treatment for gastritis?** | LAVAGE out blood clots, give a maximum dose of PPI in a 24-hour IV drip |

## MALLORY-WEISS SYNDROME

| | |
|---|---|
| **What is it?** | Post-retching, postemesis longitudinal tear (submucosa and mucosa) of the stomach near the GE junction; approximately three-fourths are in the stomach |
| **For what percentage of all upper GI bleeds does this syndrome account?** | About 10% |
| **What are the causes of a tear?** | Increased gastric pressure, often aggravated by hiatal hernia |
| **What are the risk factors?** | Retching, alcoholism (50%), more than 50% of patients have hiatal hernia |
| **What are the symptoms?** | Epigastric pain, thoracic substernal pain, emesis, hematemesis |
| **What percentage of patients will have hematemesis?** | 85% |
| **How is the diagnosis made?** | EGD |
| **What is the "classic" history?** | Alcoholic patient after binge drinking—first, vomit food and gastric contents, followed by forceful retching and bloody vomitus |

| | |
|---|---|
| **What is the treatment?** | Room temperature water lavage (90% of patients stop bleeding), electrocautery, arterial embolization, or surgery for refractory bleeding |
| **When is surgery indicated?** | When medical/endoscopic treatment fails (>6 u PRBCs infused) |
| **Can you use the Sengstaken-Blakemore tamponade balloon for treatment of Mallory-Weiss tear bleeding?** | No, it makes bleeding worse. Use the balloon only for bleeding from esophageal varices. |

## ESOPHAGEAL VARICEAL BLEEDING

| | |
|---|---|
| **What is it?** | Bleeding from formation of esophageal varices from back up of portal pressure via the coronary vein to the submucosal esophageal venous plexi secondary to portal hypertension from liver cirrhosis |
| **What is the "rule of two-thirds" of esophageal variceal hemorrhage?** | Two-thirds of patients with portal hypertension develop esophageal varices. Two-thirds of patients with esophageal varices bleed. |
| **What are the signs/symptoms?** | Liver disease, portal hypertension, hematemesis, caput medusa, ascites |
| **How is the diagnosis made?** | EGD (very important because only 50% of UGI bleeding in patients with known esophageal varices are bleeding from the varices; the other 50% have bleeding from ulcers, etc.) |
| **What is the acute medical treatment?** | Lower portal pressure with vasopressin or somatostatin |
| **In the patient with CAD, what must you give in addition to the vasopressin?** | Nitroglycerin—to prevent coronary artery vasoconstriction that may result in an MI |
| **What are the treatment options?** | Sclerotherapy or band ligation via endoscope, TIPS, liver transplant |

**What is the Sengstaken-Blakemore balloon?**

Tamponades with an esophageal balloon and a gastric balloon

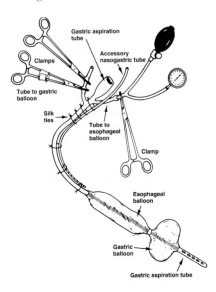

**What is the problem with shunts?**

Decreased portal pressure, but increased encephalopathy

## BOERHAAVE'S SYNDROME

**What is it?**

Postemetic esophageal rupture

**Why is the esophagus susceptible to perforation and more likely to break down an anastomosis?**

No serosa

**What is the most common location?**

Posterolateral aspect of the esophagus (on the left), 3 to 5 cm above the GE junction

**What is the cause of rupture?**

Increased intraluminal pressure, usually caused by violent retching and vomiting

**What is the associated risk factor?**

Esophageal reflux disease (50%)

| | |
|---|---|
| **What are the symptoms?** | Pain postemesis (may radiate to the back, dysphagia) |
| **What are the signs?** | Left pneumothorax, Hamman's sign, left pleural effusion, subcutaneous/mediastinal emphysema, fever, tachypnea, tachycardia, signs of infection by 24 hours, neck crepitus, widened mediastinum on CXR |
| **What is Mackler's triad?** | 1. Emesis<br>2. Lower chest pain<br>3. Cervical emphysema (sub Q air) |
| **What is Hamman's sign?** | "Mediastinal crunch or clicking" produced by the heart beating against air-filled tissues |
| **How is the diagnosis made?** | History, physical examination, CXR, esophagram with water-soluble contrast |
| **What is the treatment?** | Surgery within 24 hours to **drain** the mediastinum and surgically close the perforation and placement of pleural patch; broad-spectrum antibiotics |
| **What is the mortality rate in less than 24 hours until surgery for perforated esophagus?** | Approximately 15% |
| **What is the mortality rate if more than 24 hours until surgery for perforated esophagus?** | Approximately 33% |
| **Overall, what is the most common cause of esophageal perforation?** | Iatrogenic (most commonly cervical esophagus) |

# Chapter 41    The Stomach

## ANATOMY

**Identify the parts of the stomach:**

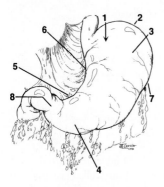

1. Cardia
2. Fundus
3. Body
4. Antrum
5. Incisura angularis
6. Lesser curvature
7. Greater curvature
8. Pylorus

**Identify the blood supply to the stomach:**

1. Left gastric artery
2. Right gastric artery
3. Right gastroepiploic artery
4. Left gastroepiploic artery
5. Short gastrics (from spleen)

**What space lies behind the stomach?**

The lesser sac; the pancreas lies behind the stomach

**What is the opening into the lesser sac?**

Foramen of Winslow

**What are the folds of gastric mucosa called?**

Rugae

## GASTRIC PHYSIOLOGY

| | |
|---|---|
| **Define the products of the following stomach cells:** | |
| Gastric parietal cells | HCl<br>Intrinsic factor |
| Chief cells | Pepsinogen (think: "a peppy chief") |
| G cells | Gastrin (think: **G** cells = **G**astrin) |
| Where are G cells located? | Antrum |
| Mucous neck cells | Bicarbonate<br>Mucus |
| **What is pepsin?** | A proteolytic enzyme that hydrolyzes peptide bonds |
| **What is intrinsic factor?** | A protein secreted by the parietal cells that combines with vitamin $B_{12}$ and allows for absorption in the terminal ileum |

## GASTROESOPHAGEAL REFLUX DISEASE (GERD)

| | |
|---|---|
| **What is it?** | Excessive reflux of gastric contents into the esophagus, "heartburn" |
| **What is pyrosis?** | Medical term for heartburn |
| **What are the causes?** | Decreased lower esophageal sphincter (LES) tone (>50% of cases)<br>Decreased esophageal motility to clear refluxed fluid<br>Gastric outlet obstruction<br>Hiatal hernia in approximately 50% of patients |
| **What are the signs/ symptoms?** | Heartburn, regurgitation, respiratory problems/pneumonia from aspiration of refluxed gastric contents; substernal pain |

**What disease must be ruled out when the symptoms of GERD are present?**

Coronary artery disease

**What tests are included in the workup?**

EGD
UGI contrast study with esophagogram
Twenty-four hour acid analysis (pH probe in esophagus)
Manometry, ECG, CXR

**What is the medical treatment?**

Small meals
PPIs (proton pump inhibitors) or $H_2$ blockers
Elevation of head at night and no meals prior to sleeping

**What are the indications for surgery?**

Intractability (failure of medical treatment)
Respiratory problems as a result of reflux and aspiration of gastric contents (e.g., pneumonia)
Severe esophageal injury (e.g., ulcers, hemorrhage, stricture, $\pm$ Barrett's esophagus)

**What is Barrett's esophagus?**

Columnar metaplasia from the normal squamous epithelium as a result of chronic irritation from reflux

**What is the major concern with Barrett's esophagus?**

Developing cancer

**What type of cancer develops in Barrett's esophagus?**

Adenocarcinoma

**What percentage of patients with GERD develop Barrett's esophagus?**

7% (5–10%)

**What percentage of patients with Barrett's esophagus will develop adenocarcinoma?**

7% lifetime (5–10%)

**Define the following
surgical options for severe
GERD:**

**LAP Nissen**

360° fundoplication—2 cm long
(laparoscopically)

**Belsey mark IV**

240° to 270° fundoplication performed
through a thoracic approach

**Hill**

Arcuate ligament repair (close large esophageal hiatus) and gastropexy to diaphragm (suture stomach to diaphragm)

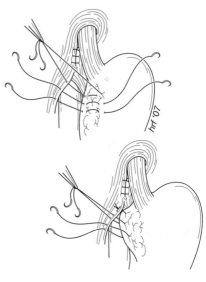

**Toupet**

Incomplete (around 200°) posterior wrap (laparoscopic) often used with severe decreased esophageal motility

**How does the Nissen wrap work?**

Controversial but thought to work by:
1. Increasing LES muscular tone
2. Elongating LES
3. Restoring angle of His
4. Decreasing distal esophageal diameter

| | |
|---|---|
| **In what percentage of patients does LAP Nissen work?** | 90% |

**What are the postoperative complications of LAP Nissen?**

1. Gas-bloat syndrome
2. Stricture
3. Dysphagia
4. Spleen injury requiring splenectomy
5. Esophageal perforation
6. Pneumothorax

**What is gas-bloat syndrome?**  Inability to burp or vomit

## GASTRIC CANCER

**What is the incidence?**  Low in United States (10/100,000); high in Japan (78/100,000)

**What are the associated risk factors?**

Diet—smoked meats, high nitrates, low fruits and vegetables, alcohol, tobacco

Environment—raised in high-risk area, poor socioeconomic status, atrophic gastritis, male gender, blood type A, previous partial gastrectomy, pernicious anemia, polyps, *Helicobacter pylori*

**What is the average age at the time of discovery?**  Older than 60 years

**What is the ratio of male to female patients?**  3:2

**Which blood type is associated with gastric cancer?**  Blood type A (there is an "**A**" in gastric but no "O" or "B" = g**A**stric = type "**A**")

**What are the symptoms?**

WEAPON
**W**eight loss
**E**mesis
**A**norexia
**P**ain/epigastric discomfort
**O**bstruction
**N**ausea

**What are the most common early symptoms?**

Mild epigastric discomfort and indigestion

**What is the most common symptom?**

Weight loss

**What are the signs?**

Anemia, melena, heme occult, epigastric mass (in advanced disease), hepatomegaly, coffee-ground emesis, Blumer's shelf, Virchow's node, enlarged ovaries, axillary adenopathy

**What does the patient with gastric cancer have if he or she has proximal colon distension?**

Colonic obstruction by direct invasion (rare)

**What is the symptom of proximal gastric cancer?**

Dysphagia (gastroesophageal junction/cardia)

**What is a Blumer's shelf?**

A solid peritoneal deposit anterior to the rectum, forming a "shelf," palpated on **rectal examination**

**What is a Virchow's node?**

Metastatic gastric cancer to the nodes in the left supraclavicular fossa

**What is Sister Mary Joseph's sign?**

Periumbilical lymph node gastric cancer metastases; presents as periumbilical mass

**What is a Krukenberg's tumor?**

Gastric cancer (or other adenocarcinoma) that has metastasized to the ovary

**What is "Irish's" node?**

Left axillary adenopathy from gastric cancer metastasis

**What is a surveillance laboratory finding?**

CEA elevated in 30% of cases (if + useful for postoperative surveillance)

**What is the initial workup?**

EGD with biopsy, endoscopic U/S to evaluate the level of invasion, CT of abdomen/pelvis for metastasis, CXR, labs

**What is the histology?**

Adenocarcinoma

**What is the differential diagnosis for gastric tumors?**
Adenocarcinoma, leiomyoma, leiomyosarcoma, lymphoma, carcinoid, ectopic pancreatic tissue, gastrinoma, benign gastric ulcer, polyp

**What are the two histologic types?**
1. Intestinal (glands)
2. Diffuse (no glands)

**What is the morphology?**
Ulcerative (75%)
Polypoid (10%)
Scirrhous (10%)
Superficial (5%)

**Are gastric cancers more common on the lesser or greater curvatures?**
Lesser ("lesser is greater")

**What is more common, proximal or distal gastric cancer?**
Proximal

**Which morphologic type is named after a "leather bottle"?**
Linitis plastica—the entire stomach is involved and looks thickened (10% of cancers)

**How do gastric adenocarcinomas metastasize?**
Hematogenously and lymphatically

**Which patients with gastric cancer are NONoperative?**
1. Distant metastasis (e.g., liver metastasis)
2. Peritoneal implants

**What is the role of laparoscopy?**
To rule out peritoneal implants and to evaluate for liver metastasis

**What is the genetic alteration seen in >50% of patients with gastric cancer?**
P53

**What is the treatment?**
Surgical resection with wide (>5 cm checked by frozen section) margins and lymph node dissection

**What operation is performed for tumor in the:**
  **Antrum?**
Distal subtotal gastrectomy

**Midbody?**

Total gastrectomy

**Proximal?**

Total gastrectomy

**What is a subtotal gastrectomy?**

Subtotal gastrectomy = 75% of stomach removed

**What is a total gastrectomy?**

The stomach is removed and a Roux-en-Y limb is sewn to the esophagus.

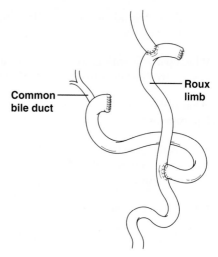

**What type of anastomosis?**

Billroth II or Roux-en-Y (never use a Billroth I)

| | |
|---|---|
| **When should splenectomy be performed?** | When the tumor directly invades the spleen/splenic hilum or with splenic hilar adenopathy |
| **Define "extended lymph node dissection."** | Extensive lymph node dissection, usually one group past the lymph node group with positive metastases |
| **What percentage of patients are inoperable at presentation?** | Approximately 10–15% |
| **What is the adjuvant treatment?** | Preoperative chemotherapy or postoperative chemotherapy and radiation |
| **What is the 5-year survival rate for gastric cancer?** | 25–50% of patients are alive 5 years after diagnosis in the United States (in Japan, 50% are alive at 5 years) |
| **Why is it thought that the postoperative survival is so much higher in Japan?** | Aggressive screening and capturing early cancers |

## GASTRIC VOLVULUS

| | |
|---|---|
| **What is it?** | Twisting of the stomach |
| **What are the symptoms?** | Brochardt's triad:<br>1. Distention of epigastrium<br>2. Cannot pass an NGT<br>3. Emesis followed by inability to vomit |
| **What is the treatment?** | Exploratory laparotomy to untwist, and gastropexy |

# Chapter 42

# Bariatric Surgery

**What is it?**

Weight reduction surgery for the morbidly obese

**Define morbid obesity.**

1. BMI >40 (basically, >100 pounds above ideal body weight) or
2. BMI >35 with a medical problem related to morbid obesity

**What is the BMI?**

Body Mass Index

**What is the formula for BMI?**

Body weight in kg divided by height in meters squared

**What is a formula for a rough estimate of BMI without using metric measures?**

$$\frac{\text{Wt (pounds)} \times 703}{(\text{Ht in inches})^2}$$

**What medical conditions are associated with morbid obesity?**

Sleep apnea, coronary artery disease, pulmonary disease, diabetes mellitus, venous stasis ulcers, arthritis, infections, sex-hormone abnormalities, HTN, breast cancer, colon cancer

**What are the current options for surgery?**

Gastric bypass (malabsorptive)
Vertical-banded gastroplasty

**Define gastric bypass.**

Stapling off of small gastric pouch (restrictive)
Roux-en-Y limb to gastric pouch

**How does gastric bypass work?**

1. Creates a small gastric reservoir
2. Causes dumping symptoms when a patient eats too much food or high-calorie foods; the food is "dumped" into the Roux-en-Y limb
3. Bypass of small bowel by Roux-en-Y limb

**Which operation works best overall?**

Gastric bypass (mean weight loss 50% of excess weight)

**What are the possible postoperative complications after weight reduction surgery?**

Gallstones (if gallbladder in situ), anastomotic leak, marginal ulcer, stenosis of pouch/anastomosis, malnutrition, incisional hernia, spleen injury, iron deficiency, $B_{12}$ deficiency

# Chapter 43     Ostomies

**Define the following terms:**

**Ostomy**

An operation that connects the GI tract to abdominal wall skin or the lumen of another hollow organ; a man-made fistula

**Stoma**

The opening of the ostomy (Gr. "mouth")

**Gastrostomy**

G-tube through the abdominal wall to the stomach for drainage or feeding

**Jejunostomy**

J-tube through the abdominal wall to the jejunum for feeding

**Kock pouch**

"Continent ileostomy"
Pouch is made of several ileal loops.
Patient must access the pouch with a tube intermittently.

**Colostomy**

Connection of colon mucosa to the abdominal wall skin for stool drainage

**End colostomy**

Proximal end of colon brought to the skin for stool drainage

**Mucus fistula**

Distal end of transected colon brought to the skin for decompression; the mucosa produces mucus, a colostomy is a fistula, and, hence, the term **mucus fistula** (proximal colon brought up as a colostomy or, if the proximal colon is removed, an ileostomy)

**Hartmann's pouch**

Distal end of transected colon stapled and dropped back into the peritoneal cavity, resulting in a blind pouch; mucus is decompressed through the anus (proximal colon is brought up as an end colostomy or, if proximal colon is removed, an end ileostomy)

**Double-barrel colostomy**

End colostomy and a mucus fistula (i.e., two barrels brought up to the skin)

**Loop colostomy**

A loop of large bowel is brought up to the abdominal wall skin and a plastic rod is placed underneath the loop. The colon is then opened and sewn to the abdominal wall skin as a colostomy.

**Ileal conduit**

Loops of stapled-off ileum made into a pouch, anastomosed to the ureters, and then brought to the abdominal wall skin to allow drainage of urine in patients who undergo removal of the bladder (cystectomy)

**Brooke ileostomy**

Ileostomy folded over itself to provide clearance from skin

| | |
|---|---|
| **Why doesn't an ileostomy or colostomy close?** | **E**pithelialization (mucosa to skin) from the acronym **FRIEND** (see Fistula chapter) |
| **Why doesn't a gastrostomy close?** | **F**oreign body (the plastic tube) from the acronym **FRIEND** |
| **If the plastic tube, G-tube, or J-tube is removed, how fast can the hole to the stomach or jejunum close?** | In a matter of hours! (Thus, if it comes out inadvertently from a well-established tract, it must be replaced immediately.) |
| **What is a "tube check"?** | A Gastrografin contrast study to confirm that a G-tube or J-tube is within the lumen of the stomach or jejunum, respectively |

# Chapter 44    Small Intestine

## SMALL BOWEL

### ANATOMY

| | |
|---|---|
| **What comprises the small bowel?** | Duodenum, jejunum, and ileum |
| **How long is the duodenum?** | Approximately 12 inches—thus the name: duodenum! |
| **What marks the end of the duodenum and the start of the jejunum?** | Ligament of Treitz |
| **What is the length of the entire small bowel?** | Approximately 6 meters (20 feet) |
| **What provides blood supply to the small bowel?** | Branches of the superior mesenteric artery |
| **What does the small bowel do?** | Major site of digestion and absorption |

| | |
|---|---|
| **What are the plicae circulares?** | Plicae means folds, circulares means circular; thus, circular folds of mucosa (A.K.A. valvulae conniventes) in small bowel lumen |
| **What are the major structural differences between the jejunum and the ileum?** | Jejunum—long vasa rectae, large plicae circulares, thicker wall<br>Ileum—shorter vasa rectae, smaller plicae circulares, thinner wall<br>(think: **I**leum = **I**nferior vasa rectae, **I**nferior plicae circulares, and **I**nferior wall thickness in comparison to the jejunum) |
| **What does the terminal ileum absorb?** | $B_{12}$, fatty acids, bile salts |

## SMALL BOWEL OBSTRUCTION

| | |
|---|---|
| **What is small bowel obstruction (SBO)?** | Mechanical obstruction to the passage of intraluminal contents |
| **What are the signs/ symptoms?** | Abdominal discomfort, cramping, nausea, abdominal distention, emesis, high-pitched bowel sounds |
| **What lab tests are performed with SBO?** | Electrolytes, CBC, type and screen, urinalysis |
| **What are classic electrolyte/ acid-base findings with proximal obstruction?** | Hypovolemic hypochloremic hypokalemia alkalosis |
| **What must be ruled out on physical exam in patients with SBO?** | Incarcerated hernia (also look for surgical scars) |
| **What major AXR findings are associated with SBO?** | Distended loops of small bowel<br>Air-fluid levels on upright film |

Air-fluid
level

**Define complete SBO.**

Complete obstruction of the lumen; usually paucity or no colon gas

**What is the danger of complete SBO?**

Closed loop strangulation of the bowel leading to bowel necrosis

**Define partial SBO.**

Incomplete SBO; some colon gas

**What is initial management of all patients with SBO?**

NPO, NGT, IVF, Foley

**What tests can differentiate partial from complete bowel obstruction?**

CT with oral contrast, small bowel follow through

**What are the ABCs of SBO?**

Causes of SBO:
1. **A**dhesions
2. **B**ulge (hernias)
3. **C**ancer and tumors

**What are other causes of SBO?**

The acronym **"GIVES BAD CRAMPS"**:
**G**allstone ileus
**I**ntussusception
**V**olvulus
**E**xternal compression
**S**MA syndrome
**B**ezoars, bowel wall hematoma
**A**bscesses
**D**iverticulitis

**C**rohn's disease
**R**adiation enteritis
**A**nnular pancreas
**M**eckel's diverticulum
**P**eritoneal adhesions
**S**tricture

| | |
|---|---|
| **What is superior mesenteric artery (SMA) syndrome?** | Seen with weight loss—SMA compresses duodenum, causing obstruction |
| **What is the treatment of complete SBO?** | Laparotomy and lysis of adhesions |
| **What is LOA?** | **L**ysis **O**f **A**dhesions |
| **What is the treatment of incomplete SBO?** | Initially, conservative treatment with close observation plus NGT decompression |
| **Intraoperatively, how can the level of obstruction be determined in patients with SBO?** | Transition from dilated bowel proximal to the decompressed bowel distal to the obstruction |
| **What is the most common indication for abdominal surgery in patients with Crohn's disease?** | SBO |
| **Can a patient have complete SBO and bowel movements and flatus?** | Yes; the bowel distal to the obstruction can clear out gas and stool. |
| **After a small bowel resection, why should the mesenteric defect always be closed?** | To prevent an internal hernia |
| **What may cause SBO if patient is on coumadin?** | Bowel wall hematoma |
| **What is the #1 cause of SBO in adults (industrialized nations)?** | Postoperative adhesions |
| **What is the #1 cause of SBO around the world?** | Hernias |

| | |
|---|---|
| **What is the #1 cause of SBO in children?** | Hernias |
| **What are the signs of strangulated bowel with SBO?** | **Fever,** severe/continuous pain, hematemesis, **shock,** gas in the bowel wall or portal vein, abdominal free air, **peritoneal signs, acidosis** (increased lactic acid) |
| **What are the clinical parameters that will lower the threshold to operate on a partial SBO?** | Increasing **WBC** **Fever** **Tachycardia**/tachypnea **Abdominal pain** |
| **What is an absolute indication for operation with partial SBO?** | Peritoneal signs, free air on AXR |
| **What classic saying is associated with complete SBO?** | "Never let the sun set or rise on complete SBO." |
| **What condition commonly mimics SBO?** | Paralytic ileus (AXR reveals gas distention throughout, including the colon) |
| **What is the differential diagnosis of paralytic (nonobstructive) ileus?** | Postoperative ileus after abdominal surgery (normally resolves in 3–5 days) Electrolyte abnormalities (hypokalemia is most common) Medications (anticholinergic, narcotics) Inflammatory intra-abdominal process Sepsis/shock Spine injury/spinal cord injury Retroperitoneal hemorrhage |
| **What tumor classically causes SBO due to "mesenteric fibrosis"?** | Carcinoid tumor |

## SMALL BOWEL TUMORS

| | |
|---|---|
| **What is the differential diagnosis of benign tumors of the small intestine?** | Leiomyoma, lipoma, lymphangioma, fibroma, adenomas, hemangiomas |

**What are the signs and symptoms of small bowel tumors?**

Abdominal pain, weight loss, obstruction (SBO), and perforation

**What is the most common benign small bowel tumor?**

Leiomyoma

**What is the most common malignant small bowel tumor?**

Adenocarcinoma

**What is the differential diagnosis of malignant tumors of the small intestine?**

1. Adenocarcinoma (50%)
2. Carcinoid (25%)
3. Lymphoma (20%)
4. Sarcomas

**What is the work up of a small bowel tumor?**

UGI with small bowel follow-through, enteroclysis, CT scan, enteroscopy

**What is the treatment for malignant small bowel tumor?**

Resection and removal of mesenteric draining lymph nodes

**What malignancy is classically associated with metastasis to small bowel?**

Melanoma

## MECKEL'S DIVERTICULUM

**What is it?**

Remnant of the omphalomesenteric duct/vitelline duct, which connects the yolk sac with the primitive midgut in the embryo

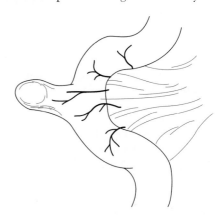

| | |
|---|---|
| **What is its claim to fame?** | Most common small bowel congenital abnormality |
| **What is the usual location?** | Within approximately 2 feet of the ileocecal valve on the **antimesenteric** border of the bowel |
| **What is the major differential diagnosis?** | Appendicitis |
| **Is it a true diverticulum?** | **Yes;** all layers of the intestine are found in the wall |
| **What is the incidence?** | Approximately 2% of the population at autopsy |
| **What is the gender ratio?** | Two times more common in **men** |
| **What is the average age at onset of symptoms?** | Most frequently in the first **2 years of life,** but can occur at any age |
| **What are the possible complications?** | **Intestinal hemorrhage** (painless)—50%; accounts for half of all lower GI bleeding in patients younger than 2 years<br>Bleeding results from ectopic gastric mucosa secreting acid → ulcer → bleeding<br>**Intestinal obstruction**—25%; most common complication in adults; includes volvulus and intussusception<br>**Inflammation** (± perforations)—20% |
| **What are the signs/ symptoms?** | Lower GI bleeding, abdominal pain, SBO |
| **What is the most common complication of Meckel's diverticulum in adults?** | Intestinal obstruction |
| **In what percentage of cases is heterotopic tissue found in the diverticulum?** | More than 50% |

**What heterotopic tissue type is most often found?**

**Gastric mucosa** (60%), but duodenal, pancreatic, and colonic mucosa are also found

**What is the "rule of 2s"?**

**2**% of patients are **symptomatic**
Found approximately **2** feet from the
    ileocecal valve
Found in **2**% of the population
Most symptoms occur before age **2** years
Ectopic tissue found in 1 of **2** patients
Most diverticula are approximately
    **2** inches long
**2** to 1 male : female ratio

**What is the role of incidental Meckel's diverticulectomy (surgical removal upon finding asymptomatic diverticulum)?**

Most experts would remove in children
(very controversial in adults).

**What is a Meckel's scan?**

Scan for ectopic gastric mucosa in
Meckel's diverticulum; uses **technetium pertechnetate** IV, which is preferentially
taken up by gastric mucosa

**What is the treatment of a Meckel's diverticulum that is causing bleeding and obstruction?**

Surgical resection, with small bowel
resection as the actual ulcer is usually
on the mesenteric wall opposite the
diverticulum!

**What is the name of the hernia associated with incarcerated Meckel's diverticulum?**

Littre's hernia (think alphabetically:
**L**ittre's, then **M**eckel's)

**In patients with guaiac-positive stools and a negative upper- and lower-GI workup, what must be ruled out?**

A small bowel tumor; evaluate with
enteroclysis (small bowel contrast study)

**What is the most common cause of small bowel bleeding?**

Small bowel angiodysplasia

# Chapter 45

# The Appendix

**What vessel provides blood supply to the appendix?**

Appendiceal artery—branch of the ileocolic artery

**Name the mesentery of the appendix.**

Mesoappendix (contains the appendiceal artery)

**How can the appendix be located if the cecum has been identified?**

Follow the taenia coli down to the appendix. The taeniae converge on the appendix.

## APPENDICITIS

**What is it?**

Inflammation of the appendix caused by **obstruction** of the appendiceal lumen, producing a closed loop with resultant inflammation that can lead to necrosis and perforation

**What are the causes?**

**Lymphoid hyperplasia, fecalith**
(A.K.A. appendicolith)
Rare—parasite, foreign body, tumor
(e.g., carcinoid)

**What is the lifetime incidence of acute appendicitis in the United States?**

Approximately 7%!

**What is the most common cause of emergent abdominal surgery in the United States?**

Acute appendicitis

**How does appendicitis classically present?**

Classic chronologic order:
1. Periumbilical pain (intermittent and crampy)
2. Nausea/vomiting
3. Anorexia
4. Pain migrates to RLQ (constant and intense pain), usually in less than 24 hours

**Why does periumbilical pain occur?**

Referred pain

**Why does RLQ pain occur?**

Peritoneal irritation

**What are the signs/ symptoms?**

Signs of peritoneal irritation may be present: guarding, muscle spasm, rebound tenderness, obturator and psoas signs, low-grade fever (high-grade if perforation occurs), RLQ hyperesthesia

**Define the following terms:**
    **Obturator sign**

Pain upon internal rotation of the leg with the hip and knee flexed; seen in patients with pelvic appendicitis

    **Psoas sign**

Pain elicited by extending the hip with the knee in full extension or by flexing the hip against resistance; seen classically $\bar{c}$ retrocecal appendicitis

    **Rovsing's sign**

Palpation or rebound pressure of the LLQ results in pain in the RLQ; seen in appendicitis

    **Valentino's sign**

RLQ pain/peritonitis from succus draining down to the RLQ from a perforated gastric or duodenal ulcer

    **McBurney's point**

Point one-third from the anterior superior iliac spine to the umbilicus (often the point of maximal tenderness)

**What is the differential diagnosis for:**

**Everyone?**

Meckel's diverticulum, Crohn's disease, perforated ulcer, pancreatitis, mesenteric lymphadenitis, constipation, gastroenteritis, intussusception, volvulus, tumors, UTI (e.g., cystitis), pyelonephritis, torsed epiploicae, cholecystitis, cecal tumor, diverticulitis (floppy sigmoid)

**Females?**

Ovarian cyst, ovarian torsion, tubo-ovarian abscess, mittelschmerz, pelvic inflammatory disease (PID), ectopic pregnancy, ruptured pregnancy

**What lab tests should be performed?**

CBC: increased WBC ($>10,000$ per $mm^3$ in $>90\%$ of cases), most often with a "left shift"

Urinalysis: to evaluate for pyelonephritis or renal calculus

**Can you have an abnormal urinalysis with appendicitis?**

Yes; mild hematuria and pyuria are common in appendicitis with pelvic inflammation, resulting in inflammation of the ureter.

**Does a positive urinalysis rule out appendicitis?**

**No;** ureteral inflammation resulting from the periappendiceal inflammation can cause abnormal urinalysis.

**What additional tests can be performed if the diagnosis is not clear?**

Spiral CT, U/S (may see a large, noncompressible appendix or fecalith), AXR

**In acute appendicitis, what classically precedes vomiting?**

Pain (in gastroenteritis, the pain classically follows vomiting)

**What radiographic studies are often performed?**

CXR: to rule out RML or RLL pneumonia, free air

AXR: abdominal films are usually nonspecific, but calcified fecalith present in about 5% of cases

**What are the radiographic signs of appendicitis on AXR?**

Fecalith, sentinel loops, **scoliosis** away from the right because of pain, mass effect (abscess), loss of psoas shadow, loss of preperitoneal fat stripe, and (very rarely) a small amount of free air if perforated

**With acute appendicitis, in what percentage of cases will a radiopaque fecalith be on AXR?**

Only approximately 5% of the time!

**What are the CT findings with acute appendicitis?**

Periappendiceal fat stranding, appendiceal diameter >6 mm, periappendiceal fluid, fecalith

**What are the preoperative medications/preparation?**

1. Rehydration with **IV fluids** (LR)
2. Preoperative **antibiotics** with anaerobic coverage (appendix is considered part of the colon)

**What is a lap appy?**

Laparoscopic appendectomy; used in most cases in women (can see adnexa) or if patient has a need to quickly return to physical activity, or is obese

**What is the treatment for *non*perforated acute appendicitis?**

Nonperforated—prompt appendectomy (prevents perforation), 24 hours of antibiotics, discharge home usually on postoperative day 1

**What is the treatment for *perforated* acute appendicitis?**

Perforated—IV fluid resuscitation and prompt appendectomy; all pus is drained with postoperative antibiotics continued for 3 to 7 days; wound is left open in most cases of perforation after closing the fascia (heals by secondary intention or delayed primary closure)

**How is an appendiceal abscess that is diagnosed preoperatively treated?**

Usually by **percutaneous** drainage of the abscess, antibiotic administration, and elective appendectomy approximately 6 weeks later (A.K.A. interval appendectomy)

**If a normal appendix is found upon exploration, should you take out the normal appendix?**

Yes

**How long after removal of a NONRUPTURED appendix should antibiotics continue postoperatively?**

For 24 hours

**Which antibiotic is used for NONPERFORATED appendicitis?**

Anaerobic coverage: Cefoxitin®, Cefotetan®, Unasyn®, Cipro® and Flagyl®

**What antibiotic is used for a PERFORATED appendix?**

**Usually triple antibiotics** (e.g., Amp/Cipro®/Clinda or a broad-spectrum penicillin such as Zosyn®)

**How long do you give antibiotics for perforated appendicitis?**

Until the patient has a normal WBC count and is afebrile, ambulating, and eating a regular diet (usually 3–7 days)

**What is the risk of perforation?**

Approximately 25% by 24 hours from onset of symptoms, approximately 50% by 36 hours, and approximately 75% by 48 hours

**What is the most common general surgical abdominal emergency in pregnancy?**

Appendicitis (about 1/1750; **appendix may be in the RUQ because of the enlarged uterus**)

**What are the possible complications of appendicitis?**

Pelvic abscess, liver abscess, free perforation, portal pylethrombophlebitis (very rare)

**What percentage of the population has a retrocecal, retroperitoneal appendix?**

Approximately 15%

**What percentage of negative appendectomies is acceptable?**

Up to 20%; taking out some normal appendixes is better than missing a case of acute appendicitis that eventually ruptures.

**Who is at risk of dying from acute appendicitis?**

Very old and very young patients

| | |
|---|---|
| **What bacteria are associated with "mesenteric adenitis" that can closely mimic acute appendicitis?** | *Yersinia enterolytica* |
| **What is an "incidental appendectomy"?** | Removal of normal appendix during abdominal operation for different procedure |
| **What are complications of an appendectomy?** | SBO, enterocutaneous fistula, wound infection, infertility with perforation in women, increased incidence of right inguinal hernia, stump abscess |
| **What is the most common postoperative complication?** | Wound infection |

## CLASSIC INTRAOPERATIVE QUESTIONS

| | |
|---|---|
| **What is the difference between a McBurney's incision and a Rocky-Davis incision?** | McBurney's is angled down (follows ext oblique fibers) and Rocky-Davis is straight across (transverse). |
| **What are the layers of the abdominal wall during a McBurney incision?** | 1. Skin<br>2. Subcutaneous fat<br>3. Scarpa's fascia<br>4. External oblique<br>5. Internal oblique<br>6. Transversus muscle<br>7. Transversalis fascia<br>8. Preperitoneal fat<br>9. Peritoneum |
| **What are the steps in laparoscopic appendectomy (lap appy)?** | 1. Identify the appendix.<br>2. Staple the mesoappendix (or coagulate).<br>3. Staple and transect the appendix at the base (or use Endoloop® and cut between).<br>4. Remove the appendix from the abdomen.<br>5. Irrigate and aspirate until clear. |

**Do you routinely get peritoneal cultures for acute appendicitis (nonperforated)?**

No

**How can you find the appendix after identifying the cecum?**

Follow the taenia down to where they converge on the appendix.

**Which way should your finger sweep trying to find the appendix?**

Lateral to medial along the lateral peritoneum—this way you will not tear the mesoappendix that lies medially!

**How do you get to a retrocecal and retroperitoneal appendix?**

Divide the lateral peritoneal attachments of the cecum.

**Why use electrocautery on the exposed mucosa on the appendiceal stump?**

To kill the mucosal cells so they do not form a mucocele

**If you find Crohn's disease in the terminal ileum, will you remove the appendix?**

Yes, if the cecal/appendiceal base is not involved

**If the appendix is normal what do you inspect intraoperatively?**

Terminal ileum: Meckel's diverticulum, Crohn's disease, intussusception
Gynecologic: Cysts, torsion, etc.
Groin: hernia, rectus sheath hematoma, adenopathy (adenitis)

**Who first described the classic history and treatment for acute appendicitis?**

Reginald Fitz

**Who performed the first appendectomy?**

Harry Hancock in 1848 (McBurney popularized the procedure in 1880s)

**Who performed the first lap appy?**

Dr. Semm (GYN) in 1983

## APPENDICEAL TUMORS

**What is the most common appendiceal tumor?**

Carcinoid tumor

**What is the treatment of appendiceal carcinoid less than 1.5 cm?**

Appendectomy (if not through the bowel wall)

**What is the treatment of appendiceal carcinoid larger than 1.5 cm?**

Right hemicolectomy

**What percentage of appendiceal carcinoids are malignant?**

Less than 5%

**What are the differential diagnoses of appendiceal tumor?**

Carcinoid, adenocarcinoma, malignant mucoid adenocarcinoma

**What type of appendiceal tumor can cause the dreaded pseudomyxoma peritonei if the appendix ruptures?**

Malignant mucoid adenocarcinoma

**What is "mittelschmerz"?**

Pelvic pain caused by ovulation

**Should one remove the normal appendix with Crohn's disease found intraoperatively?**

Yes, unless the base of the appendix is involved with Crohn's disease, the normal appendix should be removed to avoid diagnostic confusion with appendicitis in the future.

# Chapter 46

# Carcinoid Tumors

| | |
|---|---|
| **What is a carcinoid tumor?** | A tumor arising from neuroendocrine cells (APUDomas), A.K.A. **Kulchitsky cells;** basically, a tumor that secretes **serotonin** |
| **Why is it called "carcinoid"?** | The suffix "-oid" means "resembling." Thus, carcinoid resembles a carcinoma but is clinically and histologically less aggressive than most GI carcinomas. |
| **How can one remember that Kulchitsky cells are found in carcinoid tumors?** | Think: "COOL CAR" or **KUL**chitsky **CAR**cinoid |
| **What is the incidence?** | Between 0.2 and 1.0% and about 25% of all small bowel tumors |
| **What are the common sites of occurrence?** | AIR:<br>1. **A**ppendix (most common)<br>2. **I**leum<br>3. **R**ectum<br>4. Bronchus<br>Other sites: jejunum, stomach, duodenum, colon, ovary, testicle, pancreas, thymus |
| **What are the signs/ symptoms?** | Depends on location; most cases are asymptomatic; also SBO, abdominal pain, bleeding, weight loss, diaphoresis, **pellagra skin changes,** intussusception, or carcinoid syndrome, wheezing |
| **Why SBO with carcinoid?** | Classically = severe mesenteric fibrosis |
| **What are the pellagra-like symptoms?** | Remember the "3-Ds":<br>**D**ermatitis<br>**D**iarrhea<br>**D**ementia |

**What causes pellagra in carcinoid patients?**

Decreased **niacin** production

**What is carcinoid syndrome?**

Syndrome of symptoms caused by release of substances from a carcinoid tumor

**What are the symptoms of carcinoid syndrome?**

Remember the acronym "B FDR":
**B**ronchospasm

**F**lushing (skin)
**D**iarrhea
**R**ight-sided heart failure (from valve failure)

**What is a complete memory aid for carcinoid?**

Think: **B FDR** = **CAR**cinoid, or "**Be FDR** in a cool **CAR**." (COOL = **KUL**chitsky cells)

**Why does right-sided heart failure develop but not left-sided heart failure?**

The lungs act as a filter (just like the liver); thus, the left heart doesn't see all the vasoactive compounds.

**What is the incidence of carcinoid SYNDROME in patients who have a carcinoid TUMOR?**

Approximately 10%

**What released substances cause carcinoid syndrome?**

**Serotonin** and vasoactive peptides

**What is medical treatment for carcinoid syndrome?**

Octreotide IV

**What is the medical treatment of diarrhea alone?**

Odansetron (Zofran®)—serotonin **antagonist**

**How does the liver prevent carcinoid syndrome?**

By degradation of serotonin and the other vasoactive peptides when the **tumor drains into the portal vein**

**Why does carcinoid syndrome occur in some tumors and not in others?**

It occurs when **venous drainage from the tumor gains access to the systemic circulation** by avoiding hepatic degradation of the vasoactive substances.

**What tumors can produce carcinoid syndrome?**

**Liver metastases**
Retroperitoneal disease draining into paravertebral veins
Primary tumor outside the GI tract, portal venous drainage (e.g., ovary, **testicular,** bronchus), or both

**To what does the liver break down the serotonin?**

5-hydroxyindoleacetic acid (**5-HIAA**)

**What percentage of patients with a carcinoid have an elevated urine 5-HIAA level?**

50%

**What are the associated diagnostic lab findings?**

**Elevated urine 5-HIAA,** as well as elevated urine and blood **serotonin** levels

**How do you remember 5-HIAA for carcinoid?**

Think of a **5-HIGH CAR** pile up = **5-HI**AA **CAR**cinoid

**What stimulation test can often elevate serotonin levels and cause symptoms of carcinoid syndrome?**

Pentagastrin stimulation

**What are the special radiologic (scintigraphy) localization tests?**

$^{131}$I-MIBG (131 metaiodobenzylguanidine)
$^{111}$In-octreotide
PET scan utilizing $^{11}$C-labeled HTP

**How do you localize a GI carcinoid?**

Barium enema, upper GI series with small bowel follow-through, colonoscopy, abdominal CT, enteroscopy, enteroclysis, EGD

**What is the surgical treatment?**

Excision of the primary tumor and single or feasible metastasis in the liver (liver transplant is an option with unresectable liver metastasis); chemotherapy for advanced disease

**What is the medical treatment?**

Medical therapy for palliation of the carcinoid syndrome (serotonin antagonists, somatostatin analogue [**octreotide**])

**How effective is octreotide?**

It relieves diarrhea and flushing in more than 85% of cases and may shrink tumor in 10% to 20% of cases.

**What is a common antiserotonin drug?**

**Cyproheptadine**

**What is the overall prognosis?**

Two-thirds of patients are alive at 5 years.

**What is the prognosis of patients with liver metastasis or carcinoid syndrome?**

50% are alive at 3 years.

**What does carcinoid tumor look like?**

Usually intramural bowel mass; appears as **yellowish** tumor upon incision

**For appendiceal carcinoid, when is a right hemicolectomy indicated versus an appendectomy?**

If the tumor is **more than 1.5 cm,** right **hemicolectomy** is indicated; if there are no signs of serosal or cecal involvement and tumor is less than **1.5 cm, appendectomy** should be performed.

**Which primary site has the highest rate of metastasis?**

Ileal primary tumor

**Can a carcinoid tumor be confirmed malignant by looking at the histology?**

No, metastasis must be present to diagnose malignancy.

**What is the correlation between tumor size and malignancy potential?**

The vast majority of tumors less than 2 cm are benign. In tumors more than 2 cm, malignancy potential is significant.

**What treatments might you use for the patient with unresectable liver metastasis that is refractory to medical treatment?**

Chemoembolization or radiofrequency ablation

**What are the overall survival rates for carcinoid tumors at 5 years? 10 years?**

5 years = 70%; 10 years = 50%

**What are the side effects of colorectal carcinoid?**

The most common side effect is rectal bleeding +/− vague abdominal pain/discomfort.

---

# Chapter 47     Fistulas

**What is a fistula?**

An abnormal **communication** between two hollow organs or a hollow organ and the skin (i.e., two epithelial cell layers)

**What are the predisposing factors and conditions that maintain patency of a fistula?**

The acronym "HIS FRIEND":
**H**igh output fistula (> 500 cc/day)
**I**ntestinal destruction (> 50% of circumference)
**S**hort segment fistula < 2.5 cm

**F**oreign body (e.g., G-tube)
**R**adiation
**I**nfection
**E**pithelization (e.g., colostomy)
**N**eoplasm
**D**istal obstruction

## SPECIFIC TYPES OF FISTULAS

### ENTEROCUTANEOUS

| | |
|---|---|
| **What is it?** | A fistula from GI tract to skin (entero—cutaneous = **bowel to skin**) |
| **What are the causes?** | Anastomotic leak, trauma/injury to the bowel/colon, Crohn's disease, abscess, diverticulitis, inflammation/infection, inadvertent suture through bowel |
| **What is the work up?** | 1. CT to rule out abscess/inflammatory process<br>2. Fistulagram |
| **What are the possible complications?** | High-output fistulas, malnutrition, skin breakdown |
| **What is the treatment?** | NPO; TPN; drain abscesses, rule out and correct underlying causes; may feed distally (or if fistula is distal, feed elemental diet proximally); half will close spontaneously, but the other half require operation and resection of the involved bowel segment |
| **Which enterocutaneous fistula closes faster: short or long?** | A long fistula (may be counterintuitive—but true) |

### COLONIC FISTULAS

| | |
|---|---|
| **What are they?** | Include colovesical, colocutaneous, colovaginal, and coloenteric fistulas |
| **What are the most common causes?** | **Diverticulitis** (most common cause), cancer, IBD, foreign body, and irradiation |
| **What is the most common type?** | **Colovesical fistula,** which often presents with recurrent urinary tract infections; other signs include pneumaturia, dysuria, and fecaluria |
| **How is the diagnosis made?** | Via BE and cystoscopy |

| | |
|---|---|
| **What is the treatment?** | Surgery: segmental colon resection and primary anastomosis; repair/resection of the involved organ |
| **What is a cholecystenteric fistula?** | Connection between gallbladder and duodenum or other loop of small bowel due to large gallstone erosion, often resulting in SBO as the gallstone lodges in the ileocecal valve (gallstone ileus) |
| **What are the common causes of a gastrocolic fistula?** | Penetrating ulcers, **gastric** or **colonic cancer,** and Crohn's disease |
| **What are the possible complications of gastrocolic fistula?** | Malnutrition and severe **enteritis** due to reflux of colonic contents into the stomach and small bowel with subsequent bacterial overgrowth |

## PANCREATIC ENTERIC FISTULA

| | |
|---|---|
| **What is it?** | Decompression of a **pseudocyst** or **abscess** into an adjacent organ (a **rare** complication); usually done surgically or endoscopically to treat a pancreatic pseudocyst |

## EXTERNAL PANCREATIC FISTULA

| | |
|---|---|
| **What is it?** | Pancreaticocutaneous fistula; drainage of pancreatic exocrine secretions through to abdominal skin (usually through drain tract/wound) |
| **What is the treatment?** | NPO, TPN, skin protection, **octreotide** |
| **What is a "refractory" pancreatic fistula?** | Pancreaticocutaneous fistula that does not resolve with conservative medical management (the minority of cases) |
| **What is the diagnostic test for "refractory" pancreatic fistulas?** | ERCP to define site of fistula tract (i.e., tail versus head of pancreas) |
| **How is refractory tail of a pancreas fistula treated?** | Resection of the tail of the pancreas and the fistula |
| **How is refractory head of a pancreas fistula treated?** | Pancreaticojejunostomy |

BLADDER FISTULAS

**What are the specific types?**
**Vesicoenteric** (50% due to sigmoid diverticulitis); signs include pneumaturia, fecaluria
**Vesicovaginal** (most are secondary to gynecologic procedures); signs include urinary leak through vagina

# Chapter 48        Colon and Rectum

## ANATOMY

**Identify the arterial blood supply to the colon:**

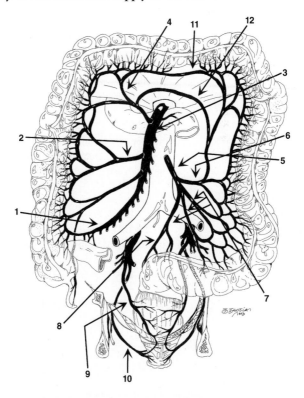

1. Ileocolic artery
2. Right colic artery
3. Superior mesenteric artery (SMA)
4. Middle colic artery
5. Inferior mesenteric artery (IMA)
6. Left colic artery
7. Sigmoidal artery
8. Superior hemorrhoidal artery (superior rectal)
9. Middle hemorrhoidal artery
10. Inferior hemorrhoidal artery
11. Marginal artery of Drummond
12. Meandering artery of Gonzalez

**What are the white lines of Toldt?**

The lateral peritoneal reflections of the ascending and descending colon

**What part of the GI tract does not have a serosa?**

Esophagus, middle and distal **rectum**

**What are the major anatomic differences between the colon and the small bowel?**

The colon has taenia coli, haustra, and appendices epiploicae (fat appendages), whereas the small intestine is smooth.

**What is the blood supply to the rectum:**
    **Proximal?**

Superior hemorrhoidal (or superior rectal) from the IMA

    **Middle?**

Middle hemorrhoidal (or middle rectal) from the hypogastric (internal iliac)

    **Distal?**

Inferior hemorrhoidal (or inferior rectal) from the pudendal artery (a branch of the hypogastric artery)

**What is the venous drainage of the rectum:**
    **Proximal?**

Via the IMV to the splenic vein, then **to the portal vein**

    **Middle?**

Via the iliac vein to the **IVC**

    **Distal?**

Via the iliac vein to the **IVC**

## COLORECTAL CARCINOMA

| | |
|---|---|
| **What is it?** | Adenocarcinoma of the colon or rectum |
| **What is the incidence?** | Most common GI cancer<br>Second most common cancer in the United States<br>Incidence increases with age starting at 40 and peaks at 70 to 80 years. |
| **How common is it as a cause of cancer deaths?** | Second most common cause of cancer deaths |
| **What is the lifetime risk of colorectal cancer?** | 6% |
| **What is the male to female ratio?** | Approximately 1:1 |
| **What are the risk factors?** | **Dietary:** Low-fiber, high-fat diets correlate with increased rates.<br>**Genetic:** Family history is important when taking history.<br>FAP, Lynch's syndrome<br>**IBD:** Ulcerative colitis > Crohn's disease, age, previous colon cancer |
| **What is Lynch's syndrome?** | **HNPCC** = **H**ereditary **N**on**P**olyposis **C**olon **C**ancer—autosomal-dominant inheritance of high risk for development of colon cancer |
| **What are current ACS recommendations for colorectal screening without family (first-degree) history of colorectal cancer?** | Annual digital rectal exam starting at age 40 (remember that approximately 10% of tumors are palpable by rectal exam!)<br>Annual test for fecal occult blood starting at age 40<br>Colonoscopy at age 50 |
| **What are the current recommendations for colorectal cancer screening if there is a history of colorectal cancer in a first-degree relative?** | Patients with a family history of colorectal cancer need a more aggressive approach: colonoscopy or air contrast barium enema (ACBE) at age 40. |

**What percentage of adults will have a guaiac-positive stool test?**

Approximately 2%

**What percentage of patients with a guaiac-positive stool test will have colon cancer?**

Approximately 10%

**What signs/symptoms are associated with the following conditions:**

**Right-sided lesions?**

Right side of bowel has a large luminal diameter, so a tumor may attain a large size before causing problems.
Microcytic anemia, occult/melena > hematochezia PR, postprandial discomfort, fatigue

**Left-sided lesions?**

Left side of bowel has smaller lumen and semisolid contents.
Change in bowel habits (small-caliber stools), colicky pain, signs of obstruction, abdominal mass, heme(+) or gross red blood
Nausea, vomiting, constipation

**From which site is melena more common?**

Right-sided colon cancer

**From which site is hematochezia more common?**

Left-sided colon cancer

**What is the incidence of rectal cancer?**

Comprises 20% to 30% of all colorectal cancer

**What are the signs/ symptoms of rectal cancer?**

Most common symptom is hematochezia (passage of red blood ± stool) or mucus; also tenesmus, feeling of incomplete evacuation of stool (because of the mass), and rectal mass.

**What is the differential diagnosis of a colon tumor/ mass?**

Adenocarcinoma, carcinoid tumor, lipoma, liposarcoma, leiomyoma, leiomyosarcoma, lymphoma, diverticular disease, ulcerative colitis, Crohn's disease, polyps

**Which diagnostic tests are helpful?**

History and physical exam (**Note: approximately 10% of cancers are palpable on rectal exam**), heme occult, CBC, barium enema, colonoscopy

**What disease does microcytic anemia signify until proven otherwise in a man or postmenopausal woman?**

Colon cancer

**What tests help find metastases?**

CXR (lung metastases), LFTs (liver metastases), abdominal CT (liver metastases), other tests based on history and physical exam (e.g., head CT for left arm weakness looking for brain metastasis)

**What is the preoperative workup for colorectal cancer?**

History, physical exam, LFTs, CEA, CBC, Chem 10, PT/PTT, type and cross 2 u PRBCs, CXR, U/A, abdominopelvic CT

**What are the means by which the cancer spreads?**

Direct extension: circumferentially and then through bowel wall to later invade other abdominoperineal organs
Hematogenous: portal circulation to liver; lumbar/vertebral veins to lungs
Lymphogenous: regional lymph nodes
Transperitoneal
Intraluminal

**Is CEA useful?**

Not for screening but for baseline and recurrence surveillance (but offers no proven survival benefit)

**What unique diagnostic test is helpful in patients with rectal cancer?**

Endorectal ultrasound (probe is placed transanally and depth of invasion and nodes are evaluated)

**How are tumors staged?**

Astler-Coller modified Dukes, and the TMN staging system

**The Dukes stages were first described for what disease?**

Rectal cancer (not colon cancer!) in 1932

**Give the Astler-Coller
modified Dukes stages:**

    **A**                              Invasion up to submucosa

    **B1**                            Invasion up to muscularis propria

    **B2**                            Invasion through wall

    **C**                              Positive nodal metastasis

    **D**                              Distant metastasis (**D** = **D**istant)

**Give the TNM stages:**

    **Stage I**                     Invades submucosa or muscularis propria (T1–2 N0 M0)

    **Stage II**                   Invades through muscularis propria or surrounding structures but with negative nodes (T3–4, N0, M0)

    **Stage III**                 **Positive nodes,** no distant metastasis (any T, N1–3, M0)

    **Stage IV**                 Positive **distant metastasis** (any T, any N, M1)

**What is the approximate
5-year survival by stage:**

    **Stage I?**                    **90%**

    **Stage II?**                  **75%**

    **Stage III?**                **50%**

    **Stage IV?**                **5%**

**What percentage of patients
with colorectal cancer are
unresectable on diagnosis?**    Approximately 10%

**What percentage of patients
with colorectal cancer
have liver metastases on
diagnosis?**    Approximately 20%

**Define the preoperative "bowel prep."**

Preoperative preparation for colon/rectal resection:
1. Golytely colonic lavage or Fleets Phospho-Soda until clear effluent per rectum
2. PO antibiotics (1 gm neomycin and 1 gm erythromycin × 3 doses)

Patient should also receive preoperative and 24-hr IV antibiotics.

**What are the common preoperative IV antibiotics?**

Cefoxitin, cefotetan, Unasyn®

**If the patient is allergic (hives, swelling), what antibiotics should be prescribed?**

IV Cipro® and Flagyl®

**What are the treatment options?**

Resection: wide surgical resection of lesion and its regional lymphatic drainage

**What decides low anterior resection (LAR) versus abdominal perineal resection (APR)?**

Distance from the anal verge, pelvis size

**What do all rectal cancer operations include?**

Total mesorectal excision—remove the rectal mesentery, including the lymph nodes

**What is the lowest LAR possible?**

Coloanal anastomosis (anastomosis normal colon directly to anus)

**What do some surgeons do with any anastomosis less than 5 cm from the anus?**

Temporary ileostomy to "protect" the anastomosis

**What surgical margins are needed for colon cancer?**

Traditionally more than 5 cm; margins must be at least 2 cm

**What is the minimal surgical margin for rectal cancer?**

2 cm

**How many lymph nodes should be resected with a colon cancer mass?**

This is controversial; some now say 17! There is increased diagnostic potential and improved prognosis with more resected nodes.

**What is the adjuvant treatment of Dukes' C colon cancer (stage III)?**

5-FU and leucovorin (or levamisole) chemotherapy (if there is nodal metastasis postoperatively)

**What is the adjuvant treatment for T3–T4 rectal cancer?**

**Preoperative radiation therapy** and 5-FU chemotherapy as a "radiosensitizer"

**What is the most common site of distant (hematogenous) metastasis from colorectal cancer?**

Liver

**What is the treatment of liver metastases from colorectal cancer?**

Resect with ≥1-cm margins and administer chemotherapy if feasible.

**What is the surveillance regimen?**

Physical exam, stool guaiac, CBC, CEA, LFTs (every 3 months for 3 years, then every 6 months for 2 years), CXR every 6 months for 2 years and then yearly, colonoscopy at years 1 and 3 postoperatively, CT scans directed by screening

**Why is follow-up so important the first 3 postoperative years?**

Approximately 90% of colorectal recurrences are within 3 years of surgery.

**What are the most common causes of colonic obstruction in the adult population?**

Colon cancer, diverticular disease, colonic volvulus

**What is the 5-year survival rate after liver resection with clean margins for colon cancer liver metastasis?**

Approximately 33% (28% to 50%)

**What is the 5-year survival rate after diagnosis of unresectable colon cancer liver metastasis?**

0%

# POLYPS

## POLYPS OF THE COLON AND RECTUM

**What are they?**

Tissue growth into bowel lumen, usually consisting of mucosa, submucosa, or both

**How are they anatomically classified?**

*Sessile* (flat)
*Pedunculated* (on a stalk)

**What are the histologic classifications of the following types:**

**Inflammatory (pseudopolyp)?**

As in Crohn's disease or ulcerative colitis

**Hamartomatous?**

Normal tissue in abnormal configuration

**Hyperplastic?**

Benign—normal cells—no malignant potential

**Neoplastic?**

Proliferation of undifferentiated cells; premalignant or malignant cells

**What are the subtypes of neoplastic polyps?**

Tubular adenomas (usually pedunculated)
Tubulovillous adenomas
Villous adenomas (usually sessile and look like broccoli heads)

**What determines malignant potential of an adenomatous polyp?**

Size
Histologic type
Atypia of cells

**What is the most common type of adenomatous polyp?**

Tubular 85%

**What is the correlation between size and malignancy?**

Polyps larger than 2 cm have a high risk of carcinoma (33%–55%).

**What about histology and cancer potential of an adenomatous polyp?**

Villous > tubovillous > tubular (think: **VILL**ous = **VILL**ain).

**What is the approximate percentage of carcinomas found in the following polyps overall:**

| | |
|---|---|
| **Tubular adenoma?** | 5% |
| **Tubulovillous adenoma?** | 20% |
| **Villous adenoma?** | 40% |

**Where are most polyps found?**  Rectosigmoid (30%)

**What are signs/symptoms?**  Bleeding (red or dark blood), change in bowel habits, mucus per rectum, electrolyte loss, totally asymptomatic

**What are the diagnostic tests?**  Best = colonoscopy
Less sensitive for small polyps = barium enema and sigmoidoscopy

**What is the treatment?**  Endoscopic resection (snared) if polyps; large sessile villous adenomas should be removed with bowel resection and lymph node resection

## POLYPOSIS SYNDROMES

### FAMILIAL POLYPOSIS

**What is another name for this condition?**  Familial adenomatous polyposis (FAP)

**What are the characteristics?**  Hundreds of adenomatous polyps within the rectum and colon that begin developing at puberty; all undiagnosed; untreated patients develop cancer by ages 40 to 50

**What is the inheritance pattern?**  Autosomal dominant (i.e., 50% of offspring)

**What is the genetic defect?**  APC (adenomatous polyposis coli) gene

**What is the treatment?**  Total proctocolectomy and ileostomy
Total colectomy and rectal mucosal removal (mucosal proctectomy) and ileoanal anastomosis

## GARDNER'S SYNDROME

| | |
|---|---|
| **What are the characteristics?** | Neoplastic polyps of the **small bowel** and **colon;** cancer by age 40 in 100% of undiagnosed patients, as in FAP |
| **What are the other associated findings?** | **Desmoid** tumors (in abdominal wall or cavity), **osteomas** of skull (seen on x-ray), **sebaceous** cysts, adrenal and thyroid tumors, retroperitoneal fibrosis, duodenal and periampullary tumors |
| **How can the findings associated with Gardner's syndrome be remembered?** | Think of a gardener planting "SOD": **S**ebaceous cysts **O**steomas **D**esmoid tumors |
| **What is a desmoid tumor?** | Tumor of the musculoaponeurotic sheath, usually of the abdominal wall; benign, but grows locally; treated by wide resection |
| **What medications may slow the growth of a desmoid tumor?** | Tamoxifen, sulindac, steroids |
| **What is the inheritance pattern?** | Varying degree of penetrance from an autosomal-dominant gene |
| **What is the treatment of colon polyps in patients with Gardner's syndrome?** | Total proctocolectomy and ileostomy Total colectomy and rectal mucosal removal (mucosal proctectomy) and ileoanal anastomosis |

## PEUTZ-JEGHERS' SYNDROME

| | |
|---|---|
| **What are the characteristics?** | Hamartomas throughout the GI tract (jejunum/ileum > colon > stomach) |
| **What is the associated cancer risk from polyps?** | Increased |
| **What is the associated cancer risk for women with Peutz-Jeghers?** | Ovarian cancer (granulosa cell tumor is most common) |
| **What is the inheritance pattern?** | Autosomal dominant |

**What are the other signs?**

Melanotic pigmentation (black/brown) of buccal mucosa (mouth), lips, digits, palms, feet (soles)
(Think: **P**eutz = **P**igmented)

**What is the treatment?**

Removal of polyps, if symptomatic (i.e., bleeding, intussusception, or obstruction) or large (> 1.5 cm)

**What are juvenile polyps?**

Benign hamartomas in the small bowel and colon; not premalignant; also known as "retention polyps"

**What is Cronkhite-Canada syndrome?**

Diffuse GI hamartoma polyps (i.e., no cancer potential) associated with malabsorption/weight loss, diarrhea, and **loss of electrolytes/protein;** signs include alopecia, nail atrophy, skin pigmentation

**What is Turcot's syndrome?**

Colon polyps with malignant **CNS tumors** (glioblastoma multiforme)

## DIVERTICULAR DISEASE OF THE COLON

### DIVERTICULOSIS

**What is diverticulosis?**

A condition in which diverticula can be found within the colon, especially the sigmoid; diverticula are actually **false diverticula** in that only mucosa and submucosa herniate through the bowel musculature; true diverticula involve all layers of the bowel wall and are rare in the colon

Diverticula

Blood vessel

**Describe the pathophysiology**

**Weakness** in the bowel wall develops at points where nutrient **blood vessels** enter between antimesenteric and mesenteric taenia; increased intraluminal pressures then cause herniation through these areas.

**What is the incidence?**

Approximately 50% to 60% in the United States by age 60, with only 10% to 20% becoming symptomatic

**What is the most common site?**

95% of people with diverticulosis have **sigmoid** colon involvement.

**Who is at risk?**

People with **low-fiber diets,** chronic constipation, and a positive family history; incidence increases with age

**What are the symptoms/ complications?**

**Bleeding:** may be massive Diverticulitis, asymptomatic (80% of cases)

**What is the diagnostic approach:**
   **Bleeding?**

Without signs of inflammation: colonoscopy

   **Pain and signs of inflammation?**

Abdominal/pelvic CT

**What is the treatment of diverticulosis?**

High-fiber diet is recommended.

**What are the indications for operation with diverticulosis?**

Complications of diverticulitis (e.g., fistula, obstruction, stricture); recurrent episodes; hemorrhage; suspected carcinoma; prolonged symptoms; abscess not drainable by percutaneous approach

**When is it safe to get a colonoscopy or barium enema/sigmoidoscopy?**

Due to risk of perforation, this is performed 6 weeks after inflammation resolves to rule out colon cancer.

## DIVERTICULITIS

| | |
|---|---|
| **What is it?** | Infection or perforation of a diverticulum |
| **What is the pathophysiology?** | **Obstruction** of diverticulum by a fecalith leading to inflammation and microperforation |
| **What are the signs/ symptoms?** | LLQ pain (cramping or steady), change in bowel habits **(diarrhea),** fever, chills, anorexia, LLQ mass, nausea/vomiting, dysuria |
| **What are the associated lab findings?** | Increased WBCs |
| **What are the associated radiographic findings?** | On x-ray: ileus, partially obstructed colon, air-fluid levels, free air if perforated<br>On abdominal/pelvic CT: swollen, edematous bowel wall; particularly helpful in diagnosing an abscess |
| **What are the associated barium enema findings?** | Barium enema should be avoided in acute cases. |
| **Is colonoscopy safe in an acute setting?** | No, there is increased risk of perforation |
| **What are the possible complications?** | Abscess, diffuse peritonitis, fistula, obstruction, perforation, stricture |
| **What is the most common fistula with diverticulitis?** | Colovesical fistula (to bladder) |
| **What is the best test for diverticulitis?** | CT scan |
| **What is the initial therapy?** | IV fluids, NPO, broad-spectrum antibiotics with anaerobic coverage, NG suction (as needed for emesis/ileus) |
| **When is surgery warranted?** | Obstruction, fistula, free perforation, abscess not amenable to percutaneous drainage, sepsis, deterioration with conservative Rx |

**What is the lifelong risk of recurrence after:**

    **First episode?**                      33%

    **Second episode?**              50%

**What are the indications for elective resection?**

Two episodes of diverticulitis. Should be considered after the **first** episode in a young, diabetic, or immunosuppressed patient

**What surgery is usually performed ELECTIVELY for recurrent bouts?**

A one-stage operation: resection of involved segment and primary anastomosis (with preoperative bowel prep)

**What type of surgery is usually performed for an acute case of diverticulitis with a complication (e.g., perforation, obstruction)?**

**Hartmann's procedure:** resection of involved segment with an end colostomy and stapled rectal stump (will need subsequent reanastomosis of colon usually after 2–3 postoperative months)

**What is the treatment of diverticular abscess?**

Percutaneous drainage; if abscess is not amenable to percutaneous drainage, then surgical approach for drainage is necessary.

**How common is massive lower GI bleeding with diverticulitis?**

Very **rare**! Massive lower GI bleeding is seen with divericu**losis,** not diverticulitis.

**What are the most common causes of massive lower GI bleeding in adults?**

Diverticulosis (especially right-sided), vascular ectasia

**What must you rule out in any patient with diverticulitis/diverticulosis?**

Colon cancer

## COLONIC VOLVULUS

**What is it?**

**Twisting of colon on itself** about its mesentery, resulting in obstruction and, if complete, vascular compromise with potential necrosis, perforation, or both

**What is the most common type of colonic volvulus?**

Sigmoid volvulus (makes sense because the sigmoid is a redundant/"floppy" structure!)

## SIGMOID VOLVULUS

**What is it?**                    Volvulus or "twist" in the sigmoid colon

**What is the incidence?**         Approximately 75% of colonic volvulus
                                   cases (think: **S**igmoid = **S**uperior)

**What are the etiologic
factors?**                         High-residue diet resulting in bulky stools
                                   and tortuous, elongated colon; chronic
                                   constipation; laxative abuse; pregnancy;
                                   seen most commonly in bedridden elderly
                                   or institutionalized patients, many of
                                   whom have history of prior abdominal
                                   surgery or distal colonic obstruction

**What are the signs/
symptoms?**                        Acute abdominal pain, progressive
                                   abdominal distention, anorexia,
                                   obstipation, cramps, nausea/vomiting

**What findings are evident
on abdominal plain film?**         Distended loop of sigmoid colon, often in
                                   the classic "bent inner tube" or "omega"
                                   sign with the loop aiming toward the RUQ

**What are the signs of necrotic
bowel in colonic volvulus?**       Free air, pneumatosis (air in bowel wall)

**How is the diagnosis made?**     Sigmoidoscopy or radiographic exam with
                                   gastrografin enema

**Under what conditions is gastrografin enema useful?**

If sigmoidoscopy and plain films fail to confirm the diagnosis; **"bird's beak"** is pathognomonic seen on enema contrast study as the contrast comes to a sharp end

**What are the signs of strangulation?**

Discolored or hemorrhagic mucosa on sigmoidoscopy, bloody fluid in the rectum, frank ulceration or necrosis at the point of the twist, peritoneal signs, fever, hypotension, ↑ WBCs

**What is the initial treatment?**

**Nonoperative:** If there is no strangulation, sigmoidoscopic reduction is successful in approximately 85% of cases; enema study will occasionally reduce (5%).

**What is the percentage of recurrence after nonoperative reduction of a sigmoid volvulus?**

Approximately 50%!

**What are the indications for surgery?**

Emergently if strangulation is suspected or nonoperative reduction unsuccessful (Hartmann's procedure); most patients should undergo resection during same hospitalization of redundant sigmoid after successful nonoperative reduction because of high recurrence rate (50%)

## CECAL VOLVULUS

**What is it?**

Twisting of the cecum upon itself and the mesentery

**What is a cecal "bascule" volvulus?**

Instead of the more common axial twist, the cecum folds upward (lies on the ascending colon).

**What is the incidence?**

Approximately 25% of colonic volvulus (i.e., much less common than sigmoid volvulus)

**What is the etiology?**

Idiopathic, poor fixation of the right colon, many patients have history of abdominal surgery

| | |
|---|---|
| **What are the signs/ symptoms?** | Acute onset of abdominal or colicky pain beginning in the RLQ and progressing to a constant pain, vomiting, obstipation, abdominal distention, and SBO; many patients will have had previous similar episodes |
| **How is the diagnosis made?** | Abdominal plain film; dilated, ovoid colon with large air/fluid level in the RLQ often forming the classic **"coffee bean"** sign with the apex aiming toward the epigastrium or LUQ (must rule out gastric dilation with NG aspiration) |
| **What diagnostic studies should be performed?** | Water-soluble contrast study (gastrografin), if diagnosis cannot be made by AXR |
| **What is the treatment?** | Emergent surgery, right colectomy with primary anastomosis or ileostomy and mucus fistula (primary anastomosis may be performed in stable patients), cecopexy is an option under optimal conditions. |
| **What are the major differences in the EMERGENT management of cecal volvulus versus sigmoid?** | Patients with cecal volvulus require **surgical** reduction, whereas the vast majority of patients with sigmoid volvulus undergo initial **endoscopic** reduction of the twist. |

# Chapter 49    **The Anus**

## ANATOMY

**Identify the following:**

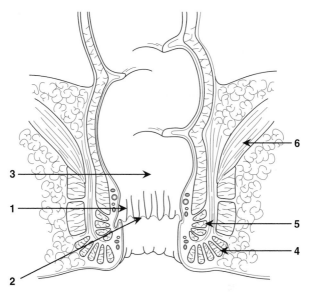

1. Anal columns
2. Dentate line
3. Rectum
4. External sphincter
5. Internal sphincter
6. Levator ani muscle

## ANAL CANCER

**What is the most common carcinoma of the anus?**

Squamous cell carcinoma (80%)
(think: **ASS** = **A**nal **S**quamous **S**uperior)

**What cell types are found in carcinomas of the anus?**

1. Squamous cell carcinoma (80%)
2. Cloacogenic (transitional cell)
3. Adenocarcinoma/melanoma/ mucoepidermal

**What is the incidence of anal carcinoma?**

Rare (1% of colon cancers incidence)

**What is anal Bowen's disease?**

Squamous cell carcinoma in situ (think: **B.S.** = **B**owen **S**quamous)

**How is Bowen's disease treated?**

With local wide excision

**What is Paget's disease of the anus?**

Adenocarcinoma in situ of the anus (think: **P.A.** = **P**aget's **A**denocarcinoma)

**How is Paget's disease treated?**

With local wide excision

**What are the risk factors for anal cancer?**

Human papilloma virus, condyloma, herpes, HIV, chronic inflammation (fistulae/Crohn's disease) immunosuppression, homosexuality in males, cervical/vaginal cancer, STDs, smoking

**What is the most common symptom of anal carcinoma?**

Anal bleeding

**What are the other signs/symptoms of anal carcinoma?**

Pain, mass, mucus per rectum, pruritus

**What percentage of patients with anal cancer are asymptomatic?**

Approximately 25%

**To what locations do anal canal cancers metastasize?**

Lymph nodes, liver, bone, lung

**What is the lymphatic drainage below the dentate line?**

Below to inguinal lymph nodes (above to pelvic chains)

**Are most patients with anal cancer diagnosed early or late?**

Late (diagnosis is often missed)

**What is the workup of a patient with suspected anal carcinoma?**

History
Physical exam: digital rectal exam, proctoscopic exam, and colonoscopy
Biopsy of mass
Abdominal/pelvic CT scan, transanal U/S
CXR
LFTs

**Define:**

**Margin cancer**

Anal verge out 5 cm onto the perianal skin

**Canal cancer**

Proximal to anal verge up to the border of the internal sphincter

**How is an anal canal epidermal carcinoma treated?**

NIGRO protocol:
1. Chemotherapy (5-FU and Mitomycin C)
2. Radiation
3. Postradiation therapy scar biopsy (6–8 weeks post XRT)

**What percentage of patients have a "complete" response with the NIGRO protocol?**

90%

**What is the 5-year survival with the NIGRO protocol?**

85%

**What is the treatment for local recurrence of anal cancer after the NIGRO protocol?**

May repeat chemotherapy/XRT or salvage APR

**How is a small (<5 cm) anal margin cancer treated?**

Surgical excision with 1-cm margins

**How is a large (>5 cm) anal margin cancer treated?**

Chemoradiation

**What is the treatment of anal melanoma?**

Wide excision or APR (especially if tumor is large) +/− XRT postoperatively

| | |
|---|---|
| **What percentage of patients with anal melanoma have an amelanotic anal tumor?** | Approximately one-third, thus making diagnosis difficult without pathology |
| **What is the prognosis of anal melanoma?** | Less than 5% 5-year survival rate |

## FISTULA IN ANO

| | |
|---|---|
| **What is it?** | Anal fistula, from rectum to perianal skin |
| **What are the causes?** | Usually anal crypt/gland infection (usually perianal abscess) |
| **What are the signs/ symptoms?** | Perianal drainage, perirectal abscess, recurrent perirectal abscess, "diaper rash," itching |
| **What disease should be considered with fistula in ano?** | Crohn's disease |
| **How is the diagnosis made?** | Exam, proctoscope |
| **What is Goodsall's rule?** | Fistulas originating **anterior** to a transverse line through the anus will course **straight** ahead and exit anteriorly, whereas those exiting **posteriorly** have a **curved** tract. |

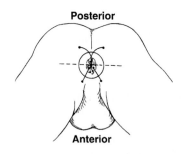

| | |
|---|---|
| **How can Goodsall's rule be remembered?** | Think of a dog with a **straight** nose (anterior) and **curved** tail (posterior) |

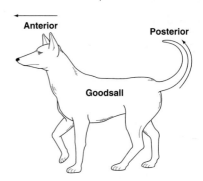

**What is the management of anorectal fistulas?**

1. Define the anatomy
2. Marsupialization of fistula tract (i.e., fillet tract open)
3. Wound care: routine Sitz baths and dressing changes
4. Seton placement if fistula is through the sphincter muscle

**What is a seton?**

A thick suture placed through fistula tract to allow slow transection of sphincter muscle; scar tissue formed will hold the sphincter muscle in place and allow for continence after transection

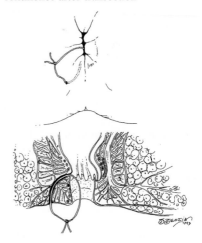

**What percentage of patients with a perirectal abscess develop a fistula in ano after drainage?**

Approximately 50%

| | |
|---|---|
| **How do you find the internal rectal opening of an anorectal fistula in the OR?** | Inject $H_2O_2$ (or methylene blue) in external opening—then look for bubbles (or blue dye) coming out of internal opening! |
| **What is a sitz bath?** | Sitting in a warm bath (usually done after bowel movement and TID) |

## PERIRECTAL ABSCESS

| | |
|---|---|
| **What is it?** | Abscess formation around the anus/rectum |
| **What are the signs/ symptoms?** | Rectal pain, drainage of pus, fever, perianal mass |
| **How is the diagnosis made?** | Physical/digital exam reveals perianal/ rectal submucosal mass/fluctuance |
| **What is the cause?** | Crypt abscess in dentate line with spread |
| **What is the treatment?** | As with all abscesses (except simple liver amebic abscess) **drainage,** Sitz bath, anal hygiene, stool softeners |
| **What is the indication for postoperative IV antibiotics for drainage?** | Cellulitis, immunosuppression, diabetes, heart valve abnormality |
| **What percentage of patients develop a fistula in ano during the 6 months after surgery?** | Approximately 50% |

## ANAL FISSURE

| | |
|---|---|
| **What is it?** | Tear or fissure in the anal epithelium |
| **What is the most common site?** | Posterior midline (comparatively low blood flow) |
| **What is the cause?** | Hard stool passage (constipation), hyperactive sphincter, disease process (e.g., Crohn's disease) |
| **What are the signs/ symptoms?** | Pain in the anus, painful (can be excruciating) bowel movement, rectal bleeding, blood on toilet tissue after bowel movement, sentinel tag, tear in the anal skin, extremely painful rectal exam, sentinel pile, hypertrophic papilla |

**What is a sentinel pile?**

Thickened mucosa/skin at the distal end of an anal fissure that is often confused with a small hemorrhoid

**What is the anal fissure triad for a chronic fissure?**

1. Fissure
2. Sentinel pile
3. Hypertrophied anal papilla

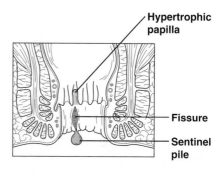

Hypertrophic papilla

Fissure

Sentinel pile

**What is the conservative treatment?**

Sitz baths, stool softeners, high fiber diet, excellent anal hygiene, topical nifedipine, Botox®

**What disease processes must be considered with a chronic anal fissure?**

Crohn's disease, anal cancer, sexually transmitted disease, ulcerative colitis, AIDS

**What are the indications for surgery?**

Chronic fissure refractory to conservative treatment

**What is one surgical option?**

Lateral internal sphincterotomy (LIS)—cut the internal sphincter to release it from spasm

**What is the "rule of 90%" for anal fissures?**

90% occur posteriorly.
90% heal with medical treatment alone.
90% of patients who undergo an LIS heal successfully.

## PERIANAL WARTS

**What are they?**

Warts around the anus/perineum

**What is the cause?**

Condyloma acuminatum (human papilloma virus)

| | |
|---|---|
| **What is the major risk?** | Squamous cell carcinoma |
| **What is the treatment if warts are small?** | Topical podophyllin, Aldara® |
| **What is the treatment if warts are large?** | Surgical resection or laser ablation |

## HEMORRHOIDS

| | |
|---|---|
| **What are they?** | Engorgement of the venous plexi of the rectum, anus, or both; with protrusion of the mucosa, anal margin, or both |
| **Why do we have "healthy" hemorrhoidal tissue?** | It is thought to be involved with fluid/air continence. |
| **What are the signs/ symptoms?** | Anal mass/prolapse, bleeding, itching, pain |
| **Which type, internal or external, is painful?** | External, below the dentate line |
| **If a patient has excruciating anal pain and history of hemorrhoids, what is the likely diagnosis?** | Thrombosed external hemorrhoid (treat by excision) |
| **What are the causes of hemorrhoids?** | Constipation/straining, portal hypertension, pregnancy |
| **What is an internal hemorrhoid?** | Hemorrhoid above the (proximal) dentate line |
| **What is an external hemorrhoid?** | Hemorrhoid below the dentate line |
| **What are the three "hemorrhoid quadrants"?** | 1. Left lateral 2. Right posterior 3. Right anterior |

### *Classification by Degrees*

| | |
|---|---|
| **Define the following terms for internal hemorrhoids:** | |
| **First-degree hemorrhoid** | Hemorrhoid that does not prolapse |

— **1st degree
hemorrhoid**

**Second-degree
hemorrhoid**

Prolapses with defecation, but returns on
its own

— **2nd degree
hemorrhoid**

**Third-degree hemorrhoid**

Prolapses with defecation or any type of
Valsalva maneuver and requires active
manual reduction (eat fiber!)

— **3rd degree
hemorrhoid**

| | |
|---|---|
| **Fourth-degree hemorrhoid** | Prolapsed hemorrhoid that cannot be reduced |
| **What is the treatment?** | High-fiber diet, anal hygiene, topical steroids, sitz baths<br>Rubber band ligation (in most cases anesthetic is not necessary for internal hemorrhoids)<br>Surgical resection for large refractory hemorrhoids |
| **What are the dreaded complications of hemorrhoidectomy?** | Exsanguination (bleeding may pool proximally in lumen of colon without any signs of external bleeding)<br>Pelvic infection (may be extensive and potentially fatal)<br>Incontinence (injury to sphincter complex)<br>Anal stricture |
| **What condition is a contraindication for hemorrhoidectomy?** | Crohn's disease |
| **Classically, what must be ruled out with lower GI bleeding believed to be caused by hemorrhoids?** | Colon cancer (colonoscopy or proctoscopy followed up with a barium enema) |

# Chapter 50    Lower GI Bleeding

| | |
|---|---|
| **What is the definition of lower GI bleeding?** | Bleeding distal to the ligament of Treitz; vast majority occurs in the colon |
| **What are the symptoms?** | **Hematochezia (bright red blood per rectum [BRBPR]),** with or without abdominal pain, melena, anorexia, fatigue, syncope, shortness of breath, shock |

**What are the signs?**

BRBPR, positive hemoccult, abdominal tenderness, hypovolemic shock, orthostasis

**What medicines should be looked for with a lower GI bleed?**

Coumadin®, aspirin, Plavix™

**What are the causes?**

Diverticulosis (usually **right**-sided in severe hemorrhage), vascular ectasia, colon cancer, hemorrhoids, trauma, hereditary hemorrhagic telangiectasia, intussusception, volvulus, ischemic colitis, IBD (especially ulcerative colitis), anticoagulation, rectal cancer, Meckel's diverticulum (with ectopic gastric mucosa), stercoral ulcer (ulcer from hard stool), infectious colitis, aortoenteric fistula, chemotherapy, irradiation injury, infarcted bowel, strangulated hernia, anal fissure

**What are the most common causes of massive lower GI bleeding?**

1. **Diverticulosis**
2. Vascular ectasia

**What lab tests should be performed?**

CBC, Chem-7, PT/PTT, type and cross

**What is the initial treatment?**

IVFs: lactated Ringer's; packed red blood cells as needed, IV × 2, Foley catheter to follow urine output, d/c aspirin, NGT

**What diagnostic tests should be performed for all lower GI bleeds?**

History, physical exam, NGT aspiration (to rule out UGI bleeding; bile or blood must be seen; otherwise, perform EGD), anoscopy/proctoscopic exam

**What must be ruled out in patients with lower GI bleeding?**

**Upper GI bleeding!** Remember, NGT aspiration is not 100% accurate (even if you get bile without blood).

**How can you have a UGI bleed with only clear succus back in the NGT?**

A duodenal bleeding ulcer can bleed distal to the pylorus with the NGT sucking normal nonbloody gastric secretions! **If there is any question, perform EGD.**

**What would an algorithm
for diagnosing and treating
lower GI bleeding look like?**

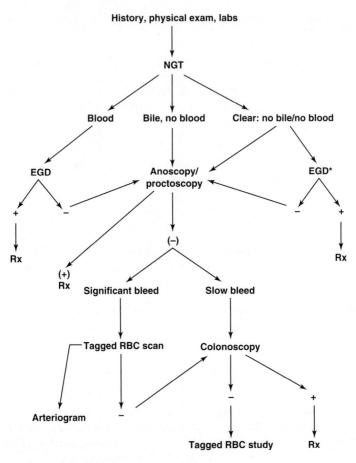

*Based on clinical suspicion

**What is the diagnostic test
of choice for localizing a
slow to moderate lower GI
bleeding source?**

Colonoscopy

**What test is performed to localize bleeding if there is too much active bleeding to see the source with a colonoscope?**

A-gram (mesenteric angiography)

**What is more sensitive for a slow, intermittent amount of blood loss: A-gram or tagged RBC study?**

Radiolabeled RBC scan is more sensitive for blood loss at a rate of ≥0.5 mL/min or intermittent blood loss because it has a longer half life (for arteriography, bleeding rate must be ≥1.0 mL/min).

**What is the colonoscopic treatment option for bleeding vascular ectasia or polyp?**

Laser or electrocoagulation; local epinephrine injection

**What is the treatment if bleeding site is KNOWN and massive or recurrent lower GI bleeding continues?**

Segmental resection of the bowel

**What is the surgical treatment of massive lower GI bleeding WITHOUT localization?**

Exploratory laparotomy with or without small intestine enteroscopy and total abdominal colectomy with primary anastomosis of ileum to rectum (ileorectostomy) as last resort

**What percentage of cases spontaneously stop bleeding?**

Between 80% and 90% stop bleeding with resuscitative measures only (at least temporarily).

**What percentage of patients require emergent surgery for lower GI bleeding?**

Only about 10%

**Does melena always signify active colonic bleeding?**

NO—the colon is very good at storing material and often will store melena/maroon stools and pass them days later (follow patient, UO, HCT, and vital signs).

**What is the therapeutic advantage of doing a colonoscopy?**

The options of injecting substance (epinephrine) or coagulating vessels is an option with C-scope to control bleeding.

| | |
|---|---|
| **What is the therapeutic advantage of doing an A-gram?** | Ability to inject vasopressin and/or embolization, with control of bleeding in >75% |

# Chapter 51

# Inflammatory Bowel Disease (IBD): Crohn's Disease and Ulcerative Colitis

| | |
|---|---|
| **What is IBD?** | **I**nflammatory **B**owel **D**isease, inflammatory disease of the GI tract |
| **What are the two inflammatory bowel diseases?** | Crohn's disease and ulcerative colitis |
| **What is another name for Crohn's disease?** | Regional enteritis |
| **What is ulcerative colitis often called?** | U.C. |
| **What is the cause of IBD?** | No one knows, but probably an autoimmune process with environmental factors contributing |
| **What is the differential diagnosis?** | Crohn's versus ulcerative colitis, infectious colitis (e.g., *C. difficile,* amebiasis, shigellosis), ischemic colitis, irritable bowel syndrome, diverticulitis, Zollinger-Ellison (Z-E) syndrome, colon cancer, carcinoid, ischemic bowel |
| **What are the extraintestinal manifestations seen in both types of IBD?** | Ankylosing spondylitis, aphthous (oral) ulcers, iritis, pyoderma gangrenosum, erythema nodosum, clubbing of fingers, |

sclerosing cholangitis, arthritis, kidney disease (nephrotic syndrome, amyloid deposits)

**How can these manifestations be remembered?**

Think of the acronym "A PIE SACK":
**A**phthous ulcers

**P**yoderma gangrenosum
**I**ritis
**E**rythema nodosum

**S**clerosing cholangitis
**A**rthritis, ankylosis spondylitis
**C**lubbing of fingers
**K**idney (amyloid deposits, nephrotic syndrome)

## COMPARISON OF CROHN'S DISEASE AND ULCERATIVE COLITIS

### INCIDENCE

**Crohn's disease:**
**Incidence**

$3-6/100,000$

**At-risk population**

High in the Jewish population, low in the African black population, similar rates between African-Americans and U.S. white population

**Sex?**

Female > male

**Distribution?**

Bimodal distribution (i.e., two peaks in incidence): peak incidence at 25 to 40 years of age; second bimodal distribution peak at 50 to 65 years of age

**Ulcerative colitis:**
**Incidence?**

$10/100,000$

**At-risk population**

High in the Jewish population, low in the African-American population
Positive family history in 20% of cases
Seen in families

**Sex?**                           Male > female

**Distribution?**                  Bimodal distribution at 20 to 35 and
                                   50 to 65 years of age

## INITIAL SYMPTOMS

**Crohn's disease?**               **Abdominal pain, diarrhea,** fever,
                                   weight loss, anal disease

**Ulcerative colitis?**            **Bloody diarrhea** (hallmark), fever,
                                   weight loss

## ANATOMIC DISTRIBUTION

**Crohn's disease?**               Classically said to involve **"mouth to
                                   anus"**
                                   Small bowel alone—20%
                                   Small bowel and colon—40%
                                   Colon alone—30%

**Ulcerative colitis?**            Colon alone (think: ulcerative **col**itis =
                                   **colon** alone)

## ROUTE OF SPREAD

**Crohn's disease?**               Small bowel, colon, or both **with "skip
                                   areas"** of normal bowel; hence, the
                                   name "regional enteritis"

**Ulcerative colitis?**            Almost always involves the rectum and
                                   spreads proximally always in a continuous
                                   route without "skip areas"

**What is "backwash" ileitis?**    Mild inflammation of the terminal
                                   ileum in ulcerative colitis; thought to be
                                   "backwash" of inflammatory mediators
                                   from the colon into the terminal ileum

## BOWEL WALL INVOLVEMENT

**Crohn's disease?**               Full thickness (transmural involvement)

**Ulcerative colitis?**            Mucosa/submucosa only

## ANAL INVOLVEMENT

| | |
|---|---|
| **Crohn's disease?** | Common (fistulae, abscesses, fissures, ulcers) |
| **Ulcerative colitis?** | Uncommon |

## RECTAL INVOLVEMENT

| | |
|---|---|
| **Crohn's disease?** | Rare |
| **Ulcerative colitis?** | 100% |

## MUCOSAL FINDINGS

| | |
|---|---|
| **Crohn's disease (6)?** | 1. Aphthoid ulcers<br>2. Granulomas<br>3. Linear ulcers<br>4. Transverse fissures<br>5. Swollen mucosa<br>6. **Full-thickness wall involvement** |
| **Ulcerative colitis (5)?** | 1. Granular, flat mucosa<br>2. Ulcers<br>3. **Crypt abscess**<br>4. Dilated mucosal vessels<br>5. **Pseudopolyps** |
| **How to remember ulcerative colitis and Crohn's anal and wall involvement?** | CAT URP:<br>**C**rohn's = **A**nal–**T**ransmural<br>**U.C.** = **R**ectum–**P**artial wall thickness |

## DIAGNOSTIC TESTS

| | |
|---|---|
| **Crohn's disease?** | Colonoscopy with biopsy, barium enema, UGI with small bowel follow-through, stool cultures |
| **Ulcerative colitis?** | Colonoscopy, barium enema, UGI with small bowel follow-through (to look for Crohn's disease), stool cultures |

## COMPLICATIONS

| | |
|---|---|
| **Crohn's disease?** | **Anal** fistula/abscess, **fistula,** stricture, perforation, **abscesses,** toxic megacolon, colovesical fistula, enterovaginal fistula, hemorrhage, **obstruction,** cancer |

| | |
|---|---|
| **Ulcerative colitis?** | **Cancer, toxic megacolon, colonic perforation, hemorrhage,** strictures, obstruction, complications of surgery |

## CANCER RISK

| | |
|---|---|
| **Crohn's disease?** | Overall increased risk, but about half that of ulcerative colitis |
| **Ulcerative colitis?** | Approximately 5% risk of developing colon cancer at 10 years; then, risk increases approximately 1% per year; thus, an incidence of about 20% after 20 years of the disease (30% at 30 years) |

## INCIDENCE OF TOXIC MEGACOLON

| | |
|---|---|
| **Crohn's disease?** | Approximately 5% |
| **Ulcerative colitis?** | Approximately 10% |

## INDICATIONS FOR SURGERY

| | |
|---|---|
| **Crohn's disease?** | Obstruction, massive bleeding, fistula, perforation, suspicion of cancer, abscess (refractory to medical treatment), toxic megacolon (refractory to medical treatment), strictures, dysplasia |
| **Ulcerative colitis?** | Toxic megacolon (refractory to medical treatment); cancer prophylaxis; massive bleeding; failure of child to mature because of disease and steroids; perforation; suspicion of or documented cancer; acute severe symptoms refractory to medical treatment; inability to wean off of chronic steroids; obstruction; dysplasia; stricture |
| **What are the common surgical options for ulcerative colitis?** | 1. Total proctocolectomy, distal rectal mucosectomy, and ileoanal pull through<br>2. Total proctocolectomy and Brooke ileostomy |

**What is "toxic megacolon"?**

**Toxic** patient: sepsis, febrile, abdominal pain

**Megacolon:** acutely and massively distended colon

**What are the medication options for treating IBD?**

**Sulfasalazine,** mesalamine (5-aminosalicylic acid)

**Steroids,** metronidazole (Flagyl®), azathioprine, 6-mercaptopurine (6-mp), infliximab

**What is infliximab?**

Antibody vs. TNF-α (tumor necrosis factor-alpha)

**What is the active metabolite of sulfasalazine?**

5'-aminosalicylate (5'-ASA), which is released in the colon

**What is the medical treatment of choice for perianal Crohn's disease?**

PO metronidazole (Flagyl®)

**What are the treatment options for long-term remission of IBD?**

6-mercaptopurine (6-mp), azathioprine, mesalamine

**What medication is used for IBD "flare-ups"?**

Steroids

**What is a unique medication route option for ulcerative colitis?**

Enemas (steroids, 5-ASA)

**Which disease has "cobblestoning" more often on endoscopic exam?**

Crohn's disease (think: **C**rohn's = **C**obblestoning)

**Which disease has pseudopolyps on colonoscopic exam?**

Ulcerative colitis; pseudopolyps are polyps of hypertrophied mucosa surrounded by mucosal atrophy

**Which disease has a "lead pipe" appearance on barium enema?**

Chronic ulcerative colitis

**Rectal bleeding/bloody diarrhea is a hallmark of which disease?**

Ulcerative colitis (rare in Crohn's disease)

**What is the most common indication for surgery in patients with Crohn's disease?**

Small bowel obstruction (SBO)

**What are the intraoperative findings of Crohn's disease?**

Mesenteric **"fat creeping"** onto the antimesenteric border of the small bowel
Shortened (and thick) mesentery
Thick bowel wall
Fistula(e)
Abscess(es)

**Why do you see fistulas and abscesses with Crohn's and not ulcerative colitis?**

Crohn's disease is **transmural.**

**What is the operation for short strictures of the small bowel in Crohn's disease?**

Stricturoplasty; basically a Heineke-Mikulicz pyloroplasty on the strictured segment (i.e., opened longitudinally and sewn closed in a transverse direction)

**Should the appendix be removed during a laparotomy for abdominal pain if Crohn's disease is discovered?**

Yes, if the cecum is not involved with active Crohn's disease

**What is pouchitis?**

Inflammation of the pouch of an ileoanal pull through; treat with metronidazole (Flagyl®)

**Do you need a frozen section for margins during a bowel resection for Crohn's disease?**

No, you need only grossly negative margins.

**What do you call it when the entire colon is involved?**

Pancolitis

# Chapter 52     **Liver**

## ANATOMY

**What is the name of the liver capsule?**

Glisson's capsule

**What is the "bare" area?**

The posterior section of the liver against the diaphragm that is "bare" without peritoneal covering

**What is Cantle's line?**

A line drawn between the gallbladder to just left of the inferior vena cava that transects the liver into the right and left lobes

**Which ligament goes from the anterior abdominal wall to the liver?**

Falciform ligament

**What does the falciform ligament contain?**

Ligamentum teres (obliterated umbilical vein)

**What is the coronary ligament?**

The peritoneal reflection on top of the liver that crowns (hence "coronary") the liver and attaches it to the diaphragm

**What are the triangular ligaments of the liver?**

The right and left lateral extents of the coronary ligament, which form triangles

**What is the origin of the hepatic arterial supply?**

From the proper hepatic artery off of the celiac trunk (celiac trunk to common hepatic artery to proper hepatic artery)

**Identify the arterial branches of the celiac trunk.**

1. Celiac trunk
2. Splenic artery
3. Left gastric artery
4. Common hepatic artery
5. Gastroduodenal artery
6. Proper hepatic artery
7. Left hepatic artery
8. Right hepatic artery

**What is the venous supply?**

**Portal vein** (formed from the splenic vein and the superior mesenteric vein)

**What is the hepatic venous drainage?**

Via the hepatic veins, which drain into the IVC (three veins: left, middle, and right)

**What sources provide oxygen to the liver?**

Portal vein blood—50%
Hepatic artery blood—50%

**From what sources does the liver receive blood?**

Portal system—75%
Hepatic artery system—25%

**What is the maximum amount of liver that can be resected while retaining adequate liver function?**

**More than 80%;** if given adequate recovery time, the original mass can be **regenerated.**

**What are the signs/ symptoms of liver disease?**

Hepatomegaly, splenomegaly, icterus, pruritus (from bile salts in skin), blanching spider telangiectasia, gynecomastia, testicular atrophy, caput medusae, dark urine, clay-colored stools, bradycardia, edema, ascites, fever, fetor hepaticus (sweet musty smell), hemorrhoids, variceal bleeding, anemia, body hair loss, liver tenderness, palmar erythema

**Which liver enzymes are made by hepatocytes?**

AST and ALT (aspartate aminotransferase and alanine aminotransferase)

**What is the source of alkaline phosphatase?**

Ductal epithelium (thus, elevated with ductal obstruction)

**What is Child's class?**

A classification system that estimates hepatic reserve in patients with hepatic failure

**What comprises the Child's classification?**

Laboratory: bilirubin, albumin
Clinical: encephalopathy, ascites, prothrombin time (PT)

**How can the criteria comprising the modified Child's classification be remembered?**

Remember the acronym: "A BEAP":
**A**scites

**B**ilirubin
**E**ncephalopathy
**A**lbumin
**P**T (prothrombin time)

**Define Child's classification:**

| | Bili | ALB | Enceph | Ascites | PT |
|---|---|---|---|---|---|
| **A** | <2 | >3.5 | none | none | <4° |
| **B** | 2–3 | 3–3.5 | minimal | easily controlled | 4–6 |
| **C** | | >3 | <3 | severe | poorly controlled | >6.0 |

(Think: as in a letter grading system, A is better than B, B is better than C)

° = over control (seconds)

**What is the operative mortality for a portocaval shunt in the following Child's classes:**

**A?**   Less than 5%

**B?**   Less than 15%

**C?**   Approximately 33%

## TUMORS OF THE LIVER

**What is the most common liver cancer?**
**Metastatic disease** outnumbers primary tumors 20:1. Primary site is usually the GI tract.

**What is the most common primary malignant liver tumor?**
Hepatocellular carcinoma (hepatoma)

**What is the most common primary benign liver tumor?**
Hemangioma

**What lab tests comprise the workup for liver metastasis?**
LFTs (AST and alkaline phosphatase are most useful), CEA for suspected primary colon cancer

**What are the associated imaging studies?**
CT, ultrasound, A-gram

**What is a right hepatic lobectomy?**
Removal of the right lobe of the liver (i.e., all tissue to the right of Cantle's line is removed)

| | |
|---|---|
| **What is a left hepatic lobectomy?** | Removal of the left lobe of the liver (i.e., removal of all the liver tissue to the left of Cantle's line) |
| **What is a right trisegmentectomy?** | Removal of all the liver tissue to the right of the falciform ligament |
| **What are the three common types of primary benign liver tumors?** | 1. Hemangioma<br>2. Hepatocellular adenoma<br>3. Focal nodular hyperplasia |
| **What are the four common types of primary malignant liver tumors?** | 1. Hepatocellular carcinoma (hepatoma)<br>2. Cholangiocarcinoma (when intrahepatic)<br>3. Angiosarcoma (associated with contrast exposure)<br>4. Hepatoblastoma (most common in infants and children) |
| **What chemical exposures are risk factors for angiosarcoma?** | **Vinyl chloride,** arsenic, thorotrast contrast |
| **What is a "hepatoma"?** | Hepatocellular carcinoma |
| **What are the other benign liver masses?** | Benign liver cyst, bile duct hamartomas, bile duct adenoma |
| **What is a liver "hamartoma"?** | White hard nodule made up of normal liver cells |

## HEPATOCELLULAR ADENOMA

| | |
|---|---|
| **What is it?** | Benign liver tumor |
| **Describe the histology.** | Normal hepatocytes without bile ducts |
| **What are the associated risk factors?** | Women, birth control pills (think: **ABC** = **A**denoma **B**irth **C**ontrol), anabolic steroids, glycogen storage disease |
| **What is the female:male ratio?** | 9:1 |
| **What is the average age of occurrence?** | Between 30 and 35 years of age |

| | |
|---|---|
| **What are the signs/ symptoms?** | Right upper quadrant pain/mass, right upper quadrant fullness, bleeding (rare) |
| **What are the possible complications?** | Rupture with bleeding (33%), necrosis, pain, risk of hepatocellular carcinoma |
| **How is the diagnosis made?** | CT, U/S, +/− biopsy (rule out hemangioma with RBC-tagged scan!) |
| **What is the treatment: Small?** | Stop birth control pills—it may regress. If does not regress, surgical resection is necessary. |
| **Large (>5 cm), bleeding, painful, or ruptured?** | Surgical resection |
| **When is the best time to resect a hepatocellular adenoma in a pregnant patient?** | Second trimester |

## FOCAL NODULAR HYPERPLASIA (FNH)

| | |
|---|---|
| **What is it?** | Benign liver tumor |
| **Describe the histology.** | Normal hepatocytes and **bile ducts (adenoma has no bile ducts)** |
| **What is the average age of occurrence?** | Approximately 40 years |
| **What are the associated risk factors?** | Female gender |
| **Are the tumors associated with birth control pills?** | Yes, but not as clearly associated as with adenoma |
| **How is the diagnosis made?** | Nuclear technetium 99 study, U/S, CT, A-gram, biopsy |
| **What is the classic CT finding?** | Liver mass with "central scar" (think: focal = central) |

| | |
|---|---|
| **What are the possible complications?** | Pain (no risk of cancer, very rarely hemorrhage) |
| **Is there a cancer risk with FNH?** | No (there is a cancer risk with adenoma) |
| **What is the treatment?** | Resection or **embolization** if patient is symptomatic; otherwise, follow if diagnosis is confirmed; stop birth control pills |
| **Why does embolization work with FNH?** | FNH tumors are usually fed by one major artery |

## HEPATIC HEMANGIOMA

| | |
|---|---|
| **What is it?** | Benign vascular tumor of the liver |
| **What is its claim to fame?** | Most common primary benign liver tumor (up to 7% of population) |
| **What are the signs/ symptoms?** | Right upper quadrant pain/mass, bruits |
| **What are the possible complications?** | Pain, congestive heart failure, coagulopathy, obstructive jaundice, gastric outlet obstruction, Kasabach-Merritt syndrome, hemorrhage (rare) |
| **Define Kasabach-Merritt syndrome?** | Hemangioma **and** thrombocytopenia and fibrinogenopenia |
| **How is the diagnosis made?** | CT with IV contrast, tagged red blood scan, MRI, ultrasound |
| **Should biopsy be performed?** | No (risk of hemorrhage with biopsy) |
| **What is the treatment?** | **Observation** (>90%) |
| **What are the indications for resection?** | Symptoms, hemorrhage, cannot make a diagnosis |

## HEPATOCELLULAR CARCINOMA

| | |
|---|---|
| **What is it?** | Most common primary malignancy of the liver |
| **By what name is it also known?** | Hepatoma |
| **What is its incidence?** | Accounts for 80% of all primary malignant liver tumors |
| **What are the geographic high-risk areas?** | Africa and Asia |
| **What are the associated risk factors?** | **Hepatitis B virus, cirrhosis, aflatoxin** (fungi toxin of *Aspergillus flavus*); Other risk factors: α-1-antitrypsin deficiency, hemochromatosis, liver fluke (*Clonorchis sinensis*), anabolic steroids, polyvinylchloride, glycogen storage disease (type I) |
| **What percentage of patients with cirrhosis will develop hepatocellular carcinoma?** | Approximately 5% |
| **What are the signs/ symptoms?** | Dull right upper quadrant pain, hepatomegaly (classic presentation: **painful hepatomegaly**), abdominal mass, weight loss, paraneoplastic syndromes, signs of portal hypertension, ascites, jaundice, fever, anemia, splenomegaly |
| **What tests should be ordered?** | Ultrasound, CT, angiography, tumor marker elevation |
| **What is the tumor marker?** | Elevated α-fetoprotein |
| **What is the most common way to get a tissue diagnosis?** | Needle biopsy with CT, ultrasound, or laparoscopic guidance |
| **What is the most common site of metastasis?** | Lungs |

**What is the treatment of hepatocellular carcinoma?** Surgical resection, if possible (e.g., lobectomy); liver transplant

**What are the treatment options if the patient is not a surgical candidate?** Percutaneous ethanol tumor injection, liquid nitrogen cryotherapy, and intra-arterial chemotherapy

**What are the indications for liver transplantation?** Cirrhosis and NO resection candidacy, as well as no distant or lymph node metastases. The tumor must be >5 cm or have three nodules, with none larger than 3 cm.

**What is the prognosis under the following conditions:**
    **Unresectable?** Almost none survive a year

    **Resectable?** Approximately 35% are alive at 5 years

**Which subtype has the best prognosis?** Fibrolamellar hepatoma (young adults)

## LIVER ABSCESSES

**What is a liver abscess?** Abscess (collection of pus) in the liver parenchyma

**What are the types of liver abscess?** Pyogenic (bacterial), parasitic (amebic), fungal

**What is the most common location of abscess in the liver?** Right lobe > left lobe

**What are the sources?** Direct spread from biliary tract infection
or
Portal spread from GI infection (e.g., appendicitis, diverticulitis)
Systemic source (bacteremia)
Liver trauma (e.g., liver gunshot wound)
Cryptogenic (unknown source)

**What are the two most common types?** **Bacterial** (most common in the United States) and amebic (most common worldwide)

## BACTERIAL LIVER ABSCESS

| | |
|---|---|
| **What are the three most common bacterial organisms affecting the liver?** | Gram negatives: *E. coli, Klebsiella,* and *Proteus* |
| **What are the most common sources/causes of bacterial liver abscesses?** | Cholangitis, diverticulitis, liver cancer, liver metastasis |
| **What are the signs/ symptoms?** | **Fever, chills, right upper quadrant pain,** leukocytosis, increased liver function tests (LFTs), jaundice, sepsis, weight loss |
| **What is the treatment?** | IV antibiotics (triple antibiotics with metronidazole), percutaneous drainage with CT or U/S guidance |
| **What are the indications for operative drainage?** | Multiple/loculated abscesses or if multiple percutaneous attempts have failed |

## AMEBIC LIVER ABSCESS

| | |
|---|---|
| **What is the etiology?** | *Entamoeba histolytica* (typically reaches liver via portal vein from intestinal amebiasis) |
| **How does it spread?** | Fecal-oral transmission |
| **What are the risk factors?** | Patients from countries south of the U.S.–Mexican border, institutionalized patients, homosexual men, alcoholic patients |
| **What are the signs/ symptoms?** | Right upper quadrant pain, fever, hepatomegaly, diarrhea<br>*Note:* chills are much less common with amebic abscesses than with pyogenic abscesses. |
| **Which lobe is most commonly involved?** | The right lobe of the liver |

| | |
|---|---|
| **Classic description of abscess contents?** | "Anchovy paste" pus |
| **How is the diagnosis made?** | Lab tests, ultrasound, CT |
| **What lab tests should be performed?** | Indirect hemagglutination titers for *Entamoeba* antibodies elevated in more than 95% of cases, elevated LFTs |
| **What is the treatment?** | Metronidazole IV |
| **What are the indications for percutaneous surgical drainage?** | Refractory to metronidazole, bacterial co-infection, or peritoneal rupture |
| **What are the possible complications of large left lobe liver amebic abscess?** | Erosion into the pericardial sac (potentially fatal!) |

## HYDATID LIVER CYSTS

| | |
|---|---|
| **What is it?** | Usually a right lobe cyst filled with *Echinococcus granulosus* |
| **What are the risk factors?** | Travel, exposure to dogs, sheep, and cattle (carriers) |
| **What are the signs/ symptoms?** | Right upper quadrant abdominal pain, jaundice, right upper quadrant mass |
| **How is the diagnosis made?** | Indirect hemagglutination antibody test (serologic testing), Casoni skin test, ultrasound, CT, radiographic imaging |
| **What are the findings on AXR?** | Possible calcified outline of cyst |
| **What are the major risks?** | Erosion into the pleural cavity, pericardial sac, or biliary tree<br>Rupture into the peritoneal cavity causing fatal anaphylaxis |
| **What is the risk of surgical removal of echinococcal (hydatid) cysts?** | Rupture or leakage of cyst contents into the abdomen may cause a fatal **anaphylactic** reaction |

| | |
|---|---|
| **When should percutaneous drainage be performed?** | Never; may cause leaking into the peritoneal cavity and anaphylaxis |
| **What is the treatment?** | **Mebendazole, followed by surgical resection;** large cysts can be drained and then injected with toxic irrigant (scoliocide) into the cyst unless aspirate is bilious (which means there is a biliary connection) followed by cyst removal |
| **Which toxic irrigations are used?** | Hypertonic saline, ethanol, or cetrimide |

## HEMOBILIA

| | |
|---|---|
| **What is it?** | Blood draining via the common bile duct into the duodenum |
| **What is the diagnostic triad?** | Triad: <br> 1. Right upper quadrant pain <br> 2. Guaiac positive/upper GI bleeding <br> 3. Jaundice |
| **What are the causes?** | Trauma, percutaneous transhepatic cholangiography (PTC), tumors |
| **How is the diagnosis made?** | EGD (blood out of the ampulla of Vater), A-gram |
| **What is the treatment?** | A-gram with embolization of the bleeding vessel |

# Chapter 53

# Portal Hypertension

**Identify the anatomy of the portal venous system.**

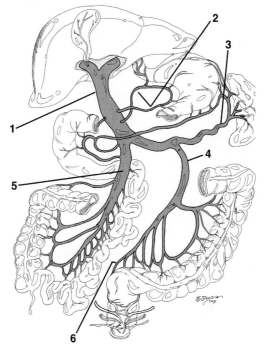

1. Portal vein
2. Coronary vein
3. Splenic vein
4. IMV (inferior mesenteric vein)
5. SMV (superior mesenteric vein)
6. Superior hemorrhoidal vein

**Describe drainage of blood from the superior hemorrhoidal vein.**

To the IMV, the splenic vein, and then the portal vein

**Where does blood drain into from the IMV?**

Into the splenic vein

| | |
|---|---|
| **Where does the portal vein begin?** | At the confluence of the splenic vein and the SMV |
| **What are the (6) potential routes of portal-systemic collateral blood flow (as seen with portal hypertension)?** | 1. Umbilical vein<br>2. Coronary vein to esophageal venous plexi<br>3. Retroperitoneal veins (veins of Retzius)<br>4. Diaphragm veins (veins of Sappey)<br>5. Superior hemorrhoidal vein to middle and inferior hemorrhoidal veins and then to the iliac vein<br>6. Splenic veins to the short gastric veins |
| **What is the pathophysiology of portal hypertension?** | Elevated portal pressure resulting from resistance to portal flow |
| **What level of portal pressure is normal?** | <10 mm Hg |
| **What is the etiology?** | **Prehepatic**—Thrombosis of portal vein/ atresia of portal vein<br>**Hepatic**—**Cirrhosis** (distortion of normal parenchyma by regenerating hepatic nodules), hepatocellular carcinoma, fibrosis<br>**Posthepatic**—Budd-Chiari syndrome: thrombosis of hepatic veins |
| **What is the most common cause of portal hypertension in the United States?** | Cirrhosis (>90% of cases) |
| **What percentage of patients with alcoholism develop cirrhosis?** | Surprisingly, less than 1 in 5 |
| **What percentage of patients with cirrhosis develop esophageal varices?** | Approximately 40% |
| **What percentage of patients with cirrhosis develop portal hypertension?** | Approximately two-thirds |

**What is the most common physical finding in patients with portal hypertension?**

Splenomegaly

**What are the associated CLINICAL findings in portal hypertension (4)?**

1. Caput medusae (engorgement of periumbilical veins)
2. Hemorrhoids
3. Splenomegaly
4. Esophageal varices

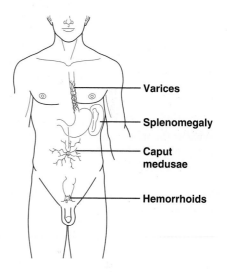

**What other physical findings are associated with cirrhosis and portal hypertension?**

Spider angioma, palmar erythema, ascites, truncal obesity and peripheral wasting, encephalopathy, asterixis (liver flap), gynecomastia, jaundice

**What is the name of the periumbilical bruit heard with caput medusae?**

Cruveilhier-Baumgarten bruit

**What constitutes the portal-systemic collateral circulation in portal hypertension in the following conditions:**
  **Esophageal varices?**

Coronary vein backing up into the azygous system

**Caput medusae?**

Umbilical vein (via falciform ligament) draining into the epigastric veins

**Retroperitoneal varices?**

Small mesenteric veins (veins of Retzius) draining retroperitoneally into lumbar veins

**Hemorrhoids?**

Superior hemorrhoidal vein (which normally drains into the inferior mesenteric vein) backing up into the middle and inferior hemorrhoidal veins

**What is the etiology?**

**Cirrhosis (90%),** schistosomiasis, hepatitis, Budd-Chiari syndrome, hemochromatosis, Wilson's disease, portal vein thrombosis, tumors, splenic vein thrombosis

**What is the most common cause of portal hypertension outside North America?**

Schistosomiasis

**What is Budd-Chiari syndrome?**

Thrombosis of the hepatic veins

**What is the most feared complication of portal hypertension?**

Bleeding from esophageal varices

**What are esophageal varices?**

Engorgement of the esophageal venous plexi secondary to increased collateral blood flow from the portal system as a result of portal hypertension

**What is the "rule of two-thirds" of portal hypertension?**

Two-thirds of patients with cirrhosis will develop portal hypertension.

Two-thirds of patients with portal hypertension will develop esophageal varices.

Two-thirds of patients with esophageal varices will bleed from the varices.

**In patients with cirrhosis and known varices who are suffering from upper GI bleeding, how often does that bleeding result from varices?**

Only about 50% of the time

**What are the signs/ symptoms?**

Hematemesis, melena, hematochezia

**What is the mortality rate from an acute esophageal variceal bleed?**

Approximately 50%

**What is the initial treatment of variceal bleeding?**

As with all upper GI bleeding: large bore IVS × 2, IV fluid, Foley catheter, type and cross blood, send labs, correct coagulopathy (vitamin K, fresh frozen plasma), +/ − intubation to protect from aspiration

**What is the diagnostic test of choice?**

**EGD (upper GI endoscopy)**
Remember, bleeding is the result of varices only half the time; must rule out ulcers, gastritis, etc.

**If esophageal varices cause bleeding, what are the initial treatment options?**

1. **Emergent endoscopic sclerotherapy:** a sclerosing substance is injected into the esophageal varices under direct endoscopic vision
2. **Endoscopic band ligation:** elastic band ligation of varices

**What are options if the patient continues to bleed after the initial treatment?**

**IV vasopressin** (and nitroglycerin, to avoid MI) or **somatostatin** (Octreotide) to achieve vasoconstriction of the mesenteric vessels; if bleeding continues, consider balloon (**Sengstaken-Blakemore tube**) tamponade of the varices, beta blocker

**What is a Sengstaken-Blakemore tube?**

A tube with a gastric and esophageal balloon for tamponading an esophageal bleed (see Chapter 40: Upper GI Bleeding)

| | |
|---|---|
| **What is the next therapy after the bleeding is controlled?** | Repeat endoscopic sclerotherapy/ banding |
| **What are the options if sclerotherapy and conservative methods fail to stop the variceal bleeding or bleeding recurs?** | Repeat sclerotherapy/banding and treat conservatively<br>TIPS<br>Surgical shunt (selective and partial)<br>Liver transplantation |
| **What is a "selective" shunt?** | A shunt that selectively decompresses the varices without decompressing the portal vein |
| **What does the acronym TIPS stand for?** | **T**ransjugular **I**ntrahepatic **P**ortosystemic **S**hunt |
| **What is a TIPS procedure?** | An angiographic radiologist places a small tube stent intrahepatically between the hepatic vein and a branch of the portal vein via a percutaneous-jugular vein route. |
| **What is a "partial shunt"?** | A shunt that directly decompresses the portal vein, but only partially |
| **What is a Warren shunt?** | Distal splenorenal shunt with ligation of the coronary vein—elective shunt procedure associated with low incidence of encephalopathy in patients postoperatively because only the splenic flow is diverted to decompress the varices |

Ligated coronary vein

Splenorenal vein anastomosis

| | |
|---|---|
| **What is a contraindication to the Warren "selective" shunt?** | Ascites |
| **Define the following shunts:** | |
|    **End-to-side portocaval shunt** | "Total shunt"—portal vein (end) to IVC (side) |
|    **Side-to-side portocaval shunt** | Side of portal vein anastomosed to side of IVC—partially preserves portal flow ("partial shunt") |
|    **Synthetic portocaval H-graft** | "Partial shunt"—synthetic tube graft from the portal vein to the IVC (good option for patients with alcoholism; associated with lower incidence of encephalopathy and easier transplantation later) |
|    **Synthetic mesocaval H-graft** | Synthetic graft from the SMV to the IVC |
| **What is the most common perioperative cause of death following shunt procedure?** | Hepatic failure, secondary to decreased blood flow (accounts for two-thirds of deaths) |

**What is the major postoperative morbidity after a shunt procedure?**

Increased incidence of hepatic encephalopathy because of decreased portal blood flow to the liver and decreased clearance of toxins/metabolites from the blood

**What medication is infused to counteract the coronary artery vasoconstriction of IV vasopressin?**

Nitroglycerin IV drip

**What lab value roughly correlates with degree of encephalopathy?**

Serum ammonia level (Note: thought to correlate with but not cause encephalopathy)

**What medications are used to treat hepatic encephalopathy?**

Lactulose PO, with or without neomycin PO

# Chapter 54    Biliary Tract

## ANATOMY

**Name structures 1 through 8 (below) of the biliary tract.**

1. Intrahepatic ducts
2. Left hepatic duct
3. Right hepatic duct
4. Common hepatic duct
5. Gallbladder
6. Cystic duct
7. Common bile duct
8. Ampulla of Vater

**Which is the proximal and which is the distal bile duct?**

Proximal is close to the liver. (Bile and the liver is analogous to blood and the heart; they both flow distally.)

**What is the name of the node in Calot's triangle?**

Calot's node

**What are the small ducts that drain bile directly into the gallbladder from the liver?**

Ducts of Luschka

**Which artery is susceptible to injury during cholecystectomy?**

Right hepatic artery, because of its proximity to the cystic artery and Calot's triangle

**What is the name of the valves of the gallbladder?**

Spiral valves of Heister

**Where is the infundibulum of the gallbladder?**

Near the cystic duct

**Where is the fundus of the gallbladder?**

At the end of the gallbladder

**What is "Hartmann's pouch"?**

The gallbladder infundibulum

**What are the boundaries of the triangle of Calot?**

The 3 C's:
1. **C**ystic duct
2. **C**ommon hepatic duct
3. **C**ystic artery

| | |
|---|---|
| **"Dr. Blackbourne, are you absolutely sure that the Triangle of Calot includes the cystic artery and not the liver edge?"** | Yes, look up *Gastroenterology*, 2002; 123(5):1440. |

## PHYSIOLOGY

| | |
|---|---|
| **What is the source of alkaline phosphatase?** | Bile duct epithelium; expect alkaline phosphatase to be elevated in bile duct obstruction |
| **What is in bile?** | Cholesterol, lecithin (phospholipid), bile acids, and bilirubin |
| **What does bile do?** | Emulsify fats |
| **What is the enterohepatic circulation?** | Circulation of bile acids from liver to gut and back to the liver |
| **Where are most of the bile acids absorbed?** | In the terminal ileum |
| **What stimulates gallbladder emptying?** | Cholecystokinin and vagal input |
| **What is the source of cholecystokinin?** | Duodenal mucosal cells |
| **What stimulates the release of cholecystokinin?** | Fat, protein, amino acids, and HCl |
| **What inhibits its release?** | Trypsin and chymotrypsin |

**What are its actions?**

Gallbladder emptying
Opening of ampulla of Vater
Slowing of gastric emptying
Pancreas acinar cell growth and release
of exocrine products

## PATHOPHYSIOLOGY

**At what level of serum total bilirubin does one start to get jaundiced?**

Greater than 2.5

**Classically, what is thought to be the anatomic location where one first finds evidence of jaundice?**

Under the tongue

**With good renal function, how high can the serum total bilirubin go?**

Very rarely, greater than 20

**What are the signs and symptoms of obstructive jaundice?**

Jaundice
Dark urine
Clay-colored stools (acholic stools)
Pruritus (itching)
Loss of appetite
Nausea

**What causes the itching in obstructive jaundice?**

Bile salts in the dermis (not bilirubin!)

**Define the following terms:**
    **Cholelithiasis**

Gallstones in gallbladder

**Cholethiasis**

hrf '07

**Choledocholithiasis**　　Gallstone in common bile duct

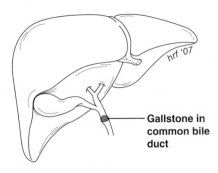

Gallstone in
common bile
duct

**Cholecystitis**　　Inflammation of gallbladder

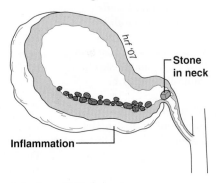

Stone
in neck

Inflammation

**Cholangitis**　　Infection of biliary tract

**Cholangiocarcinoma**　　Adenocarcinoma of bile ducts

**Klatskin's tumor**　　Cholangiocarcinoma of bile duct at the
junction of the right and left hepatic
ducts

**Biliary colic**　　Pain from gallstones, usually from a stone
at cystic duct. The pain is located in the
RUQ, epigastrium, or right subscapular
region of the back. It usually lasts
minutes to hours but eventually goes
away. It is often postprandial, especially
after fatty foods.

**Biloma**　　Intraperitoneal bile fluid collection

| | |
|---|---|
| **Choledochojejunostomy** | Anastomosis between common bile duct and jejunum |
| **Hepaticojejunostomy** | Anastomosis of hepatic ducts or common hepatic duct to jejunum |

## DIAGNOSTIC STUDIES

| | |
|---|---|
| **What is the initial diagnostic study of choice for evaluation of the biliary tract/gallbladder/cholelithiasis?** | Ultrasound! |
| **Define the following diagnostic studies:** | |
|     **ERCP** | **E**ndoscopic **R**etrograde **C**holangio**P**ancreatography |
|     **PTC** | **P**ercutaneous **T**ranshepatic **C**holangiogram |
|     **IOC** | **I**ntra**O**perative **C**holangiogram (done laparoscopically or open to rule out choledocholithiasis) |
|     **HIDA/PRIDA scan** | Radioisotope study; isotope concentrated in liver and secreted into bile; will demonstrate cholecystitis, bile leak, or CBD obstruction |
| **How does the HIDA scan reveal cholecystitis?** | Non-opacification of the gallbladder from obstruction of the cystic duct |
| **How often will plain x-ray films see gallstones?** | 10% to 15% |

## BILIARY SURGERY

| | |
|---|---|
| **What is a cholecystectomy?** | Removal of the gallbladder laparoscopically or through a standard Kocher incision |
| **What is a "lap chole"?** | A **LAP**aroscopic **CHOLE**cystectomy |

**What is the Kocher incision?**  Right subcostal incision

**What is a sphincterotomy?**  Cut through sphincter of Oddi to allow passage of gallstones from the common bile duct; most often done at ERCP; also known as papillotomy

**How should postoperative biloma be treated after a lap chole?**
1. Percutaneous drain bile collection
2. ERCP with placement of biliary stent past leak (usually cystic duct remnant leak)

**What is the treatment of major CBD injury after a lap chole?**  Choledochojejunostomy

## OBSTRUCTIVE JAUNDICE

**What is it?**  Jaundice (hyperbilirubinemia >2.5) from obstruction of bile flow to the duodenum

**What is the differential diagnosis of *proximal* bile duct obstruction?**
Cholangiocarcinoma
Lymphadenopathy
Metastatic tumor
Gallbladder carcinoma
Sclerosing cholangitis
Gallstones
Tumor embolus
Parasites
Postsurgical stricture
Hepatoma
Benign bile duct tumor

| | |
|---|---|
| **What is the differential diagnosis of *distal* bile duct obstruction?** | Choledocholithiasis (**gallstones**)<br>Pancreatic carcinoma<br>Pancreatitis<br>Ampullary carcinoma<br>Lymphadenopathy<br>Pseudocyst<br>Postsurgical stricture<br>Ampulla of Vater dysfunction/stricture<br>Lymphoma<br>Benign bile duct tumor<br>Parasites |
| **What is the initial study of choice for obstructive jaundice?** | Ultrasound |
| **What lab results are associated with obstructive jaundice?** | Elevated alkaline phosphatase, elevated bilirubin with or without elevated LFTs |

## CHOLELITHIASIS

| | |
|---|---|
| **What is it?** | The formation of gallstones |
| **What is the incidence?** | About 10% of U.S. population will develop gallstones. |
| **What are the "Big 4" risk factors?** | The "four Fs": **F**emale, **F**at, **F**orty, **F**ertile (multiparity) |
| **What are other less common risk factors for gallstones?** | Oral contraceptives<br>Bile stasis<br>Chronic hemolysis (pigment stones)<br>Cirrhosis<br>Infection<br>Native American heritage<br>Rapid weight loss/gastric bypass<br>Obesity<br>Inflammatory bowel disease (IBD)<br>Terminal ileal resection<br>Total parenteral nutrition (TPN)<br>Vagotomy<br>Advanced age<br>Hyperlipidemia<br>Somatostatin therapy |

| | |
|---|---|
| **What are the types of stones?** | Cholesterol stones (75% of all stones) and pigment stones (25% of all stones) |
| **What are the types of pigmented stones?** | Black stones (contain calcium bilirubinate) and brown stones (associated with biliary tract infection) |
| **What are the causes of black-pigmented stones?** | Cirrhosis, hemolysis |
| **What is the pathogenesis of cholesterol stones?** | Secretion of bile **supersaturated** with cholesterol (relatively decreased amounts of lecithin and bile salts); then, cholesterol precipitates out and forms solid crystals, then gallstones |
| **Is hypercholesterolemia a risk factor for gallstone formation?** | No (but hyperlipidemia is) |
| **What are the signs and symptoms?** | Symptoms of: biliary colic, cholangitis, choledocholithiasis, gallstone, pancreatitis |
| **Is biliary colic pain really "colic"?** | No, symptoms usually last for hours; therefore, colic is a misnomer! |
| **What percentage of patients with gallstones are Asymptomatic?** | Eighty percent of patients with cholelithiasis are Asymptomatic! |
| **What is thought to cause biliary colic?** | Gallbladder contraction against a stone temporarily at the gallbladder/cystic duct junction; a stone in the cystic duct; or a stone passing through the cystic duct |
| **What is Boas' sign?** | The referred right subscapular pain of biliary colic |
| **What are the five major complications of gallstones?** | Acute cholecystitis<br>Choledocholithiasis<br>Gallstone pancreatitis<br>Gallstone ileus<br>Cholangitis |
| **How is cholelithiasis diagnosed?** | History<br>Physical examination<br>**Ultrasound** |

**How often does ultrasound detect cholelithiasis?**

More than 98% of the time!

**How often does ultrasound detect choledocholithiasis?**

About 33% of the time . . . not a very good study for choledocholithiasis!

**How are symptomatic or complicated cases of cholelithiasis treated?**

By cholecystectomy

**What are the possible complications of a lap chole?**

Common bile duct injury; right hepatic duct/artery injury; cystic duct leak; biloma (collection of bile)

**What are the indications for cholecystectomy in the asymptomatic patient?**

Sickle-cell disease
Calcified gallbladder (porcelain gallbladder)
The patient is a child

**Define IOC.**

**I**ntra**O**perative **C**holangiogram (dye in bile duct by way of the cystic duct with fluoro/x-ray)

**What are the indications for an IOC?**

1. Jaundice
2. Hyperbilirubinemia
3. Gallstone pancreatitis (resolved)
4. Elevated alkaline phosphatase
5. Choledocholithiasis on ultrasound
6. To define anatomy

**What is choledocholithiasis?**

Gallstones in the bile ducts

**What is the management of choledocholithiasis?**

1. ERCP with papillotomy and basket/ balloon retrieval of stones (pre- or postoperatively)
2. Laparoscopic transcystic duct or trans common bile duct retrieval
3. Open common bile duct exploration

**What medication may dissolve a cholesterol gallstone?**

Chenodeoxycholic acid, ursodeoxycholic acid (Actigall®); but if medication is stopped, gallstones recur

**What is the major feared complication of ERCP?**

Pancreatitis

## ACUTE CHOLECYSTITIS

| | |
|---|---|
| **What is the pathogenesis of acute cholecystitis?** | Obstruction of cystic duct leads to inflammation of the gallbladder; about 95% of cases result from calculi, and about 5% from acalculous obstruction. |
| **What are the risk factors?** | Gallstones |
| **What are the signs and symptoms?** | **Unrelenting** RUQ pain or tenderness<br>**Fever**<br>Nausea/vomiting<br>Painful palpable gallbladder in 33%<br>Positive Murphy's sign<br>Right subscapular pain (referred)<br>Epigastric discomfort (referred) |
| **What is Murphy's sign?** | Acute pain and **inspiratory arrest** elicited by palpation of the RUQ during inspiration |
| **What are the complications of acute cholecystitis?** | Abscess<br>Perforation<br>Choledocholithiasis<br>Cholecystenteric fistula formation<br>Gallstone ileus |
| **What lab results are associated with acute cholecystitis?** | Increased WBC; may have:<br>Slight elevation in alkaline phosphatase, LFTs<br>Slight elevation in amylase, T. Bili |
| **What is the diagnostic test of choice for acute cholecystitis?** | Ultrasound |
| **What are the signs of acute cholecystitis on ultrasound?** | Thickened gallbladder wall (thicker than 3 mm)<br>Pericholecystic fluid<br>Distended gallbladder<br>Gallstones present/cystic duct stone<br>Sonographic Murphy's sign (pain on inspiration after placement of ultrasound probe over gallbladder) |

**What is the difference between acute cholecystitis and biliary colic?**

Biliary colic has temporary pain. Acute cholecystitis has pain that does not resolve, usually with elevated WBCs, fever, and signs of acute inflammation on U/S.

**What is the treatment of acute cholecystitis?**

IVFs, antibiotics, and cholecystectomy early

**What are the steps in lap chole (6)?**

1. Dissection of peritoneum overlying the cystic duct and artery
2. Clipping of cystic artery and transect
3. Division of cystic duct between clips
4. Dissection of gallbladder from the liver bed
5. Cauterization; irrigation; suction, to obtain hemostasis of the liver bed
6. Removal of the gallbladder through the umbilical trocar site

**How is an IOC performed?**

By:
1. Placing a clip on the cystic duct–gallbladder junction
2. Cutting a small hole in the distal cystic duct so as to cannulate
3. Injecting half-strength contrast and taking an x-ray or fluoro

**What percentage of patients have an accessory cystic artery?**

10%

**Why should the gallbladder specimen be opened in the operating room?**

Looking for gallbladder cancer

## ACUTE ACALCULOUS CHOLECYSTITIS

**What is it?**

Acute cholecystitis without evidence of stones

**What is the pathogenesis?**

It is believed to result from sludge and gallbladder disuse and **biliary stasis,** perhaps secondary to absence of cholecystokinin stimulation (decreased contraction of gallbladder).

| | |
|---|---|
| **What are the risk factors?** | Prolonged fasting<br>TPN<br>Trauma<br>Multiple transfusions<br>Dehydration<br>Often occurs in prolonged postoperative or ICU setting |
| **What are the diagnostic tests of choice?** | 1. **Ultrasound;** sludge and inflammation usually present with acute acalculous cholecystitis<br>2. HIDA scan |
| **What are the findings on HIDA scan?** | Nonfilling of the gallbladder |
| **What is the management of acute acalculous cholecystitis?** | Cholecystectomy, or cholecystostomy tube if the patient is unstable (placed percutaneously by radiology or open surgery) |

## CHOLANGITIS

| | |
|---|---|
| **What is it?** | Bacterial infection of the biliary tract from obstruction (either partial or complete); potentially life-threatening |
| **What are the common causes?** | **Choledocholithiasis**<br>Stricture (usually postoperative)<br>Neoplasm (usually ampullary carcinoma)<br>Extrinsic compression (pancreatic pseudocyst/pancreatitis)<br>Instrumentation of the bile ducts (e.g., PTC/ERCP)<br>Biliary stent |
| **What is the most common cause of cholangitis?** | Gallstones in common bile duct (choledocholithiasis) |
| **What are the signs and symptoms?** | **Charcot's triad:** fever/chills, RUQ pain, and jaundice<br>**Reynold's pentad:** Charcot's triad plus altered mental status and shock |
| **What lab results are associated with cholangitis?** | Increased WBC, bilirubin, and alkaline phosphatase, positive blood cultures |

**Which organisms are most commonly isolated with cholangitis?**

Gram-negative organisms (*E. coli, Klebsiella, Pseudomonas, Enterobacter, Proteus, Serratia*) are the most common.

Enterococci are the most common gram-positive bacteria.

Anaerobes are less common (*B. fragilis* most frequent).

Fungi are even less common (*Candida*).

**What are the diagnostic tests of choice?**

Ultrasound and contrast study (e.g., ERCP or IOC) after patient has "cooled off" with IV antibiotics

**What is suppurative cholangitis?**

Severe infection with sepsis—"pus under pressure"

**What is the management of cholangitis?**

**Nonsuppurative:** IVF and antibiotics, with definitive treatment later (e.g., lap chole +/− ERCP)

**Suppurative:** IVF, antibiotics, and decompression; decompression can be obtained by ERCP with papillotomy, PTC with catheter drainage, or laparotomy with T-tube placement

## SCLEROSING CHOLANGITIS

**What is it?**

Multiple inflammatory fibrous thickenings of bile duct walls resulting in biliary strictures

**What is its natural history?**

Progressive obstruction possibly leading to cirrhosis and liver failure; 10% of patients will develop cholangiocarcinoma

**What is the etiology?**

Unknown, but probably autoimmune

**What is the major risk factor?**

Inflammatory bowel disease

**What type of IBD is the most common risk factor?**

Ulcerative colitis ($\approx 66\%$)

| | |
|---|---|
| **What are the signs and symptoms of sclerosing cholangitis?** | The same as the signs of obstructive jaundice:<br>    Jaundice<br>    Itching (pruritus)<br>    Dark urine<br>    Clay-colored stools<br>    Loss of energy<br>    Weight loss<br>    (Many patients are asymptomatic.) |
| **What are the complications?** | Cirrhosis<br>Cholangiocarcinoma (10%)<br>Cholangitis<br>Obstructive jaundice |
| **How is it diagnosed?** | Elevated alkaline phosphatase, and PTC or ERCP revealing "beads on a string" appearance on contrast study |
| **What are the management options?** | Hepatoenteric anastomosis (if primarily extrahepatic ducts are involved) and resection of extrahepatic bile ducts because of the risk of cholangiocarcinoma<br>Transplant (if primarily intrahepatic disease or cirrhosis)<br>Endoscopic balloon dilations |
| **What percentage of patients with IBD develop sclerosing cholangitis?** | Less than 5% |

## GALLSTONE ILEUS

| | |
|---|---|
| **What is it?** | Small bowel obstruction from a large gallstone (>2.5 cm) that has eroded through the gallbladder and into the duodenum/small bowel |
| **What is the classic site of obstruction?** | The ileocecal valve (but may cause obstruction in the duodenum, sigmoid colon) |

**What are the classic findings of gallstone ileus?**

Air in the hepatic bile ducts

SBO with air fluid levels

Gallstone in ileocecal valve

**What is the population at risk?**

Gallstone ileus is most commonly seen in **women older than 70 years.**

**What are the signs/ symptoms?**

Symptoms of SBO: distention, vomiting, hypovolemia, RUQ pain

**What is the differential diagnosis?**

Other causes of SBO (**A, B, C: A**dhesions, **B**ulge/hernia, **C**ancer)

**Gallstone ileus causes what percentage of cases of SBO?**

Less than 1%

**What are the diagnostic tests of choice?**

**Abdominal x-ray:** occasionally reveals radiopaque gallstone in the bowel; **40% of patients show air in the biliary tract,** small bowel distention, and air fluid levels secondary to ileus

UGI: used if diagnosis is in question; will show cholecystenteric fistula and the obstruction

**Abdominal CT:** reveals air in biliary tract, SBO +/− gallstone in intestine

**What is the management?**

Surgery: enterotomy with removal of the stone ± interval cholecystectomy (interval-delayed)

## CARCINOMA OF THE GALLBLADDER

| | |
|---|---|
| **What is it?** | Malignant neoplasm arising in the gallbladder, vast majority are **adenocarcinoma (90%)** |
| **What are the risk factors?** | **Gallstones, porcelain gallbladder,** cholecystenteric fistula |
| **What is the female:male ratio?** | 4:1 |
| **What is the most common site of gallbladder cancer on the gallbladder?** | 60% in fundus |
| **What is a porcelain gallbladder?** | Calcified gallbladder |
| **What percentage of patients with a porcelain gallbladder will have gallbladder cancer?** | Approximately 50% |
| **What is the incidence?** | **About 1% of all gallbladder specimens** |
| **What are the symptoms?** | Biliary colic, weight loss, anorexia; many patients are asymptomatic until late; may present as acute cholecystitis |
| **What are the signs?** | Jaundice (from invasion of the common duct or compression by involved pericholedochal lymph nodes), RUQ mass, palpable gallbladder (advanced disease) |
| **What are the diagnostic tests of choice?** | Ultrasound, abdominal CT, ERCP |
| **What is the route of spread?** | Contiguous spread to the liver is most common. |
| **What is the management under the following conditions?** | |
|     **Confined to mucosa** | Cholecystectomy |

| | |
|---|---|
| **Confined to muscularis/serosa** | Radical cholecystectomy: cholecystectomy and wedge resection of overlying liver, and lymph node dissection ± chemotherapy/XRT |
| **What is the main complication of a lap chole for gallbladder cancer?** | Trocar site tumor implants (so if known preoperatively, perform open cholecystectomy) |

## CHOLANGIOCARCINOMA

| | |
|---|---|
| **What is it?** | Malignancy of the extrahepatic or intrahepatic ducts—**primary bile duct cancer** |
| **What is the histology?** | Almost all are adenocarcinomas |
| **What is the average age of the patient?** | About 65 years, affects males and females equally |
| **What are the signs and symptoms?** | The signs and symptoms of biliary obstruction: jaundice, **pruritus, dark urine, clay-colored stools, cholangitis** |
| **What is the most common location?** | Proximal bile duct |
| **What are the risk factors?** | Choledochal cysts<br>Ulcerative colitis<br>Thorotrast contrast dye (used in 1950s)<br>Sclerosing cholangitis<br>Liver flukes (clonorchiasis)<br>Toxin exposures (e.g., Agent Orange) |
| **What is a Klatskin tumor?** | Tumor that involves the junction of the right and left hepatic ducts |

**What are the diagnostic tests of choice?**

Ultrasound, CT, ERCP/PTC with biopsy/brushings for cytology, MRCP

**What is an MRCP?**

An MRI with visualization of pancreatic and bile ducts

**What is the management of proximal bile duct cholangiocarcinoma?**

Resection with Roux-en-Y hepaticojejunostomy (anastomose bile ducts to jejunum) ± unilateral hepatic lobectomy

**What is the management of distal common bile duct cholangiocarcinoma?**

Whipple procedure

## MISCELLANEOUS CONDITIONS

**What is a porcelain gallbladder?**

**Calcified gallbladder** seen on abdominal x-ray; results from chronic cholelithiasis/cholecystitis with calcified scar tissue in gallbladder wall; **cholecystectomy** required because of the strong association of **gallbladder carcinoma** with this condition

**What is hydrops of the gallbladder?**

Complete obstruction of the cystic duct by a gallstone, with filling of the gallbladder with fluid (not bile) from the gallbladder mucosa

**What is Gilbert syndrome?**

Inborn error in liver bilirubin uptake and glucuronyl transferase resulting in hyperbilirubinemia (think: **G**ilberts = **G**lucuronyl)

| | |
|---|---|
| **What is Courvoisier's gallbladder?** | Palpable, **nontender** gallbladder (unlike acute cholecystitis) associated with cancer of the head of the pancreas; able to distend because it has not been "scarred down" by gallstones |
| **What is Mirizzi's syndrome?** | Common hepatic duct obstruction as a result of **extrinsic** obstruction from a gallstone impacted in the cystic duct |

# Chapter 55     Pancreas

**Identify the regions of the pancreas.**

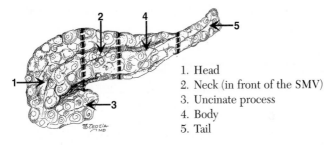

1. Head
2. Neck (in front of the SMV)
3. Uncinate process
4. Body
5. Tail

| | |
|---|---|
| **What structure is the tail of the pancreas said to "tickle"?** | The spleen |
| **Name the two pancreatic ducts.** | 1. Wirsung duct<br>2. Santorini duct |
| **Which duct is the main duct?** | The duct of Wirsung is the major duct (think: **S**antorini = **S**mall duct). |
| **How is blood supplied to the head of the pancreas?** | 1. Celiac trunk → gastroduodenal → Anterior superior pancreaticoduodenal artery<br>Posterior superior pancreaticoduodenal artery |

2. Superior mesenteric artery →
Anterior inferior pancreaticoduodenal artery
Posterior inferior pancreaticoduodenal artery
3. Splenic artery →
Dorsal pancreatic artery

**Why must the duodenum be removed if the head of the pancreas is removed?**

They share the same blood supply (gastroduodenal artery).

**What is the endocrine function of the pancreas?**

Islets of Langerhans
α-cells: glucagon
β-cells: insulin

**What is the exocrine function of the pancreas?**

Digestive enzymes: amylase, lipase, trypsin, chymotrypsin, carboxypeptidase

**What maneuver is used to mobilize the duodenum and pancreas and evaluate the entire pancreas?**

Kocher maneuver: incise the lateral attachments of the duodenum and then lift the pancreas to examine the posterior surface

# PANCREATITIS

## ACUTE PANCREATITIS

**What is it?**

Inflammation of the pancreas

**What are the most common etiologies in the United States?**

1. Alcohol abuse (50%)
2. Gallstones (30%)
3. Idiopathic (10%)

**What acronym represents the other causes of pancreatitis?**

"**I GET SMASHED**":
**I**diopathic

**G**allstones
**E**thanol
**T**rauma

**S**corpion bite
**M**umps (viruses)
**A**utoimmune
**S**teroids

**H**yperlipidemia
**E**RCP
**D**rugs

| | |
|---|---|
| **What are the symptoms?** | Epigastric pain (frequently radiates to back); nausea and vomiting |
| **What are the signs of pancreatitis?** | Epigastric tenderness<br>Diffuse abdominal tenderness<br>Decreased bowel sounds (adynamic ileus)<br>Fever<br>Dehydration/shock |
| **What is the differential diagnosis?** | Gastritis/PUD<br>Perforated viscus<br>Acute cholecystitis<br>SBO<br>Mesenteric ischemia/infarction<br>Ruptured AAA<br>Biliary colic<br>Inferior MI/pneumonia |
| **What lab tests should be ordered?** | CBC<br>LFT<br>Amylase/lipase<br>Type and cross<br>ABG<br>Calcium<br>Chemistry<br>Coags<br>Serum lipids |
| **What are the associated diagnostic findings?** | Lab—High amylase, high lipase, high WBC<br>AXR—Sentinel loop, colon cutoff, possibly gallstones (only 10% visible on x-ray)<br>U/S—Phlegmon, cholelithiasis<br>CT—Phlegmon, pancreatic necrosis |
| **What is the most common sign of pancreatitis on AXR?** | Sentinel loop(s) |

**What is the treatment?**

NPO
IVF
NGT if vomiting
+/− TPN vs. postpyloric tube feeds
$H_2$ blocker/PPI
Analgesia (Demerol®, not morphine—
  less sphincter of Oddi spasm)
Correction of coags/electrolytes
+/− Alcohol withdrawal prophylaxis
"Tincture of time"

**Are postpyloric tube feeds safe in acute pancreatitis?**

YES

**What are the possible complications?**

Pseudocyst
Abscess/infection
Pancreatic necrosis
Splenic/mesenteric/portal vessel rupture
  or thrombosis
Pancreatic ascites/pancreatic pleural
  effusion
Diabetes
ARDS/sepsis/MOF
Coagulopathy/DIC
Encephalopathy
Severe hypocalcemia

**What is the prognosis?**

Based on Ranson's criteria

**What are Ranson's criteria for the following stages:**
  **At presentation?**

1. Age >55
2. WBC >16,000
3. Glc >200
4. AST >250
5. LDH >350

  **During the initial 48 hours?**

1. Base deficit >4
2. BUN increase >5 mg/dL
3. Fluid sequestration >6 L
4. Serum $Ca^{2+}$ <8
5. Hct decrease >10%
6. $PO_2$ (ABG) <60 mm Hg
   (Amylase value is NOT one of Ranson's
   criteria!)

**What is the mortality per positive criteria:**

| | |
|---|---|
| **0 to 2?** | Less than 5% |
| **3 to 4?** | Approximately 15% |
| **5 to 6?** | Approximately 40% |
| **7 to 8?** | Approximately 100% |

**How can the admission Ranson criteria be remembered?**

"GA LAW (Georgia law)":
**G**lucose >200
**A**ge >55

**L**DH >350
**A**ST >250
**W**BC >16,000
("Don't mess with the pancreas and don't mess with the Georgia law.")

**How can Ranson's criteria at less than 48 hours be remembered?**

"C HOBBS (Calvin and Hobbes)":
**C**alcium <8 mg/dL

**H**ct drop of >10%
**O**2 <60 (PaO2)
**B**ase deficit >4
**B**un >5 increase
**S**equestration >6 L

**How can the AST versus LDH values in Ranson's criteria be remembered?**

Alphabetically: A before L and 250 before 350
Therefore, AST >250 and LDH >350

**What is the etiology of hypocalcemia with pancreatitis?**

Fat saponification: fat necrosis binds to calcium

**What complication is associated with splenic vein thrombosis?**

Gastric varices (treatment with splenectomy)

**Can TPN with lipids be given to a patient with pancreatitis?**

Yes, if the patient does not suffer from hyperlipidemia (triglycerides <300)

**What is the least common cause of acute pancreatitis (and possibly the most commonly asked cause on rounds!)**

Scorpion bite (found on the island of Trinidad)

## CHRONIC PANCREATITIS

| | |
|---|---|
| **What is it?** | Chronic inflammation of the pancreas region causing destruction of the parenchyma, fibrosis, and calcification, resulting in loss of endocrine and exocrine tissue |
| **What are the subtypes?** | 1. Chronic calcific pancreatitis<br>2. Chronic obstructive pancreatitis (5%) |
| **What are the causes?** | Alcohol abuse (most common; 70% of cases)<br>Idiopathic (15%)<br>Hypercalcemia (hyperparathyroidism)<br>Hyperlipidemia<br>Familial (found in families without any other risk factors)<br>Trauma<br>Iatrogenic<br>Gallstones |
| **What are the symptoms?** | Epigastric and/or back pain, weight loss, steatorrhea |
| **What are the associated signs?** | Type 1 diabetes mellitus (up to one-third)<br>Steatorrhea (up to one-fourth), weight loss |
| **What are the signs of pancreatic exocrine insufficiency?** | Steatorrhea (fat malabsorption from lipase insufficiency—stools float in water)<br>Malnutrition |
| **What are the signs of pancreatic endocrine insufficiency?** | Diabetes (glucose intolerance) |
| **What are the common pain patterns?** | Unrelenting pain<br>Recurrent pain |
| **What is the differential diagnosis?** | PUD, biliary tract disease, AAA, pancreatic cancer, angina |
| **What percentage of patients with chronic pancreatitis have or will develop pancreatic cancer?** | Approximately 2% |

| | |
|---|---|
| **What are the appropriate lab tests?** | Amylase/lipase<br>72-hour fecal fat analysis<br>Glc tolerance test (IDDM) |
| **Why may amylase/lipase be normal in a patient with chronic pancreatitis?** | Because of extensive pancreatic tissue loss ("burned-out pancreas") |
| **What radiographic tests should be performed?** | CT—Has greatest sensitivity for gland enlargement/atrophy, calcifications, masses, pseudocysts<br>KUB—Calcification in the pancreas<br>ERCP—Ductal irregularities with dilation and stenosis (Chain of Lakes), pseudocysts |
| **What is the medical treatment?** | Discontinuation of alcohol use—can reduce attacks, though parenchymal damage continues secondary to ductal obstruction and fibrosis<br>Insulin for type 1 diabetes mellitus<br>Pancreatic enzyme replacement<br>Narcotics for pain (watch for addiction) |
| **What is the surgical treatment?** | Puestow—longitudinal pancreaticojejunostomy (pancreatic duct **must be dilated**)<br>Duval—distal pancreaticojejunostomy<br>Near-total pancreatectomy |
| **What is the Frey procedure?** | Longitudinal pancreaticojejunostomy with core resection of the pancreatic head |
| **What is the indication for surgical treatment of chronic pancreatitis?** | Severe, prolonged/refractory pain |
| **What are the possible complications of chronic pancreatitis?** | Insulin dependent diabetes mellitus<br>Steatorrhea<br>Malnutrition<br>Biliary obstruction<br>Splenic vein thrombosis<br>Gastric varices |

Pancreatic pseudocyst/abscess
Narcotic addiction
Pancreatic ascites/pleural effusion
Splenic artery aneurysm

## GALLSTONE PANCREATITIS

| | |
|---|---|
| **What is it?** | Acute pancreatitis from a gallstone in or passing through the ampulla of Vater (the exact mechanism is unknown) |
| **How is the diagnosis made?** | Acute pancreatitis and cholelithiasis and/or choledocholithiasis and no other cause of pancreatitis (e.g., no history of alcohol abuse) |
| **What radiologic tests should be performed?** | U/S to look for gallstones<br>CT to look at the pancreas, if symptoms are severe |
| **What is the treatment?** | Conservative measures and early interval cholecystectomy (laparoscopic cholecystectomy or open cholecystectomy) and intraoperative cholangiogram (IOC) 3 to 5 days (after pancreatic inflammation resolves) |
| **Why should early interval cholecystectomy be performed on patients with gallstone pancreatitis?** | Pancreatitis will recur in approximately 33% of patients within 8 weeks (so always perform early interval cholecystectomy and IOC in 3 to 5 days when pancreatitis resolves). |
| **What is the role of ERCP?** | 1. Cholangitis<br>2. Refractory choledocholithiasis |

## HEMORRHAGIC PANCREATITIS

| | |
|---|---|
| **What is it?** | Bleeding into the parenchyma and retroperitoneal structures with extensive pancreatic necrosis |
| **What are the signs?** | Abdominal pain, shock/ARDS, Cullen's sign, Grey Turner's sign, Fox's sign |

**Define the following terms:**

| | |
|---|---|
| Cullen's sign | **Bluish discoloration of the periumbilical area** from retroperitoneal hemorrhage tracking around to the anterior abdominal wall through fascial planes |
| Grey Turner's sign | **Ecchymosis or discoloration of the flank** in patients with retroperitoneal hemorrhage from dissecting blood from the retroperitoneum (think: Grey Turner = turn side to side = flank [side] hematoma) |
| Fox's sign | **Ecchymosis of the inguinal ligament** from blood tracking from the retroperitoneum and collecting at the inguinal ligament |

**What are the significant lab values?**

Increased amylase/lipase
Decreased Hct
Decreased calcium levels

**What radiologic test should be performed?**

CT scan with IV contrast

## PANCREATIC ABSCESS

**What is it?**

Infected peripancreatic purulent fluid collection

**What are the signs/ symptoms?**

Fever, unresolving pancreatitis, epigastric mass

**What radiographic tests should be performed?**

Abdominal CT with needle aspiration → send for Gram stain/culture

**What are the associated lab findings?**

Positive Gram stain and culture of bacteria

**Which organisms are found in pancreatic abscesses?**

Gram negative (most common):
  *Escherichia coli, Pseudomonas, Klebsiella*
Gram positive: *Staphylococcus aureus, Candida*

| | |
|---|---|
| **What is the treatment?** | Antibiotics and percutaneous drain placement or operative debridement and placement of drains |

## PANCREATIC NECROSIS

| | |
|---|---|
| **What is it?** | Dead pancreatic tissue, usually following acute pancreatitis |
| **How is the diagnosis made?** | Abdominal CT with IV contrast; dead pancreatic tissue does not take up IV contrast and is not enhanced on CT scan (i.e., doesn't "light up") |
| **What is the treatment?** | Surgical debridement and drain placement IF there is infected necrosis or patient is severely ill and refractory to medical management |

## PANCREATIC PSEUDOCYST

| | |
|---|---|
| **What is it?** | Encapsulated collection of pancreatic fluid |

**Non-communicating pseudocyst**

**Communicating pseudocyst**

hrf '07

| | |
|---|---|
| **What makes it a "pseudo" cyst?** | Wall is formed by inflammatory fibrosis, NOT epithelial cell lining |
| **What is the incidence?** | Approximately 1 in 10 after alcoholic pancreatitis |
| **What are the associated risk factors?** | Acute pancreatitis < chronic pancreatitis from alcohol |

**What is the most common cause of pancreatic pseudocyst in the United States?**

Chronic alcoholic pancreatitis

**What are the symptoms?**

Epigastric pain/mass
Emesis
Mild fever
Weight loss
Should be suspected when a patient with acute pancreatitis fails to resolve pain

**What are the signs?**

Palpable epigastric mass, tender epigastrium, ileus

**What lab tests should be performed?**

Amylase/lipase
Bilirubin
CBC

**What are the diagnostic findings?**

Lab—High amylase, leukocytosis, high bilirubin (if there is obstruction)
U/S—Fluid-filled mass
CT—Fluid-filled mass, good for showing multiple cysts
ERCP—Radiopaque contrast material fills cyst if there is a communicating pseudocyst (i.e., pancreatic duct communicates with pseudocyst)

**What is the differential diagnosis of a pseudocyst?**

Cystadenocarcinoma, cystadenoma

**What are the possible complications of a pancreatic pseudocyst?**

Infection, bleeding into the cyst, fistula, pancreatic ascites, gastric outlet obstruction, SBO, biliary obstruction

**What is the treatment?**

Drainage of the cyst or observation

**What is the waiting period before a pseudocyst should be drained?**

It takes 6 weeks for pseudocyst walls to "mature" or become firm enough to hold sutures and most will resolve in this period of time if they are going to.

| | |
|---|---|
| **What percentage of pseudocysts resolve spontaneously?** | Approximately 50% |
| **What is the treatment for pseudocyst with bleeding into cyst?** | Angiogram amd embolization |
| **What is the treatment for pseudocyst with infection?** | Percutaneous external drainage/IV antibiotics |
| **What size pseudocyst should be drained?** | Most experts say: Pseudocysts larger than 5 cm have a small chance of resolving and have a higher chance of complications Calcified cyst wall Thick cyst wall |
| **What are two treatment options for pancreatic pseudocyst?** | 1. Percutaneous aspiration/drain 2. Operative drainage |
| **What are the surgical options for the following conditions:** | |
| **Pseudocyst adherent to the stomach?** | Cystogastrostomy (drain into the stomach) |
| **Pseudocyst adherent to the duodenum?** | Cystoduodenostomy (drain into the duodenum) |
| **Pseudocyst not adherent to the stomach or duodenum?** | Roux-en-Y cystojejunostomy (drain into the Roux limb of the jejunum) |
| **Pseudocyst in the tail of the pancreas?** | Resection of the pancreatic tail with the pseudocyst |
| **What is the other endoscopic option for drainage of a pseudocyst?** | **Endoscopic** cystogastrostomy |
| **What must be done during a surgical drainage procedure for a pancreatic pseudocyst?** | **Biopsy** of the cyst wall to rule out a cystic carcinoma (e.g., cystadenocarcinoma) |

**What is the most common cause of death due to pancreatic pseudocyst?**

Massive hemorrhage into the pseudocyst

## PANCREATIC CARCINOMA

**What is it?**

Adenocarcinoma of the pancreas arising from duct cells

**What are the associated risk factors?**

**Smoking** 3× **risk,** diabetes mellitus, heavy alcohol use, chronic pancreatitis, diet high in fried meats, previous gastrectomy

**What is the male to female ratio?**

3:2

**What is the African-American to white ratio?**

2:1

**What is the average age?**

Older than 60 years

**What are the different types?**

More than 80% are duct cell adenocarcinomas; other types include cystadenocarcinoma and acinar cell carcinoma.

**What percentage arise in the pancreatic head?**

**Two-thirds** arise in the pancreatic **head; one-third** arise in the **body and tail.**

**Why are most pancreatic cancers in the tail nonresectable?**

These tumors grow without symptoms until it is too late and they have already spread—head of the pancreas tumors draw attention earlier because of biliary obstruction.

**What are the signs/ symptoms of tumors based on location:**
    **Head of the pancreas?**

**Painless jaundice** from obstruction of common bile duct; weight loss; abdominal pain; back pain; weakness; **pruritus** from bile salts in skin; anorexia; **Courvoisier's sign;** acholic stools; dark urine; diabetes

| | |
|---|---|
| **Body or tail?** | Weight loss and pain (90%); migratory thrombophlebitis (10%); jaundice (<10%); nausea and vomiting; fatigue |
| **What are the most common symptoms of cancer of the pancreatic HEAD?** | 1. Weight loss (90%)<br>2. Pain (75%)<br>3. Jaundice (70%) |
| **What is "Courvoisier's sign"?** | Palpable, nontender distended gallbladder |
| **What percentage of patients with cancers of the pancreatic HEAD have Courvoisier's sign?** | 33% |
| **What is the classic presentation of pancreatic cancer in the head of the pancreas?** | Painless jaundice |
| **What metastatic lymph node described classically for gastric cancer can be found with metastatic pancreatic cancer?** | Virchow's node; Sister Mary Joseph's nodule |
| **What are the associated lab findings?** | Increased direct bilirubin and alkaline phosphatase (as a result of biliary obstruction)<br>Increased LFTs<br>Elevated pancreatic tumor markers |
| **Which tumor markers are associated with pancreatic cancer?** | CA-19-9 |
| **What does CA-19-9 stand for?** | Carbohydrate Antigen 19-9 |
| **What diagnostic studies are performed?** | Abdominal CT, U/S, cholangiography (ERCP to rule out choledocholithiasis and cell brushings), endoscopic U/S with biopsy |

**What are the pancreatic cancer STAGES:**

**Stage I?**

Tumor is limited to pancreas, with no nodes or metastases.

**Stage II?**

Tumor extends into bile duct, peripancreatic tissues, or duodenum; there are no nodes or metastases.

**Stage III?**

Same findings as stage II plus **positive nodes**

**Stage IVA?**

Tumor extends to stomach, colon, spleen, or major vessels, with any nodal status and no metastases.

**Stage IVB?**

**Distant metastases** (any nodal status, any tumor size) are found.

**What is the treatment based on location:**

**Head of the pancreas?**

Whipple procedure (pancreaticoduodenectomy)

**Body or tail?**

Distal resection

**What factors signify inoperability?**

Vascular encasement (portal vein, SMA), hepatic artery
Liver metastasis
Peritoneal implants
Distant lymph node metastasis (periaortic/celiac nodes)
Distant metastasis

**Should patients undergo preoperative biliary drainage (e.g., ERCP)?**

No (exceptions for symptoms/ preoperative XRT, trials, etc.)

**Define the Whipple procedure (pancreaticoduodenectomy).**

Cholecystectomy
Truncal vagotomy
Antrectomy
Pancreaticoduodenectomy—removal of head of pancreas and duodenum
Choledochojejunostomy—anastomosis of common bile duct to jejunum

Pancreaticojejunostomy—anastomosis of distal pancreas remnant to jejunum
Gastrojejunostomy—anastomosis of stomach to jejunum

**What is the complication rate after a Whipple procedure?**

Approximately 25%

**What mortality rate is associated with a Whipple procedure?**

Approximately 3%

**What is the "pylorus-preserving Whipple"?**

No antrectomy; anastomose duodenum to jejunum

**What are the possible post-Whipple complications?**

Delayed gastric emptying (if antrectomy is performed); **anastomotic leak** (from the bile duct or pancreatic anastomosis), causing pancreatic/biliary fistula; wound infection; postgastrectomy syndromes; sepsis; pancreatitis

**Why must the duodenum be removed if the head of the pancreas is resected?**

They share the same blood supply.

**What is the postoperative adjuvant therapy?**

Chemotherapy

**What is the palliative treatment if the tumor is inoperable and biliary obstruction is present?**

PTC or ERCP and placement of stent across obstruction

**What is the prognosis at 1 year after diagnosis?**

Dismal; 90% of patients die within 1 year of diagnosis

**What is the survival after resection at 5 years?**

Survival rate is 20% at 5 years after resection.

## MISCELLANEOUS

| | |
|---|---|
| **What is an annular pancreas?** | Pancreas encircling the duodenum; if obstruction is present, bypass, **do not resect** |
| **What is pancreatic divisum?** | Failure of the two pancreatic ducts to fuse; the normally small duct (small = **S**antorini) of Santorini acts as the main duct in pancreatic divisum (think: the two pancreatic ducts are **D**ivided = **D**ivisum) |
| **What is heterotopic pancreatic tissue?** | Heterotopic pancreatic tissue usually found in the stomach, intestine, duodenum |
| **What is a Puestow procedure?** | Longitudinal filleting of the pancreas/pancreatic duct with a side-to-side anastomosis with the small bowel |
| **What medication decreases output from a pancreatic fistula?** | Somatostatin (GI-inhibitory hormone) |
| **Which has a longer half life: amylase or lipase?** | Lipase; therefore, amylase may be normal and lipase will remain elevated longer |
| **What is the WDHA syndrome?** | A pancreatic **VIP**oma (**V**asoactive **I**ntestinal **P**olypeptide tumor) Also known as Verner-Morrison syndrome Tumor secretes VIP, which causes: **W**atery **D**iarrhea **H**ypokalemia **A**chlorhydria (inhibits gastric acid secretion) |
| **What is the Whipple triad of pancreatic insulinoma?** | 1. Hypoglycemia (Glc <50) 2. Symptoms of hypoglycemia: mental status changes/vasomotor instability 3. Relief of symptoms with administration of glucose |

| | |
|---|---|
| **What is the most common islet cell tumor?** | Insulinoma |
| **What pancreatic tumor is associated with gallstone formation?** | Somatostatinoma (inhibits gallbladder contraction) |
| **What is the triad found with pancreatic somatostatinoma tumor?** | 1. Gallstones<br>2. Diabetes<br>3. Steatorrhea |
| **What are the two classic findings with pancreatic glucagonoma tumors?** | 1. Diabetes<br>2. Dermatitis/rash (necrotizing migratory erythema) |

# Chapter 56     The Breast

## ANATOMY OF THE BREAST AND AXILLA

| | |
|---|---|
| **Name the boundaries of the axilla for dissection:** | |
|    **Superior boundary** | Axillary vein |
|    **Posterior boundary** | Long thoracic nerve |
|    **Lateral boundary** | Latissimus dorsi muscle |
|    **Medial boundary** | Lateral to, deep to, or medial to pectoral minor muscle, depending on level of nodes taken |
| **What four nerves must the surgeon be aware of during an axillary dissection?** | 1. **Long thoracic nerve**<br>2. **Thoracodorsal nerve**<br>3. Medial pectoral nerve<br>4. Lateral pectoral nerve |

**Describe the location of these nerves and the muscle each innervates:**

**Long thoracic nerve**

Courses along lateral chest wall in midaxillary line on serratus anterior muscle; innervates serratus anterior muscle

**Thoracodorsal nerve**

Courses lateral to long thoracic nerve on latissimus dorsi muscle; innervates latissimus dorsi muscle

**Medial pectoral nerve**

Runs **lateral** to or through the pectoral minor muscle, actually **lateral** to the lateral pectoral nerve; innervates the pectoral minor and pectoral major muscles

**Lateral pectoral nerve**

Runs **medial** to the medial pectoral nerve (names describe orientation from the brachial plexus!); innervates the pectoral major

**Identify the nerves in the axilla on the illustration below.**

1. Thoracodorsal nerve
2. Long thoracic nerve
3. Medial pectoral nerve
4. Lateral pectoral nerve
5. Axillary vein

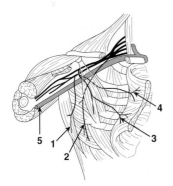

**What is the name of the deformity if you cut the long thoracic nerve in this area?**

"Winged scapula"

**What is the name of the CUTANEOUS nerve that crosses the axilla in a transverse fashion? (Many surgeons try to preserve this nerve.)**

Intercostobrachial nerve

**What is the name of the large vein that marks the upper limit of the axilla?**

Axillary vein

**What is the lymphatic drainage of the breast?**

Lateral: axillary lymph nodes
Medial: parasternal nodes that run with
    internal mammary artery

**What are the levels of axillary lymph nodes?**

Level I (low): lateral to pectoral minor
Level II (middle): deep to pectoral minor
Level III (high): medial to pectoral minor
In breast cancer, a higher level of
    involvement has a worse prognosis,
    but the level of involvement is less
    important than the number of posi-
    tive nodes. (Think: Levels I, II, and
    III are in the same superior–inferior
    anatomic order as the LeFort facial
    fractures and the trauma neck zones;
    *I dare you to forget!*)

**What are Rotter's nodes?**

Nodes between the pectoralis major
and minor muscles; not usually removed
unless they are enlarged or feel
suspicious intraoperatively

**What are the suspensory breast ligaments called?**

Cooper's ligaments

**What is the mammary "milk line"?**

The embryological line from shoulder
to thigh where "supernumerary" breast
areolar and/or nipples can be found

**What is the "tail of Spence"?**

The "tail" of breast tissue that tapers into
the axilla

**Which hormone is mainly responsible for breast milk production?**

Prolactin

## BREAST CANCER

| | |
|---|---|
| **What is the incidence of breast cancer?** | **12% lifetime risk** |
| **What percentage of women with breast cancer have no known risk factor?** | 75%! |
| **What percentage of all breast cancers occur in women younger than 30 years?** | Approximately 2% |
| **What percentage of all breast cancers occur in women older than 70 years?** | 33% |
| **What are the major breast cancer susceptibility genes?** | **BRCA1** and **BRCA2** (easy **BR** = breast and **CA** = cancer) |
| **What is the most common motivation for medicolegal cases involving the breast?** | Failure to diagnose a breast carcinoma |
| **What is the "TRIAD OF ERROR" for misdiagnosed breast cancer?** | 1. Age < 45 years<br>2. Self-diagnosed mass<br>3. Negative mammogram<br>More than 75% of cases of **MISDIAGNOSED** breast cancer have these three characteristics. |
| **What are the history risk factors for breast cancer?** | "N.A.A.C.P.":<br>**N**ulliparity<br>**A**ge at menarche (younger than 13 years)<br>**A**ge at menopause (older than 55 years)<br>**C**ancer of the breast (in self or family)<br>**P**regnancy with first child (older than 30 years) |
| **What are physical/anatomic risk factors for breast cancer?** | "CHAFED LIPS":<br>**C**ancer in the breast (3% synchronous contralateral cancer)<br>**H**yperplasia (moderate/florid) (2 × risk) |

**A**typical hyperplasia (4×)
**F**emale (100 × male risk)
**E**lderly
**D**CIS

**L**CIS
**I**nherited genes (BRCA I and II)
**P**apilloma (1.5×)
**S**clerosing adenosis (1.5×)

**What is the relative risk
of hormone replacement
therapy?**

1–1.5

**Is "run of the mill"
fibrocystic disease a risk
factor for breast cancer?**

No

**What are the possible
symptoms of breast cancer?**

No symptoms
Mass in the breast
Pain **(most are painless)**
Nipple discharge
Local edema
Nipple retraction
Dimple
Nipple rash

**Why does skin retraction
occur?**

Tumor involvement of Cooper's ligaments
and subsequent traction on ligaments
pull skin inward.

**What are the signs of breast
cancer?**

Mass (1 cm is usually the smallest lesion
    that can be palpated on examination)
Dimple
Nipple rash
Edema
Axillary/supraclavicular nodes

**What is the most common
site of breast cancer?**

Approximately one-half of cancers
develop in the upper outer quadrants.

**What are the major types
of invasive carcinoma?**

Invasive ductal carcinoma (90%)
Invasive lobular carcinoma (10%)
Inflammatory carcinoma

**What is the most common type of breast cancer?**

Infiltrating ductal carcinoma

**What is the differential diagnosis?**

Fibrocystic disease of the breast
Fibroadenoma
Intraductal papilloma
Duct ectasia
Fat necrosis
Abscess
Radial scar
Simple cyst

**Describe the appearance of the edema of the dermis in inflammatory carcinoma of the breast.**

Peau d'orange (orange peel)

**What are the screening recommendations for breast cancer:**

**Breast exam recommendations?**

Self-exam of breasts monthly
Ages 20 to 40 years: breast exam every 2 to 3 years by a physician
Older than 40 years: Annual breast exam by physician

**Mammograms?**

Recommendations are controversial, but most experts say:
Baseline mammogram between 35 and 40 years
Mammogram every year or every other year for ages 40 to 50
Mammogram yearly after age 50

**When is the best time for breast self-exams?**

One week after menstrual period

**Why is mammography a more useful diagnostic tool in older women than in younger?**

Breast tissue undergoes fatty replacement with age, making masses more visible. Younger women have more fibrous tissue, which makes mammograms harder to interpret.

**What are the radiographic tests for breast cancer?**

Mammography and breast ultrasound, MRI

**What is the classic picture of breast cancer on mammogram?**

Spiculated mass

**Which option is best to evaluate a breast mass in a woman younger than 30 years?**

Breast ultrasound

**What are the methods for obtaining tissue for pathologic examination?**

Fine needle aspiration (FNA), core biopsy (larger needle core sample), mammotome stereotactic biopsy, and open biopsy. Open biopsy can be incisional (cutting a **piece** of the mass) or excisional (cutting out the **entire** mass).

**What are the indications for biopsy?**

Persistent mass after aspiration
Solid mass
Blood in cyst aspirate
Suspicious lesion by mammography/U/S/ MRI
Bloody nipple discharge
Ulcer or dermatitis of nipple
Patient's concern of persistent breast abnormality

**What is the process for performing a biopsy when a nonpalpable mass is seen on mammogram?**

Stereotactic (mammotome) biopsy or needle localization biopsy

**What is a needle loc biopsy (NLB)?**

Needle localization by radiologist, followed by biopsy. Removed breast tissue must be checked by mammogram to ensure all of the suspicious lesion has been excised.

**What is a mammotome biopsy?**

Mammogram-guided computerized stereotatic core biopsies (mammatome)

**What is obtained first, the mammogram or the biopsy?**

The mammogram is obtained first; otherwise, tissue extraction (core or open) may alter the mammographic findings. (Fine needle aspiration may be done prior to the mammogram because the fine needle usually will not affect the mammographic findings.)

**What would be suspicious mammographic findings?**

Mass, microcalcifications, stellate/ spiculated mass

**What is the "workup" for a breast mass?**

1. Clinical breast exam
2. Mammogram or breast ultrasound
3. Fine needle aspiration, core biopsy, or open biopsy

**How do you proceed if the mass appears to be a cyst?**

Aspirate it with a needle.

**Is the fluid from a breast cyst sent for cytology?**

Not routinely; bloody fluid should be sent for cytology

**When do you proceed to open biopsy for a breast cyst?**

1. In the case of a second cyst recurrence
2. Bloody fluid in the cyst
3. Palpable mass after aspiration

**What is the preoperative staging workup in a patient with breast cancer?**

Bilateral mammogram (cancer in one breast is a risk factor for cancer in the contralateral breast!)
CXR (to check for lung metastasis)
LFTs (to check for liver metastasis)
Serum calcium level, alkaline phosphatase. (If these tests indicate bone metastasis/"bone pain" proceed to bone scan.)
Other tests, depending on signs/ symptoms (e.g., head CT if patient has focal neurologic deficit, to look for brain metastasis)

**What hormone receptors must be checked for in the biopsy specimen?**

**Estrogen and progesterone receptors.** This is **key for determining adjuvant treatment.** This information must be obtained on all specimens (including fine needle aspirates).

| | |
|---|---|
| **What staging system is used for breast cancer?** | TMN: tumor/metastases/nodes (AJCC) |

**Describe the staging (simplified):**

| | |
|---|---|
| **Stage I** | Tumor ≤2 cm in diameter without metastases, **no nodes** |
| **Stage IIA** | Tumor ≤2 cm in diameter with mobile axillary nodes **or** <br> Tumor 2 to 5 cm in diameter, no nodes |
| **Stage IIB** | Tumor 2 to 5 cm in diameter with mobile axillary nodes **or** <br> Tumor larger than 5 cm **with no nodes** |
| **Stage IIIA** | Tumor larger than 5 cm with mobile axillary nodes **or** <br> Any size tumor with **fixed** axillary nodes, no metastases |
| **Stage IIIB** | Peau d'orange (skin edema) or <br> Chest wall invasion/fixation or <br> Inflammatory cancer or <br> Breast skin ulceration or <br> Breast skin satellite metastases or <br> Any tumor and + ipsilateral **internal mammary** lymph nodes |
| **Stage IV** | **Distant metastases** (including ipsilateral supraclavicular nodes) |

| | |
|---|---|
| **What are the sites of metastases?** | Lymph nodes (most common) <br> Lung/pleura <br> Liver <br> Bones <br> Brain |
| **What are the major treatments of breast cancer?** | Modified radical mastectomy <br> Lumpectomy and radiation <br> (Both treatments either with or without postop chemotherapy/tamoxifen) |
| **What are the indications for modified radical postmastectomy radiation therapy?** | 1. >4 lymph nodes, **plus** <br> 2. Chest wall involvement by tumor |

**What breast carcinomas are candidates for lumpectomy and radiation?**

Stage I and stage II (tumors <5 cm)

**What is the treatment of inflammatory carcinoma of the breast?**

**Chemotherapy first!** Then often followed by radiation, mastectomy, or both

**What is a lumpectomy and radiation?**

Lumpectomy (segmental mastectomy: removal of a **part** of the breast); axillary node dissection; and course of radiation therapy **after** operation, over a period of several weeks

**What is the major absolute contraindication to lumpectomy and radiation?**

Pregnancy

**What are other contraindications to lumpectomy and radiation?**

Previous radiation to the chest
Positive margins
Collagen vascular disease
Extensive DCIS (often seen as diffuse microcalcification)
**Relative contraindications:**
Lesion that cannot be seen on the mammograms (i.e., early recurrence will be missed on follow-up mammograms)
Very small breast (no cosmetic advantage)

**What is a modified radical mastectomy?**

Breast, axillary nodes (level II, I), and nipple–areolar complex are removed.
Pectoralis major and minor muscles are **not** removed (Auchincloss modification).
Drains are placed to drain lymph fluid.

**Where are the drains placed with an MRM?**

1. Axilla
2. Chest wall (breast bed)

**When should the drains be removed?**

<30 cc/day drainage

**What are the potential complications after a modified radical mastectomy?**

Ipsilateral arm lymphedema, infection, and injury to nerves, skin flap necrosis, hematoma/seroma, phantom breast syndrome

**During an axillary dissection, should the patient be paralyzed?**

NO, because the nerves (long thoracic/ thoracodorsal) are stimulated with resultant muscle contraction to help identify them

**How can the long thoracic and thoracodorsal nerves be identified during an axillary dissection?**

The nerves can be stimulated with a forceps, which results in contraction of the latissimus dorsi (thoracodorsal nerve) or anterior serratus (long thoracic nerve).

**When do you remove the drains after an axillary dissection?**

When there is less than 30 cc of drainage per day, or on postoperative day 14 (whichever comes first)

**What is a "sentinel" node biopsy?**

Instead of removing all the axillary lymph nodes, the **primary** draining or "sentinel" lymph node is removed.

**How is the "sentinel" lymph node found?**

Inject blue dye or technetium-labeled sulfur colloid

**What follows a positive sentinel node biopsy?**

Removal of the rest of the axillary lymph nodes

**What do you do with a mammotome biopsy that returns as "atypical hyperplasia"?**

Open needle loc biopsy as many will have DCIS or invasive cancer

**How does tamoxifen work?**

It binds estrogen receptors.

**What is the treatment for local recurrence in breast after lumpectomy and radiation?**

"Salvage" mastectomy (axillary dissection already completed)

**Can tamoxifen prevent breast cancer?**

**Yes.** In the Breast Cancer Prevention Trial of 13,000 women, tamoxifen reduced the risk of breast cancer by 50% in women who had a 1.7% 5-year risk of developing breast cancer.

**What are common options for breast reconstruction?**

TRAM flap, implant, latissimus dorsi flap

**What is a TRAM flap?**

Transverse Rectus Abdominis Myocutaneous flap

**What are side effects of tamoxifen?**

**Endometrial cancer** (2.5 relative risk), DVT, pulmonary embolus, cataracts, hot flashes, mood swings

**In high-risk women, is there a way to reduce the risk of developing breast cancer?**

Yes, tamoxifen for 5 years will lower the risk by up to 50%. But with an increased risk of endometrial cancer and clots, it must be an individual patient determination.

**Give the common adjuvant therapy for the following patients with breast cancer. (These are rough guidelines; check for current guidelines, as they are always changing.) (ER = estrogen receptor):**

    **Premenopausal, node +, ER −**

Chemotherapy

    **Premenopausal, node +, ER +**

Chemotherapy and tamoxifen

| | |
|---|---|
| **Premenopausal, node –, ER +** | Tamoxifen |
| **Postmenopausal, node +, ER +** | Tamoxifen, +/– chemotherapy |
| **Postmenopausal, node +, ER –** | Chemotherapy, +/– tamoxifen |
| **What type of chemotherapy is usually used for breast cancer?** | CMF (cyclophosphamide, methotrexate, 5-fluorouracil) or CAF (cyclophosphamide, Adriamycin, 5-fluorouracil) |
| **Chemotherapy for high-risk tumors with negative lymph nodes should be considered. What makes a tumor "HIGH RISK"?** | High risk: > 2 cm in size Lymphatic/vascular invasion Nuclear grade (high) S phase (high) ER negative |

## DCIS

| | |
|---|---|
| **What does DCIS stand for?** | **D**uctal **C**arcinoma **I**n **S**itu |
| **What is DCIS also known as?** | Intraductal carcinoma |
| **Describe DCIS.** | Cancer cells in the duct without invasion (in situ: cells do not penetrate the basement membrane) |
| **What are the signs/symptoms?** | Usually none; usually nonpalpable |
| **What are the mammographic findings?** | Microcalcifications |
| **How is the diagnosis made?** | Core or open biopsy |
| **What is the most aggressive histologic type?** | Comedo |
| **What is the risk of lymph node metastasis with DCIS?** | Less than 2% (usually when microinvasion is seen) |
| **What is the major risk with DCIS?** | Subsequent development of infiltrating ductal carcinoma in the **same breast** |

**What is the treatment for DCIS in the following cases:**

**Tumor less than 1 cm (low grade)?**

Remove with 1 cm margins +/− XRT

**Tumor >1 cm?**

Perform lumpectomy with 1 cm margins and radiation **or** total mastectomy (**no** axillary dissection).

**What is a total (simple) mastectomy?**

Removal of the breast and nipple without removal of the axillary nodes (always remove nodes with invasive cancer)

**When must a simple mastectomy be performed for DCIS?**

Diffuse breast involvement (e.g., diffuse microcalcifications), >1 cm and contraindication to radiation

**What is the role of axillary node dissection with DCIS?**

No role in true DCIS (i.e., without micro-invasion); some perform a sentinel lymph node dissection for high-grade DCIS

**What is adjuvant for DCIS?**

1. Tamoxifen
2. Postlumpectomy XRT

**What is the role of tamoxifen in DCIS?**

Tamoxifen for 5 years will lower the risk up to 50%, but with increased risk of endometrial cancer and clots; it must be an individual patient determination.

**What is a memory aid for the breast in which DCIS breast cancer arises?**

Cancer arises in the **same** breast as DCIS. (Think: **DCIS** = **D**irectly in same breast)

## LCIS

**What is LCIS?**

**L**obular **C**arcinoma **I**n **S**itu (carcinoma cells in the lobules of the breast without invasion)

**What are the signs/symptoms?**

There are none.

**What are the mammographic findings?**

There are none.

**How is the diagnosis made?**

LCIS is found **incidentally** on biopsy.

**What is the major risk?**

Carcinoma of **either** breast

**Which breast is most at risk for developing an invasive carcinoma?**

Equal risk in both breasts! (Think of LCIS as a **risk marker** for future development of cancer in either breast.)

**What percentage of women with LCIS develop an invasive breast carcinoma?**

About 30% in the 20 years after diagnosis of LCIS!

**What type of invasive breast cancer do patients with LCIS develop?**

Most commonly, **infiltrating ductal carcinoma, with equal distribution** in the contralateral and ipsilateral breasts

**What medication may lower the risk of developing breast cancer in LCIS?**

Tamoxifen for 5 years will lower the risk up to 50%, but with an increased risk of endometrial cancer and clots; it must be an individual patient determination.

**What is the treatment of LCIS?**

Close follow-up (or bilateral simple mastectomy in high-risk patients)

**What is the major difference in the subsequent development of invasive breast cancer with DCIS and LCIS?**

LCIS cancer develops in *either* breast; DCIS cancer develops in the ipsilateral breast.

**What is the most common cause of bloody nipple discharge in a young woman?**

Intraductal papilloma

**What is the most common breast tumor in patients younger than 30 years?**

Fibroadenoma

**What is Paget's disease of the breast?**

Scaling rash/dermatitis of the nipple caused by invasion of skin by cells from a ductal carcinoma

**What are the common options for breast reconstruction after a mastectomy?**

Saline implant
TRAM flap

| | |
|---|---|
| **What is a memory aid for which breast LCIS breast cancer can arise?** | Think: **LCIS** = **L**iberally **i**n **e**ither breast |

## MALE BREAST CANCER

| | |
|---|---|
| **What is the incidence of breast cancer in men?** | <1% of all breast cancer cases (1/150) |
| **What is the average age at diagnosis?** | 65 years of age |
| **What are the risk factors?** | Increased estrogen<br>Radiation<br>Gynecomastia from increased estrogen<br>Estrogen therapy<br>Klinefelter's syndrome (XXY)<br>BRCA2 carriers |
| **What type of breast cancer do men develop?** | Nearly 100% of cases are ductal carcinoma. (Men do not usually have breast lobules.) |
| **What are the signs/ symptoms of breast cancer in men?** | Breast mass (most are painless), breast skin changes (ulcers, retraction), and nipple discharge (usually blood or a blood-tinged discharge) |
| **What is the most common presentation?** | Painless breast mass |
| **How is breast cancer in men diagnosed?** | Biopsy and mammogram |
| **What is the treatment?** | 1. Mastectomy<br>2. Sentinel LN dissection of clinically negative axilla<br>3. Axillary dissection if clinically positive axillary LN |

## BENIGN BREAST DISEASE

| | |
|---|---|
| **What is the most common cause of green, straw-colored, or brown nipple discharge?** | Fibrocystic disease |

| | |
|---|---|
| **What is the most common cause of breast mass after breast trauma?** | Fat necrosis |
| **What is Mondor's disease?** | Thrombophlebitis of superficial breast veins |
| **What must be ruled out with spontaneous galactorrhea (+/– amenorrhea)?** | Prolactinoma (check pregnancy test and prolactin level) |

## CYSTOSARCOMA PHYLLODES

| | |
|---|---|
| **What is it?** | It is a mesenchymal tumor arising from breast lobular tissue; most are benign. "Sarcoma" is a misnomer, as the vast majority are benign (1% of breast cancers) |
| **What is the usual age of the patient with this tumor?** | Older than 30 years (usually older than the patient with fibroadenoma; 35–55 years of age) |
| **What are the signs/ symptoms?** | Mobile, smooth breast mass that resembles a fibroadenoma on exam, mammogram/ultrasound |
| **How is it diagnosed?** | Through core biopsy or excision |
| **What is the treatment?** | If benign, wide local excision; if malignant, simple total mastectomy |
| **What is the role of axillary dissection with cystosarcoma phyllodes tumor?** | Only if clinically palpable axillary nodes, as the malignant form rarely spreads to nodes (most common site of metastasis is the lung) |
| **Is there a role for chemotherapy with cystosarcoma phyllodes?** | Consider chemotherapy if large tumor >5 cm and "stromal overgrowth" |

## FIBROADENOMA

| | |
|---|---|
| **What is it?** | Benign tumor of the breast consisting of stromal overgrowth, collagen arranged in "swirls" |

| | |
|---|---|
| **What is the clinical presentation of a fibroadenoma?** | A solid, mobile, **well-circumscribed** round breast mass, usually <40 years of age |
| **How is fibroadenoma diagnosed?** | Negative needle aspiration looking for fluid; ultrasound; core biopsy |
| **What is the treatment?** | Surgical resection for large or growing lesions; small fibroadenomas can be observed closely |
| **What is this "tumor's" claim to fame?** | It is the most common breast tumor in women younger than 30 years. |

## FIBROCYSTIC DISEASE

| | |
|---|---|
| **What is it?** | A common benign breast condition consisting of fibrous (rubbery) and cystic changes in the breast |
| **What are the signs/ symptoms?** | Breast pain or tenderness that varies with the menstrual cycle; cysts; and fibrous ("nodular") fullness |
| **How is it diagnosed?** | Through breast exam, history, and aspirated cysts (usually straw-colored or green fluid) |
| **What is the treatment for symptomatic fibrocystic disease?** | **Stop caffeine**<br>Pain medications (NSAIDs)<br>Vitamin E, evening primrose oil (danazol and OCP as last resort) |
| **What is done if the patient has a breast cyst?** | Needle drainage: if aspirate is bloody or a palpable mass remains after aspiration, an open biopsy is performed. If the aspirate is straw-colored or green, the patient is followed closely; then, if there is recurrence, a second aspiration is performed. A re-recurrence usually requires open biopsy. |

## MASTITIS

| | |
|---|---|
| **What is it?** | Superficial infection of the breast (cellulitis) |
| **In what circumstance does it most often occur?** | Breast-feeding |
| **What bacteria are most commonly the cause?** | *Staphylococcus aureus* |
| **How is mastitis treated?** | Stop breast-feeding and use a breast pump instead; apply heat; administer antibiotics |
| **Why must the patient with mastitis have close follow-up?** | To make sure that she does not have inflammatory breast cancer! |

## BREAST ABSCESS

| | |
|---|---|
| **What are the causes?** | Mammary ductal ectasia (stenosis of breast duct) and mastitis |
| **What is the most common bacteria?** | Nursing = *Staphylococcus aureus* Nonlactating = mixed infection |
| **What is the treatment of breast abscess?** | Antibiotics (e.g., dicloxacillin) Needle or open drainage with cultures taken Resection of involved ducts if recurrent Breast pump if breast-feeding |
| **What is lactational mastitis?** | Infection of the breast during breast-feeding—most commonly caused by **S. aureus.** Treat with antibiotics and follow for abscess formation. |
| **What must be ruled out with a breast abscess in a nonlactating woman?** | Breast cancer! |

## MALE GYNECOMASTIA

| | |
|---|---|
| **What is it?** | Enlargement of the male breast |
| **What are the causes?** | **Medications** Illicit drugs (marijuana) |

Liver failure
Increased estrogen
Decreased testosterone

**What is the major
differential diagnosis in the
older patient?**

Male breast cancer

**What is the treatment?**

Stop or change medications; correct
underlying cause if there is a hormonal
imbalance; and perform biopsy or
subcutaneous mastectomy (i.e., leave
nipple) if refractory to conservative
measures and time.

# Chapter 57     Endocrine

## ADRENAL GLAND

### ANATOMY

**Where is the drainage of the
*left* adrenal vein?**

Left renal vein

**Where is the drainage of the
*right* adrenal vein?**

Inferior vena cava (IVC)

### NORMAL ADRENAL PHYSIOLOGY

**What is CRH?**

**Corticotropin-releasing hormone:**
released from anterior hypothalamus and
causes release of ACTH from anterior
pituitary

**What is ACTH?**

**AdrenoCorticoTropic hormone:**
released normally by anterior pituitary,
which in turn causes adrenal gland to
release cortisol

**What feeds back to inhibit
ACTH secretion?**

Cortisol

## CUSHING'S SYNDROME

| | |
|---|---|
| **What is Cushing's syndrome?** | Excessive **cortisol** production (think: **C**ushing's-**C**ortisol) |
| **What is the most common cause?** | Iatrogenic (i.e., prescribed prednisone) |
| **What is the second most common cause?** | Cushing's disease (most common noniatrogenic cause) |
| **What is Cushing's disease?** | Cushing's syndrome caused by excess production of ACTH by anterior **pituitary** |
| **What is an ectopic ACTH source?** | A tumor not found in the pituitary that secretes ACTH, which in turn causes adrenal gland to release cortisol without the normal negative feedback loop |
| **What are the signs/ symptoms of Cushing's syndrome?** | Truncal obesity, hirsutism, "moon" facies, acne, "buffalo hump," purple striae, hypertension, diabetes, weakness, depression, easy bruising, myopathy |
| **How can cortisol levels be indirectly measured over a short duration?** | By measuring urine cortisol or the breakdown product of cortisol, 17-hydroxycorticosteroid (**17-OHCS**), in the urine |
| **What is a direct test of serum cortisol?** | Serum cortisol level (highest in the morning and lowest at night in healthy patients) |
| **What initial tests should be performed in Cushing's syndrome?** | Electrolytes<br>Serum cortisol<br>Urine-free cortisol, urine 17-OHCS<br>Low-dose dexamethasone suppression test |
| **What is the low-dose dexamethasone suppression test?** | Dexamethasone is a synthetic cortisol that results in negative feedback on ACTH secretion and subsequent cortisol secretion in healthy patients. Patients with **Cushing's syndrome** do **not** suppress their cortisol secretion. |
| **After the dexamethasone test, what is next?** | Check ACTH levels |

**Can plasma ACTH levels be checked directly?**

Yes

**What is the work up in a patient suspected of having Cushing's syndrome?**

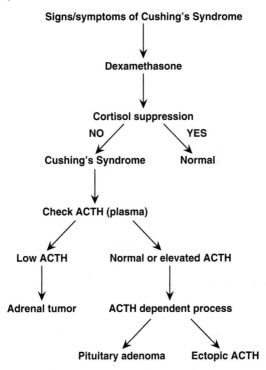

**In ACTH-dependent Cushing's syndrome, how do you differentiate between a pituitary vs. an ectopic ACTH source?**

High dose dexamethasone test:
**Pituitary source**—Cortisol is suppressed
**Ectopic ACTH source**—No cortisol suppression

**Summarize the "Cushing's syndrome" lab values found in the majority of patients with the following conditions:**

**Healthy patients**

Normal cortisol and ACTH, suppression with low-dose or high-dose dexamethasone (<1/2)

| | |
|---|---|
| **Cushing's disease (pituitary ACTH hypersecretion)** | High cortisol and ACTH, no suppression with low-dose dexamethasone, suppression with high-dose dexamethasone |
| **Adrenal tumor** | High cortisol, low ACTH, no suppression with low-dose or high-dose dexamethasone |
| **Ectopic ACTH-producing tumor** | High cortisol and ACTH, no suppression with low-dose or high-dose dexamethasone |

**What is the most common site of ectopic ACTH-producing tumor?**

More than two-thirds are oat cell tumors of the lung (#2 is carcinoid)

**How are the following tumors treated:**

**Adrenal adenoma?**

Adrenalectomy (almost always **unilateral**)

**Adrenal carcinoma?**

Surgical excision (only one-third of cases are operable)

**Ectopic ACTH-producing tumor?**

Surgical excision, if feasible

**Cushing's *disease*?**

Transphenoidal adenomectomy

**What medication must be given to a patient who is undergoing surgical correction of Cushing's syndrome?**

Cortisol (usually hydrocortisone until PO is resumed)

**Give the mechanism of action:**

**Ketoconazole (an antifungal)**

Inhibits 11 beta-hydroxylase, c17-20 lyase, and cholesterol side chain cleavage

**Aminoglutethimide (an anticonvulsant)**

Inhibits cleavage of cholesterol side chains

| | |
|---|---|
| **Mitotane** | Inhibits 11 beta-hydroxylase and cholesterol side chain cleavage; causes irreversible adrenocortical cells (and thus can be used for "medical adrenalectomy") |
| **Metyrapone** | Inhibits 11 beta-hydroxylase |

**What medications inhibit cortisol production?**

1. Ketoconazole
2. Metyrapone
3. Aminoglutethimide
4. Mitotane

**What is a complication of BILATERAL adrenalectomy?**

Nelson's syndrome—occurs in 10% of patients after bilateral adrenalectomy

**What is Nelson's syndrome?**

Functional pituitary adenoma producing excessive ACTH and mass effect producing visual disturbances, hyperpigmentation, amenorrhea, with elevated ACTH levels

Think: **N**elson = **N**uclear reaction in the pituitary

## ADRENAL INCIDENTALOMA

**What is an incidentaloma?**

A tumor found in the adrenal gland **incidentally** on a CT scan performed for an unrelated reason

**What is the incidence of incidentalomas?**

4% of all CTs (9% of autopsies)

**What is the most common cause of incidentaloma?**

Nonfunctioning adenoma (>75% of cases)

**What is the differential diagnosis of incidentaloma?**

Nonfunctioning adenoma
Pheochromocytoma
Adrenocortical carcinoma
Aldosteronoma
Metastatic diagnosis
Nodular hyperplasia

**What is the risk factor for carcinoma?**

Solid tumor more than 6 cm in diameter

**What is the treatment?**

Controversial for smaller/medium-sized tumors, but almost all surgeons would agree that resection is indicated for solid incidentalomas more than 6 cm in diameter because of risk of cancer

**What are the indications for removal of adrenal incidentaloma less than 6 cm?**

MRI T2 signal >2
**Hormonally active** = hyperfunctioning tumor
Enlarging cystic lesion
Does not look like an adenoma

**What tumor must be ruled out prior to biopsy or surgery for any adrenal mass?**

Pheochromocytoma

## PHEOCHROMOCYTOMA

**What is it?**

Tumor of the adrenal **MEDULLA** and sympathetic ganglion (from chromaffin cell lines) that produces **catecholamines** (norepinephrine > epinephrine)

**What is the incidence?**

It is the cause of hypertension in approximately 1/500 hypertensive patients (≈ 10% of U.S. population has hypertension).

**Which age group is most likely to be affected?**

Any age (children and adults); average age is 40 to 60 years

**What are the associated risk factors?**

MEN-II, family history, Von Recklinghausen disease, Von Hippel-Lindau disease

**What are the signs/symptoms?**

"Classic" triad:
1. **Palpitations**
2. **Headache**
3. **Episodic diaphoresis**
Also, hypertension (50%), pallor → flushing, anxiety, weight loss, tachycardia, hyperglycemia

| | |
|---|---|
| **How can the pheochromocytoma SYMPTOMS triad be remembered?** | Think of the first three letters in the word **PHE**ochromocytoma: **P**alpitations **H**eadache **E**pisodic diaphoresis |
| **What is the most common sign of pheochromocytoma?** | Hypertension |
| **What is the differential diagnosis?** | Renovascular hypertension, menopause, migraine headache, carcinoid syndrome, preeclampsia, neuroblastoma, anxiety disorder with panic attacks, hyperthyroidism, insulinoma |
| **What diagnostic tests should be performed?** | Urine screen: vanillylmandelic acid **(VMA), metanephrine,** and normetanephrine (all breakdown products of the catechols) Urine/serum **epinephrine/ norepinephrine** levels |
| **What are the other common lab findings?** | Hyperglycemia (epinephrine increases glucose, norepinephrine decreases insulin) Polycythemia (resulting from intravascular volume depletion) |
| **What is the most common site of a pheochromocytoma?** | **Adrenal** >90% |
| **What are the other sites for pheochromocytoma?** | Organ of Zuckerkandl, thorax (mediastinum), bladder, scrotum |
| **What are the tumor localization tests?** | CT, MRI, $^{131}$**I-MIBG,** PET scan, Octreo Scan ($^{111}$In-pentetreotide scan) |
| **What does $^{131}$I-MIBG stand for?** | **M**eta**I**odo**B**enzyl**G**uanidine |
| **How to remember MIBG and pheochromocytoma?** | Think: **MIBG** = **M**y **B**ig = and thus "My Big Pheo" = MIBG Pheo |

**How does the $^{131}$I-MIBG scan work?**

$^{131}$I-MIBG is a norepinephrine analog that collects in adrenergic vesicles and, thus, in pheochromocytomas.

**What is the role of PET scan?**

**P**ositron **E**mission **T**omography is helpful in localizing pheochromocytomas that do not accumulate MIBG.

**What is the scan for imaging adrenal cortical pheochromocytoma?**

NP-59 (a cholesterol analog)

**What is the localizing option if a tumor is not seen on CT, MRI, or I-MIBG?**

IVC venous sampling for catecholamines (gradient will help localize the tumor)

**What is the tumor site if epinephrine is elevated?**

It must be adrenal or near the adrenal gland (e.g., organs of Zuckerkandl), because nonadrenal tumors lack the capability to methylate norepinephrine to epinephrine.

**What percentage of patients have malignant tumors?**

Approximately 10%

**Can histology be used to determine malignancy?**

No; only distant metastasis or invasion can determine malignancy.

**What is the classic pheochromocytoma "rule of 10's"?**

**10% malignant**
**10% bilateral**
**10% in children**
**10% multiple tumors**
**10% extra-adrenal**

**What is the preoperative/ medical treatment?**

**Increase intravascular volume** with α-blockade (e.g., phenoxybenzamine or prazosin) to allow reduction in catecholamine-induced vasoconstriction and resulting volume depletion; treatment should start as soon as diagnosis is made. +/− beta blockers

**How can you remember phenoxybenzamine as a medical treatment of pheochromocytoma?**

**PHE**ochromocytoma = **PHE**noxybenzamine

| | |
|---|---|
| **What is the surgical treatment?** | Tumor resection with early ligation of venous drainage (lower possibility of catecholamine release/crisis by tying off drainage) and minimal manipulation |
| **What are the possible perioperative complications?** | Anesthetic challenge: hypertensive crisis with manipulation (treat with nitroprusside), hypotension with total removal of the tumor, cardiac dysrhythmias |
| **In the patient with pheochromocytoma, what must be ruled out?** | MEN type II (almost all cases are bilateral) |
| **What are the organs of Zuckerkandl?** | Embryonic chromaffin cells around the abdominal aorta (near the inferior mesenteric artery) that normally atrophy during childhood but are the most common site of extra-adrenal pheochromocytoma |

## CONN'S SYNDROME

| | |
|---|---|
| **What is it?** | Primary hyper**aldosteronism** due to high aldosterone production |
| **How do you remember what Conn's syndrome is?** | **Con**n's disease = **HYPERAL**dosterone = "**CON HYPER AL**" |

**What are the common sources?**

**Adrenal adenoma** or **adrenal hyperplasia;** aldosterone is abnormally secreted by an adrenal adenoma (two-thirds) > hyperplasia > carcinoma

**What is the normal physiology for aldosterone secretion?**

BP in the renal afferent arteriole is low. Low sodium and hyperkalemia cause **renin** secretion from juxtaglomerular cells.
Renin then converts angiotensinogen to angiotensin I.
Angiotensin converting enzyme in the lung then converts angiotensin I to angiotensin II.
Angiotensin II then causes the adrenal glomerulosa cells to secrete **aldosterone.**

**What is the normal physiologic effect of aldosterone?**

Aldosterone causes sodium retention for exchange of potassium in the kidney, resulting in fluid retention and increased BP.

**What are the signs/ symptoms?**

**Hypertension,** headache, polyuria, weakness

**What are the two classic clues of Conn's syndrome?**

1. Hypertension
2. Hypokalemia

**Classically, what kind of hypertension?**

Diastolic hypertension

**What are the renin levels with Conn's syndrome?**

Normal or decreased!

**What percent of all patients with hypertension have Conn's syndrome?**

1%

**What diagnostic tests should be ordered?**

1. Plasma aldosterone concentration
2. Plasma renin activity

**What ratio of these diagnostic tests is associated with primary hyperaldosteronism?**

Aldosterone to renin ratio of >30

| | |
|---|---|
| **What is secondary hyperaldosteronism?** | Hyperaldosteronism resulting from abnormally high renin levels (renin increases angiotensin/aldosterone) |
| **What diagnostic tests should be performed?** | CT, adrenal venous sampling for aldosterone levels, saline infusion |
| **What is the saline infusion test?** | Saline infusion will decrease aldosterone levels in normal patients but not in Conn's syndrome. |
| **What is the preoperative treatment?** | Spironolactone |
| **What is spironolactone?** | An antialdosterone medication (works at the kidney tubule) |
| **What are the causes of Conn's syndrome?** | Adrenal adenoma (66%)<br>Bilateral idiopathic adrenal hyperplasia (30%)<br>Adrenal cancer (<1%) |
| **What is the treatment of the following conditions:** | |
|     **Adenoma?** | Unilateral adrenalectomy (laparoscopic) |
|     **Unilateral hyperplasia?** | Unilateral adrenalectomy (laparoscopic) |
|     **Bilateral hyperplasia?** | Spironolactone (no surgery) |
| **What are the renin levels in patients with PRIMARY hyperaldosteronism?** | Normal or low (key point!) |

## ADDISON'S DISEASE

| | |
|---|---|
| **What is it?** | Acute adrenal insufficiency |
| **What are the electrolyte findings?** | HYPERkalemia, hyponatremia |
| **How do you remember what ADDISON's disease is?** | Think: **ADD**ison's disease = **AD**renal **D**own |

## INSULINOMA

| | |
|---|---|
| **What is it?** | Insulin-producing tumor arising from β cells |
| **What is the incidence?** | Number one islet cell neoplasm; half of β cell tumors of the pancreas produce insulin |
| **What are the associated risks?** | Associated with MEN-I syndrome (ppp = pituitary, pancreas, parathyroid tumors) |
| **What are the signs/ symptoms?** | **Sympathetic nervous system symptoms resulting from hypoglycemia:** palpitations, diaphoresis, tremulousness, irritability, weakness |
| **What are the neurologic symptoms?** | Personality changes, confusion, obtundation, seizures, coma |
| **What is Whipple's triad?** | 1. Hypoglycemic symptoms produced by fasting<br>2. Blood glucose <50 mg/dL during symptomatic attack<br>3. Relief of symptoms by administration of glucose |
| **What is the differential diagnosis?** | Reactive hypoglycemia<br>Functional hypoglycemia with gastrectomy<br>Adrenal insufficiency<br>Hypopituitarism<br>Hepatic insufficiency<br>Munchausen syndrome (insulin self-injections)<br>Nonislet cell tumor causing hypoglycemia<br>Surreptitious administration of insulin or OHAs |
| **What lab tests should be performed?** | Glucose and insulin levels during fast; C-peptide and proinsulin levels (if self-injection of insulin is a concern, as insulin injections have **no** proinsulin or C-peptides) |

| | |
|---|---|
| **What diagnostic tests should be performed?** | Fasting hypoglycemia with inappropriately high levels of insulin<br>**72-hour fast,** then check glucose and insulin levels every 6 hours (monitor very closely because patient can develop hypoglycemic crisis) |
| **What is the diagnostic fasting insulin to glucose ratio?** | >0.4 |
| **What localizing tests should be performed?** | CT, A-gram, endoscopic U/S, venous catheterization (to sample blood along portal and splenic veins to measure insulin and localize tumor), intraoperative U/S |
| **What is the medical treatment?** | Diazoxide, to suppress insulin release |
| **What is the surgical treatment?** | Surgical resection |
| **What is the prognosis?** | Approximately 80% of patients have a benign solitary adenoma that is cured by surgical resection. |

## GLUCAGONOMA

| | |
|---|---|
| **What is it?** | Glucagon-producing tumor |
| **Where is it located?** | Pancreas (usually in the tail) |
| **What are the symptoms?** | **Necrotizing migratory erythema** (usually below the waist), glossitis, stomatitis, diabetes |
| **What are the skin findings?** | Necrotizing migratory erythema is a red often psoriatic-appearing rash with serpiginous borders over the trunk and limbs. |
| **What are the associated lab findings?** | Hyperglycemia, low amino acid levels, high glucagon levels |
| **What is the classic finding on CBC?** | Anemia |

| | |
|---|---|
| **What is the classic nutritional finding?** | Low amino acid levels |
| **What stimulation test is used for glucagonoma?** | Tolbutamide stimulation test: IV tolbutamide results in elevated glucagon levels |
| **What test is used for localization?** | CT |
| **What is the medical treatment of necrotizing migratory erythema?** | Somatostatin, IV amino acids |
| **What is the treatment?** | Surgical resection |

## SOMATOSTATINOMA

| | |
|---|---|
| **What is it?** | Pancreatic tumor that secretes somatostatin |
| **What is the diagnostic triad?** | **DDD**<br>1. **D**iabetes<br>2. **D**iarrhea<br>3. **D**ilation of the gallbladder with gallstones |
| **What is used to make the diagnosis?** | CT scan and somatostatin level |
| **What is the treatment?** | Resection (do not enucleate) |
| **What is the medical treatment if the tumor is unresectable?** | Streptozocin, dacarbazine, or doxorubicin |

## ZOLLINGER-ELLISON SYNDROME (ZE SYNDROME)

| | |
|---|---|
| **What is it?** | **Gastrinoma:** Non-β islet cell tumor of the pancreas (or other locale) that produces gastrin, causing gastric hypersecretion of HCl acid, resulting in GI **ulcers** |
| **What is the incidence?** | 1/1000 in patients with peptic ulcer disease, but nearly 2% in patients with **recurrent ulcers** |

| | |
|---|---|
| **What is the associated syndrome?** | MEN-I syndrome |
| **What percentage of patients with ZE have MEN-I syndrome?** | Approximately 25% (75% of cases of ZE are "sporadic") |
| **What percentage of patients with MEN-I will have ZE syndrome?** | Approximately 50% |
| **With gastrinoma, what lab tests should be ordered to screen for MEN-I?** | 1. Calcium level<br>2. Parathyroid hormone level |
| **What are the signs/ symptoms?** | Peptic ulcers, diarrhea, weight loss, abdominal pain |
| **What causes the diarrhea?** | Massive acid hypersecretion and destruction of digestive enzymes |
| **What are the signs?** | **PUD:** epigastric pain, hematemesis, melena, hematochezia, GERD, diarrhea, **recurrent ulcers,** ulcers in unusual locations (e.g., proximal jejunum) |
| **What are the possible complications?** | GI hemorrhage/perforation, gastric outlet obstruction/stricture, metastatic disease |
| **What is the differential diagnosis of increased gastrin?** | Postvagotomy<br>Gastric outlet obstruction<br>G-cell hyperplasia<br>Pernicious anemia<br>Atrophic gastritis<br>Short gut syndrome<br>Renal failure<br>$H_2$ blocker, PPI |
| **Which patients should have a gastrin level checked?** | Those with recurrent ulcer; ulcer in unusual position (e.g., jejunum) or refractory to medical management; before any operation for ulcer |

| | |
|---|---|
| **What lab tests should be performed?** | Fasting gastrin level<br>Postsecretin challenge gastrin level<br>Calcium (screen for MEN-I)<br>Chem 7 |
| **What are the associated gastrin levels?** | NL fasting = 100 pg/ml<br>ZES fasting = 200–1000 pg/ml<br>Basal acid secretion; (ZES >15 mEq/hr, nl <10mEq/hr) |
| **What is the secretin stimulation test?** | IV secretin is administered and the gastrin level is determined. Patients with ZE have a paradoxic increase in gastrin. |
| **What are the classic secretin stimulation results?** | **Lab results with secretin challenge:**<br>NL—Decreased gastrin<br>ZE—Increased gastrin (increased by > 200 pg/ml) |
| **How can you remember the diagnostic stimulation test for ZE?** | Think: "Secret ZE GAS": **SECRET**in = **ZE GAS**trin |
| **What tests are used to evaluate ulcers?** | EGD, UGI, or both |
| **What tests are used to localize the tumor?** | **Octreotide scan** (somatostatin receptor scan), abdominal CT, MRI, endoscopic ultrasonography (EUS) |
| **What is the most common site?** | Pancreas |
| **What is the most common NONpancreatic site?** | Duodenum |
| **What are some other sites?** | Stomach, lymph nodes, liver, kidney, ovary |
| **Define "Passaro's triangle."** | A.K.A. "gastrinoma triangle," a triangle drawn from the following points:<br>1. Cystic duct/CBD junction<br>2. Junction of the second and third portions of the duodenum<br>3. Neck of the pancreas |

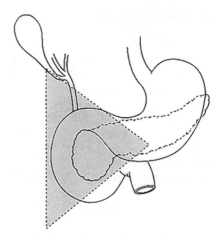

**What percent of gastrinomas are in Passaro's triangle?**

≈ 80%

**What is the next step if the tumor cannot be localized?**

Exploratory surgery (if tumor is not in pancreas, open duodenum and look), proximal gastric vagotomy if not found

**What is the medical treatment?**

$H_2$ blockers, omeprazole, somatostatin

**What is the surgical treatment needed for each of the following:**
    **Tumor in head of pancreas?**

1. Enucleation of tumor
2. Whipple procedure if main pancreatic duct is involved

    **Tumor in body or tail of pancreas?**

Distal pancreatectomy

    **Tumor in duodenum?**

Local resection

    **Unresectable tumor?**

High selective vagotomy

**What percentage have malignant tumors?**

Two-thirds

**What is the most common site of metastasis?**

Liver

| | |
|---|---|
| **What is the treatment of patients with liver metastasis?** | Excision, if technically feasible |
| **What is the surgical option if gastrinoma is in duodenum/ head of pancreas and is too large for local resection?** | Whipple procedure |
| **What is the prognosis with the following procedures:** | |
| **Complete excision?** | 90% 10-year survival |
| **Incomplete excision?** | 25% 10-year survival |

## MULTIPLE ENDOCRINE NEOPLASIA

| | |
|---|---|
| **What is it also known as?** | MEN syndrome |
| **What is it?** | Inherited condition of propensity to develop multiple endocrine tumors |
| **How is it inherited?** | Autosomal dominant (but with a significant degree of variation in penetrance) |
| **Which patients should be screened for MEN?** | All family members of patients diagnosed with MEN |

### MEN TYPE I

| | |
|---|---|
| **What is the common eponym?** | Wermer's syndrome (think: Wermer = Winner = # 1 = type **1**) |
| **What is the gene defect in MEN type I?** | Chromosome 11 (think **11** = **1**) |
| **What are the most common tumors and their incidences?** | "PPP": **P**arathyroid hyperplasia ($\approx 90\%$) **P**ancreatic islet cell tumors ($\approx 66\%$) Gastrinoma: ZE syndrome (50%) Insulinoma (20%) **P**ituitary tumors ($\approx 50\%$) |

| | |
|---|---|
| **How can tumors for MEN-I be remembered?** | Think: type 1 = primary, primary, primary = **PPP** = **p**arathyroid, **p**ancreas, **pi**tuitary |
| **How can the P's associated with MEN-I be remembered?** | All the P's are followed by a vowel: PA, PA, PI |
| **What percentage of patients with MEN-I have parathyroid hyperplasia?** | Approximately 90% |
| **What percentage of patients with MEN-I have a gastrinoma?** | Approximately 50% |
| **What other tumors (in addition to PPP) are associated with MEN-I?** | Adrenal (30%) and thyroid (15%) adenomas |

## MEN TYPE IIA

| | |
|---|---|
| **What is the common eponym?** | Sipple's syndrome (think: Sipple = Second = # 2 = type **2**) |
| **What is the gene defect in MEN type II?** | RET (think re**T** = **T**wo) |
| **What are the most common tumors and their incidences?** | "MPH": **M**edullary thyroid carcinoma (100%) Calcitonin secreted **P**heochromocytoma (>33%) Catecholamine excess **H**yperparathyroidism (about 50%) Hypercalcemia |
| **How can the tumors involved with MEN-II be remembered?** | Think: type 2 = 2 **MPH** or 2 **M**iles **P**er **H**our = **MPH** = **M**edullary, **P**heochromocytoma, **H**yperparathyroid |
| **How can the P of MPH be remembered?** | Followed by the consonant "H"— PHEOCHROMOCYTOMA (remember, the P's of MEN-I are followed by vowels) |

| | |
|---|---|
| **What percentage of patients with MEN-IIA have medullary carcinoma of the thyroid?** | 100% |

## MEN TYPE IIB

| | |
|---|---|
| **What are the most common abnormalities, their incidences, and symptoms?** | "MMMP": **M**ucosal neuromas (100%)—in the nasopharynx, oropharynx, larynx, and conjunctiva **M**edullary thyroid carcinoma ($\approx$ 85%)—more aggressive than in MEN-IIa **M**arfanoid body habitus (long/lanky) **P**heochromocytoma ($\approx$ 50%) and found bilaterally |
| **How can the features of MEN-IIB be remembered?** | MMMP (think: **3M P**lastics) |
| **How can you remember that MEN-IIB is marfanoid habitus?** | Think: "**To be** marfanoid" = **II B** marfanoid |
| **What is the anatomic distribution of medullary thyroid carcinoma in MEN-II?** | **Almost always bilateral;** sporadic cases are almost always **unilateral!** |
| **What are the physical findings/signs of MEN-IIB?** | Mucosal neuromas (e.g., mouth, eyes) Marfanoid body habitus Pes cavus/planum (large arch of foot/flatfooted) Constipation |
| **What is the most common GI complaint of patients with MEN-IIB?** | **Constipation** resulting from ganglioneuromatosis of GI tract |
| **What percentage of pheochromocytomas in MEN-IIA/B are bilateral?** | Approximately 70% (but found bilaterally in only 10% of all patients diagnosed with pheochromocytoma) |

**What is the major difference between MEN-IIA and MEN-IIB?**

MEN-IIA = parathyroid hyperplasia
MEN-IIB = **no** parathyroid hyperplasia
   (and neuromas, marfanoid habitus,
   pes cavus [extensive arch of foot], etc.)

**What type of parathyroid disease is associated with MEN-I and MEN-IIA?**

**Hyperplasia** (treat with removal of all parathyroid tissue with autotransplant of some of the parathyroid tissue to the forearm)

**What percentage of patients with ZE have MEN-I?**

Approximately 25%

# Chapter 58     Thyroid Gland

## THYROID DISEASE

### ANATOMY

**Identify the following structures:**

1. Pyramidal lobe
2. Right lobe
3. Isthmus
4. Left lobe

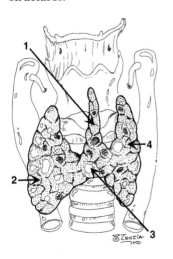

**Define the arterial blood
supply to the thyroid.**

**Two arteries:**
1. Superior thyroid artery (first branch
   of the external carotid artery)
2. Inferior thyroid artery (branch of the
   thyrocervical trunk) (IMA artery rare)

**What is the venous drainage
of the thyroid?**

**Three veins:**
1. Superior thyroid vein
2. **Middle** thyroid vein
3. Inferior thyroid vein

| | |
|---|---|
| **Name the thyroid lobe appendage coursing toward the hyoid bone from around the thyroid isthmus.** | Pyramidal lobe |
| **What percentage of patients have a pyramidal lobe?** | Approximately 50% |
| **What veins do you first see after opening the platysma muscle when performing a thyroidectomy?** | Anterior jugular veins |
| **Name the lymph node group around the pyramidal thyroid lobe.** | Delphian lymph node group |
| **What is the thyroid isthmus?** | Midline tissue border between the left and right thyroid lobes |
| **Which ligament connects the thyroid to the trachea?** | Ligament of Berry |
| **What is the IMA (not I.M.A.) artery?** | A small inferior artery to the thyroid from the aorta or innominate artery |
| **What percentage of patients have an IMA artery?** | Approximately 3% |
| **Name the most posterior extension of the lateral thyroid lobes.** | Tubercle of Zuckerkandl |
| **Which paired nerves must be carefully identified during a thyroidectomy?** | The **recurrent laryngeal nerves,** which are found in the tracheoesophageal grooves and dive behind the cricothyroid muscle; damage to these nerves paralyzes laryngeal abductors and causes hoarseness if unilateral and airway obstruction if bilateral. |
| **What other nerve is at risk during a thyroidectomy and what are the symptoms?** | **Superior laryngeal nerve;** if damaged, patient will have a deeper and quieter voice (unable to hit high pitches) |

| | |
|---|---|
| **What is the name of the famous opera singer whose superior laryngeal nerve was injured during thyroidectomy?** | **Urban legend** has it that it was Amelita Galli-Curci, but no objective data support such a claim (ANN SURG 233:588. April 2001). |

## PHYSIOLOGY

| | |
|---|---|
| **What is TRH?** | **T**hyrotropin-**R**eleasing **H**ormone released from the hypothalamus; causes release of TSH |
| **What is TSH?** | **T**hyroid-**S**timulating **H**ormone released by the anterior pituitary; causes release of thyroid hormone from the thyroid |
| **What are the thyroid hormones?** | T3 and T4 |
| **What is the most active form of thyroid hormone?** | T3 |
| **What is a negative feedback loop?** | T3 and T4 feed back negatively on the anterior pituitary (causing decreased release of TSH in response to TRH). |
| **What is the most common site of conversion of T4 to T3?** | Peripheral (e.g., liver) |
| **What is Synthroid® (levothyroxine): T3 or T4?** | T4 |
| **What is the half-life of Synthroid® (levothyroxine)?** | 7 days |
| **What do parafollicular cells secrete?** | Calcitonin |

## THYROID NODULE

| | |
|---|---|
| **What percentage of people have a thyroid nodule?** | About 5% |

| | |
|---|---|
| **What is the differential diagnosis of a thyroid nodule?** | Multinodular goiter<br>Adenoma<br>Hyperfunctioning adenoma<br>Cyst<br>Thyroiditis<br>Carcinoma/lymphoma<br>Parathyroid carcinoma |
| **Name three types of nonthyroidal neck masses.** | 1. Inflammatory lesions (e.g., abscess, lymphadenitis)<br>2. Congenital lesions (i.e., thyroglossal duct [midline], branchial cleft cyst [lateral])<br>3. Malignant lesions: lymphoma, metastases, squamous cell carcinoma |
| **What studies can be used to evaluate a thyroid nodule?** | U/S—solid or cystic nodule<br>**Fine needle aspirate** (FNA) → cytology<br>$^{123}$I scintiscan—hot or cold nodule |
| **What is the DIAGNOSTIC test of choice for thyroid nodule?** | FNA |
| **What is the percentage of false negative results on FNA for thyroid nodule?** | Approximately 5% |
| **What is meant by a hot versus a cold nodule?** | Nodule uptake of IV $^{131}$I or $^{99}$mT<br>**Hot**—Increased $^{123}$I uptake = functioning/hyperfunctioning nodule<br>**Cold**—Decreased $^{123}$I uptake = nonfunctioning nodule |
| **What are the indications for a $^{123}$I scintiscan?** | 1. Nodule with multiple "nondiagnostic" FNA with low TSH<br>2. Nodule with thyrotoxicosis and low TSH |
| **What is the role of thyroid suppression of a thyroid nodule?** | Diagnostic and therapeutic; administration of thyroid hormone suppresses TSH secretion, and up to half of the benign thyroid nodules will disappear! |

**In evaluating thyroid nodule, which of the following suggest thyroid carcinoma:**

**History?**

1. Neck radiation
2. Family history (thyroid cancer, MEN-II)
3. Young age (especially children)
4. Male > female

**Signs?**

1. Single nodule
2. Cold nodule
3. Increased calcitonin levels
4. Lymphadenopathy
5. Hard, immobile nodule

**Symptoms?**

1. Voice change (vocal cord paralysis)
2. Dysphagia
3. Discomfort (in neck)
4. Rapid enlargement

**What is the most common cause of thyroid enlargement?**

Multinodular goiter

**What are indications for surgery with multinodular goiter?**

Cosmetic deformity, compressive symptoms, cannot rule out cancer

**What is Plummer's disease?**

Toxic multinodular goiter

## MALIGNANT THYROID NODULES

**What percentage of cold thyroid nodules are malignant?**

Approximately 25% in adults

**What percentage of multinodular masses are malignant?**

Approximately 1%

**What is the treatment of a patient with a history of radiation exposure, thyroid nodule, and negative FNA?**

Most experts would remove the nodule surgically (because of the high risk of radiation).

| | |
|---|---|
| **What should be done with thyroid cyst aspirate?** | Send to cytopathology |

## THYROID CARCINOMA

| | |
|---|---|
| **Name the FIVE main types of thyroid carcinoma and their relative percentages.** | 1. Papillary carcinoma: 80% (**P**opular = **P**apillary) <br> 2. Follicular carcinoma: 10% <br> 3. Medullary carcinoma: 5% <br> 4. Hürthle cell carcinoma: 4% <br> 5. Anaplastic/undifferentiated carcinoma: 1% to 2% |
| **What are the signs/ symptoms?** | Mass/nodule, lymphadenopathy; most are **euthyroid** |
| **What comprises the workup?** | **FNA,** Thyroid U/S, TSH, calcium level, CXR, +/− scintiscan $^{123}$I |
| **What oncogenes are associated with thyroid cancers?** | *Ras* gene family and RET proto-oncogene |

## PAPILLARY ADENOCARCINOMA

| | |
|---|---|
| **With what condition is it associated?** | Gardner's syndrome and neck irradiation |
| **What are the associated histologic findings?** | Psammoma bodies (remember, **P** = **P**sammoma = **P**apillary, which constitute 80% of thyroid tumors; therefore, **P**apillary = **P**opular) |
| **Describe the route and rate of spread.** | Most spread via lymphatics (cervical adenopathy); spread occurs slowly. |
| $^{131}$**I uptake?** | Good uptake |
| **What is the 10-year survival rate?** | Approximately 95% |
| **What is the treatment for: <br>   &lt;1.5 cm and no history <br>   of neck radiation <br>   exposure?** | Options: <br> 1. Thyroid lobectomy and isthmectomy <br> 2. Near-total thyroidectomy <br> 3. Total thyroidectomy |

| | |
|---|---|
| >1.5 cm, bilateral, + cervical node mets OR history of radiation exposure? | Total thyroidectomy |
| **What is the treatment for:** | |
| Lateral palpable cervical lymph nodes? | Modified neck dissection (ipsilateral) |
| Central? | Central neck dissection |
| **Do positive cervical nodes affect the prognosis?** | NO! |
| **What postoperative medication should be administered?** | Thyroid hormone replacement, to suppress TSH |
| **What is a postoperative treatment option for papillary carcinoma?** | Postoperative $^{131}$I scan can locate residual tumor and distant metastasis that can be treated with ablative doses of $^{131}$I. |
| **What are the "P's" of papillary thyroid cancer?** | **P**apillary cancer: <br> **P**opular (most common type) <br> **P**sammoma bodies <br> **P**alpable lymph nodes (spreads most commonly by lymphatics, seen in up to one-third of patients) <br> **P**ositive $^{131}$I uptake <br> **P**ositive prognosis <br> **P**ostoperative $^{131}$I scan to diagnose/treat metastases |

## FOLLICULAR ADENOCARCINOMA

| | |
|---|---|
| **What percentage of thyroid cancers does it comprise?** | Approximately 10% |
| **Describe the nodule consistency.** | Rubbery, encapsulated |
| **What is the route of spread?** | Hematogenous, more aggressive than papillary adenocarcinoma |
| **What is the male:female ratio?** | 1:3 |

| | |
|---|---|
| $^{131}$I uptake? | Good uptake |
| **What is the overall 10-year survival rate?** | Approximately 85% |
| **Can the diagnosis be made by FNA?** | No; tissue structure is needed for a diagnosis of cancer. |
| **What histologic findings define malignancy in follicular cancer?** | Capsular or blood vessel invasion |
| **What is the most common site of distant metastasis?** | Bone |
| **What is the treatment for follicular cancer?** | Total thyroidectomy |
| **What is the postoperative treatment option if malignant?** | Postoperative $^{131}$I scan for diagnosis/treatment |
| **What are the "F's" of follicular cancer?** | Follicular cancer: Far-away metastasis (spreads hematogenously) Female (3 to 1 ratio) FNA . . . NOT (FNA CANNOT diagnose cancer) Favorable prognosis |

## HÜRTHLE CELL THYROID CANCER

| | |
|---|---|
| **What is it?** | Thyroid cancer of Hürthle cells |
| **What percentage of thyroid cancers does it comprise?** | Approximately 5% |
| **What is the cell of origin?** | Follicular cells |
| $^{131}$I uptake? | No uptake |
| **How is the diagnosis made?** | FNA can identify cells, but malignancy can be determined only by tissue histology (like follicular cancer). |

| | |
|---|---|
| **What is the route of metastasis?** | Lymphatic > hematogenous |
| **What is the treatment?** | Total thyroidectomy |

## MEDULLARY CARCINOMA

| | |
|---|---|
| **What percentage of all thyroid cancers does it comprise?** | Approximately 5% |
| **With what other conditions is it associated?** | MEN type II; autosomal-dominant genetic transmission |
| **Histology?** | Amyloid (a**M**yloid = **M**edullary) |
| **What does it secrete?** | Calcitonin |
| **What is the appropriate stimulation test?** | Pentagastrin (causes an increase in calcitonin) |
| **Describe the route and rate of spread.** | Lymphatic and hematogenous distant metastasis |
| **How is the diagnosis made?** | FNA |
| **$^{131}$I uptake?** | Poor uptake |
| **What is the prognosis?** | Ten-year survival rate is 50%; cure rate is 95% when occult tumors are found in MEN family members being screened for elevated calcitonin. If detected when clinically palpable, cure rate is <20%. |
| **What is the treatment?** | Total thyroidectomy and **median lymph node dissection** Modified neck dissection, if lateral cervical nodes are positive |
| **What are the "M's" of medullary carcinoma?** | **M**edullary cancer: **M**EN II a**M**yloid **M**edian lymph node dissection **M**odified neck dissection if lateral nodes are positive |

## ANAPLASTIC CARCINOMA

| | |
|---|---|
| **What is it also known as?** | Undifferentiated carcinoma |
| **What is it?** | An undifferentiated cancer arising in approximately 75% of previously differentiated thyroid cancers (most commonly, follicular carcinoma) |
| **What percentage of all thyroid cancers does it comprise?** | Approximately 2% |
| **What is the gender preference?** | Women > men |
| **What are the associated histologic findings?** | Giant cells, spindle cells |
| $^{131}$**I uptake?** | Very poor uptake |
| **How is the diagnosis made?** | FNA (large tumor) |
| **What is the major differential diagnosis?** | Thyroid lymphoma (much better prognosis!) |
| **What is the treatment of the following disorders:** | |
| **Small tumors?** | Total thyroidectomy ± external beam x-ray therapy |
| **Airway compromise?** | Debulking surgery and tracheostomy |
| **What is the prognosis?** | Dismal, because most patients are at stage IV at presentation (3% alive at 5 years) |

## MISCELLANEOUS

| | |
|---|---|
| **What laboratory value must be followed postoperatively after a thyroidectomy?** | **Calcium** decreased secondary to parathyroid damage; during lobectomy, the parathyroids must be spared and their blood supply protected; if blood supply is compromised intraoperatively, they can be autografted into the sternocleidomastoid muscle or forearm |

| | |
|---|---|
| **What is the differential diagnosis of postoperative dyspnea after a thyroidectomy?** | Neck hematoma (remove sutures and clot at the **bedside**)<br>**Bilateral** recurrent laryngeal nerve damage |
| **What is a "lateral aberrant rest" of the thyroid?** | A misnomer; it is **papillary** cancer of a lymph node from metastasis. |

## BENIGN THYROID DISEASE

| | |
|---|---|
| **What is the most common cause of hyperthyroidism?** | Graves' disease |
| **What is Graves' disease?** | Diffuse goiter with hyperthyroidism, exophthalmos, and pretibial myxedema |
| **What is the etiology?** | Caused by circulating **antibodies** that stimulate TSH receptors on follicular cells of the thyroid and cause deregulated production of thyroid hormones (i.e., hyperthyroidism) |
| **What is the female:male ratio?** | 6:1 |
| **What specific physical finding is associated with Graves'?** | Exophthalmos |
| **How is the diagnosis made?** | Increased T3, T4, and anti-TSH receptor antibodies, decreased TSH, global uptake of $^{131}I$ radionuclide |
| **Name treatment option modalities for Graves' disease.** | 1. **Medical blockade:** iodide, propranolol, propylthiouracil (PTU), methimazole, Lugol's solution (potassium iodide)<br>2. **Radioiodide ablation:** most popular therapy<br>3. **Surgical resection:** (bilateral subtotal thyroidectomy) |
| **What are the possible indications for surgical resection?** | Suspicious nodule; if patient is noncompliant or refractory to medicines, pregnant, a child, or if patient refuses radioiodide therapy |

| | |
|---|---|
| **What is the major complication of radioiodide or surgery for Graves' disease?** | Hypothyroidism |
| **What does PTU stand for?** | **P**ropyl**T**hio**U**racil |
| **How does PTU work?** | 1. Inhibits incorporation of iodine into T4/T3 (by blocking peroxidase oxidation of iodide to iodine)<br>2. Inhibits peripheral conversion of T4 to T3 |
| **How does methimazole work?** | Inhibits incorporation of iodine into T4/T3 **only** (by blocking peroxidase oxidation of iodide to iodine) |

## TOXIC MULTINODULAR GOITER

| | |
|---|---|
| **What is it A.K.A.?** | Plummer's disease |
| **What is it?** | **Multiple** thyroid nodules with one or more nodules producing thyroid hormone, resulting in hyperfunctioning thyroid (hyperthyroidism or a "toxic" thyroid state) |
| **How is the hyperfunctioning nodule(s) localized?** | $^{131}$I radionuclide scan |
| **What is the treatment?** | Surgically remove hyperfunctioning nodule(s) with lobectomy or near total thyroidectomy |
| **What is Pemberton's sign?** | A large goiter causes plethora of head with raising of both arms. |

## THYROIDITIS

| | |
|---|---|
| **What are the features of acute thyroiditis?** | Painful, swollen thyroid; fever; overlying skin erythema; dysphagia |
| **What is the cause of ACUTE thyroiditis?** | Bacteria (usually *Streptococcus* or *Staphylococcus*), usually caused by a thyroglossal fistula or anatomic variant |

| | |
|---|---|
| **What is the treatment of ACUTE thyroiditis?** | Antibiotics, drainage of abscess, needle aspiration for culture; most patients need definitive surgery later to remove the fistula |
| **What are the features of subacute thyroiditis?** | Glandular swelling, tenderness, often follows URI, elevated ESR |
| **What is the cause of subacute thyroiditis?** | Viral infection |
| **What is the treatment of subacute thyroiditis?** | Supportive: NSAIDS, ± steroids |
| **What is De Quervain's thyroiditis?** | Just another name for subacute thyroiditis caused by a virus (think: De QuerVain:Virus) |
| **How can the differences between etiologies of ACUTE and SUBACUTE thyroiditis be remembered?** | Alphabetically: **A** before **S, B** before **V** (i.e., **A**cute before **S**ubacute and **B**acterial before **V**iral and thus: **A**cute = **B**acterial and **S**ubacute = **V**iral) |
| **What are the common causative bacteria in acute suppurative thyroiditis?** | *Streptococcus* or *Staphylococcus* |
| **What are the two types of chronic thyroiditis?** | 1. Hashimoto's thyroiditis<br>2. Riedel's thyroiditis |
| **What are the features of Hashimoto's (chronic) thyroiditis?** | Firm and rubbery gland, 95% in women, lymphocyte invasion |
| **What is the claim to fame of Hashimoto's disease?** | Most common cause of hypothyroidism in the United States |
| **What is the etiology of Hashimoto's disease?** | Autoimmune (think: Hashim**OTO** = **AUTO**; thus, Hashimoto = autoimmune) |
| **What lab tests should be performed to diagnose Hashimoto's disease?** | Antithyroglobulin and microsomal antibodies |

**What is Riedel's thyroiditis?**

Benign inflammatory thyroid enlargement **with fibrosis** of thyroid
Patients present with painless, large thyroid.
Fibrosis may involve surrounding tissues.

# Chapter 59    Parathyroid

## ANATOMY

**How many parathyroids are there?**

Usually **four** (two superior and two inferior)

**What percentage of patients have five parathyroid glands?**

Approximately 5% (think 5 = 5)

**What percentage of patients have three parathyroid glands?**

Approximately 10%

**What is the usual position of the inferior parathyroid glands?**

Posterior and lateral behind the thyroid and below the inferior thyroid artery

**What is the most common site of an "extra" gland?**

Thymus gland

**What percentage of patients have a parathyroid gland in the mediastinum?**

Approximately 1%

**If only three parathyroid glands are found at surgery, where can the fourth one be hiding?**

Thyroid gland
Thymus/mediastinum
Carotid sheath
Tracheoesophageal groove
Behind the esophagus

**What is the embryologic origin of the following structures:**

    **Superior parathyroid glands?**      Fourth pharyngeal pouch

    **Inferior parathyroid glands?**      Third pharyngeal pouch (counterintuitive)

**What supplies blood to the parathyroid glands?**      Inferior thyroid artery

**What percentage of patients have all four parathyroid glands supplied by the inferior thyroid arteries exclusively?**      Approximately 80%

**What is DiGeorge's syndrome?**      Congenital absence of the parathyroid glands and the thymus

**What is the most common cause of hypercalcemia in hospitalized patients?**      Cancer

**What is the most common cause of hypercalcemia in outpatients?**      Hyperparathyroidism

## PHYSIOLOGY

**What cell type produces PTH?**      Chief cells

**What are the major actions of parathyroid hormone (PTH)?**      **Increases** blood **calcium** levels (takes from bone breakdown, GI absorption, increased resorption from kidney, excretion of phosphate by kidney), **decreases** serum phosphate

**How does vitamin D work?**      Increases intestinal absorption of calcium and phosphate

**Where is calcium absorbed?**      Duodenum and proximal jejunum

## HYPERPARATHYROIDISM (HPTH)

**Define primary HPTH.**
Increased secretion of PTH by parathyroid gland(s); marked by elevated calcium, low phosphorus

**Define secondary HPTH.**
Increased serum PTH resulting from calcium wasting caused by **renal failure or decreased GI calcium absorption,** rickets or osteomalacia; calcium levels are usually **low**

**Define tertiary HPTH.**
Persistent HPTH after correction of secondary hyperparathyroidism; results from autonomous PTH secretion not responsive to the normal negative feedback due to elevated $Ca^{++}$ levels

**What are the methods of imaging the parathyroids?**
Surgical operation
Ultrasound
**Sestamibi scan**
$^{201}$TI(technetium)—thallium subtraction scan
CT/MRI
A-gram (rare)
Venous sampling for PTH (rare)

**What are the indications for a localizing preoperative study?**
**Reoperation** for recurrent hyperparathyroidism

**What is the most common cause of primary HPTH?**
Adenoma ($>85\%$)

**What are the etiologies of primary HPTH and percentages?**
**Adenoma** ($\sim 85\%$)
Hyperplasia ($\sim 10\%$)
Carcinoma ($\sim 1\%$)

**What is the incidence of primary HPTH in the United States?**
Approximately $1/1000-4000$

**What are the risk factors for primary HPTH?**
Family history, MEN-I and MEN-IIa, irradiation

**What are the signs/ symptoms of primary HPTH hypercalcemia?**

"Stones, bones, groans, and psychiatric overtones":

**Stones:** Kidney stones

**Bones:** Bone pain, pathologic fractures, subperiosteal resorption

**Groans:** Muscle pain and weakness, pancreatitis, gout, constipation

**Psychiatric overtones:** Depression, anorexia, anxiety

**Other symptoms:** Polydipsia, weight loss, HTN (10%), polyuria, lethargy

**What is the "33 to 1" rule?**

Most patients with primary HPTH have a ratio of serum ($Cl^-$) to phosphate $\geq 33$.

**What plain x-ray findings are classic for HPTH?**

Subperiosteal bone resorption (usually in hand digits; said to be "pathognomonic" for HPTH!)

**How is primary HPTH diagnosed?**

Labs—elevated PTH (hypercalcemia, $\downarrow$ phosphorus, $\uparrow$ chloride); urine calcium should be checked for familial hypocalciuric hypercalcemia

**What is familial hypocalciuric hypercalcemia?**

Familial (autosomal-dominant) inheritance of a condition of **asymptomatic** hypercalcemia and low urine calcium, with or without elevated PTH; in contrast, hypercalcemia from HPTH results in high levels of urine calcium

Surgery to remove parathyroid glands is not indicated for this diagnosis.

**How many of the glands are USUALLY affected by the following conditions:**

    **Hyperplasia?**

Four

    **Adenoma?**

One

    **Carcinoma?**

One

**What percentage of adenomas are not single but are found in more than one gland?**

Approximately 5%

**What is the differential diagnosis of hypercalcemia?**

"CHIMPANZEES":

**C**alcium overdose
**H**yperparathyroidism (1°/2°/3°),
    **H**yperthyroidism, **H**ypocalciuric
    **H**ypercalcemia (familial)
**I**mmobility/iatrogenic (thiazide diuretics)
**M**etastasis/milk alkali syndrome (rare)
**P**aget's disease (bone)
**A**ddison's disease/acromegaly
**N**eoplasm (colon, lung, breast, prostate,
    multiple myeloma)
**Z**ollinger-Ellison syndrome
**E**xcessive vitamin D
**E**xcessive vitamin A
**S**arcoid

**What is the initial medical treatment of hypercalcemia (1° HPTH)?**

Medical—IV fluids, furosemide—**NOT** thiazide diuretics

**What is the definitive treatment of HPTH in the following cases:**

    **Primary HPTH resulting from HYPERPLASIA?**

Neck exploration removing all parathyroid glands and leaving at least 30 mg of parathyroid tissue placed in the forearm muscles (nondominant arm, of course!)

    **Primary HPTH resulting from parathyroid ADENOMA?**

Surgically remove adenoma (send for frozen section) and biopsy all abnormally enlarged parathyroid glands (some experts biopsy all glands).

    **Primary HPTH resulting from parathyroid CARCINOMA?**

Remove carcinoma, ipsilateral thyroid lobe, and all enlarged lymph nodes.

    **Secondary HPTH?**

Correct calcium and phosphate; perform renal transplantation (no role for parathyroid surgery).

| | |
|---|---|
| **Tertiary HPTH?** | Correct calcium and phosphate; perform surgical operation to remove all parathyroid glands and reimplant 30 to 40 mg in the forearm if **REFRACTORY** to medical management. |
| **Why place 30 to 40 mg of sliced parathyroid gland in the forearm?** | To retain parathyroid function. If HPTH recurs, remove some of the parathyroid gland from the easily accessible forearm. |
| **What must be ruled out in the patient with HPTH from hyperplasia?** | MEN type I and MEN type IIa |
| **What carcinomas are commonly associated with hypercalcemia?** | **Breast cancer metastases,** prostate cancer, kidney cancer, lung cancer, pancreatic cancer, multiple myeloma |
| **What is the most likely diagnosis if a patient has a PALPABLE neck mass, hypercalcemia, and elevated PTH?** | Parathyroid carcinoma (vast majority of other causes of primary HPTH have nonpalpable parathyroids) |

## PARATHYROID CARCINOMA

| | |
|---|---|
| **What is it?** | Primary carcinoma of the parathyroid gland |
| **What is the number of glands usually affected?** | One |
| **What are the signs/ symptoms?** | Hypercalcemia, elevated PTH, **PALPABLE** parathyroid gland (50%), pain in neck, recurrent laryngeal nerve paralysis (change in voice), hypercalcemic crisis (usually associated with calcium levels >13) |
| **What is the common tumor marker?** | Human chorionic gonadotrophin |
| **What is the treatment?** | Surgical resection of parathyroid mass with ipsilateral thyroid lobectomy, ipsilateral lymph node resection |

| | |
|---|---|
| **What percentage of all cases of primary HPTH are caused by parathyroid carcinoma?** | 1% |

## POSTOPERATIVE COMPLICATIONS OF PARATHYROIDECTOMY

| | |
|---|---|
| **What are the possible postoperative complications after a parathyroidectomy?** | Recurrent nerve injury (unilateral: voice change; bilateral: airway obstruction), neck hematoma (open at bedside if breathing is compromised), hypocalcemia, superior laryngeal nerve injury |
| **What is "hungry bone syndrome"?** | Severe hypocalcemia seen after surgical correction of HPTH as chronically calcium-deprived bone aggressively absorbs calcium |
| **What are the signs/ symptoms of postoperative hypocalcemia?** | Perioral tingling, paresthesia, positive Chvostek's sign, positive Trousseau's sign, positive tetany |
| **What is the treatment of hypoparathyroidism?** | Acute: IV calcium<br>Chronic: PO calcium, and vitamin D |

# Chapter 60

# Spleen and Splenectomy

| | |
|---|---|
| **Which arteries supply the spleen?** | The splenic artery, a branch of the celiac trunk, and the short gastric arteries that arise from the gastroepiploic arteries |
| **What is the venous drainage of the spleen?** | The **portal** vein, via the splenic vein and the left gastroepiploic vein |
| **What is said to "tickle" the spleen?** | The tail of the pancreas |

**What percentage of people have an accessory spleen?**

Approximately 20%

**What percentage of the total body platelets are stored in the spleen?**

33%

**What are the functions of the human spleen?**

Filters abnormal RBCs (does NOT store RBCs like canine spleen!), stores platelets, produces tuftsin and properdin (opsins), produces antibodies (especially IGM) and is site of phagocytosis

**What is "delayed splenic rupture"?**

A subcapsular hematoma or pseudoaneurysm may rupture some time after blunt trauma, causing "delayed splenic rupture." Rupture classically occurs about 2 weeks after the injury and presents with shock/abdominal pain.

**What are the signs/symptoms of ruptured/injured spleen?**

Hemoperitoneum and Kehr's sign, LUQ abdominal pain, Ballance's sign

**What is Kehr's sign?**

Left shoulder pain seen with splenic rupture

**What is Balance's sign?**

LUQ dullness to percussion

**What is Seagesser's sign?**

Phrenic nerve compression causing neck tenderness in splenic rupture

**How is a spleen injury diagnosed?**

Abdominal CT, **if the patient is stable;** DPL or FAST exam if the patient is unstable

**What is the treatment?**

1. Nonoperative in a stable patient with an isolated splenic injury without hilar involvement/complete rupture
2. If patient is unstable, DPL/FAST laparotomy with splenorrhaphy or splenectomy
3. Embolization is an option in selected patients

**What is a splenorrhaphy?**

Splenic salvage operation: wrapping vicral mesh, aid of topical hemostatic agents or partial splenectomy (VAST majority of pediatric patients undergo nonoperative treatment for blunt spleen injury)

**What are the other indications for splenectomy:**
**Malignant diseases?**

Hodgkin's staging not conclusive by CT (rare)
Splenic tumors (primary/metastatic/locally invasive)
Hypersplenism caused by other leukemias/nonHodgkin's lymphomas

**Anemias?**

Medullary fibrosis with myeloid metaplasia
Hereditary elliptocytosis
Sickle-cell anemia (rare, most autosplenectomize)
Pyruvate kinase deficiency
Autoimmune hemolytic anemia
Hereditary spherocytosis
Thalassemias (e.g., β-thalassemia major A.K.A. Cooley's)

**Thrombocytopenia?**

ITP (idiopathic thrombocytopenic purpura)
TTP (thrombotic thrombocytopenic purpura)

**Miscellaneous indications?**

Variceal bleeding with splenic vein thrombosis, Gaucher's disease, splenic abscess, refractory splenic cysts, hypersplenism, Felty's syndrome

**Is G6PD deficiency an indication for splenectomy?**

NO

**What are the possible postsplenectomy complications?**

Thrombocytosis, subphrenic abscess, atelectasis, pancreatitis gastric dilation, and **overwhelming postsplenectomy sepsis (OPSS)**

**What causes OPSS?**

Increased susceptibility to fulminant bacteremia, meningitis, or pneumonia because of loss of splenic function

**What is the incidence of OPSS in adults?**

<1%

**What is the incidence and overall mortality of OPSS in children?**

1% to 2% with 50% mortality rate

**What is the typical presentation of OPSS?**

Fever, lethargy, common cold, sore throat, URI followed by confusion, shock, and coma with death ensuing within 24 hours in up to 50% of patients

**What are the common organisms associated with OPSS?**

**Encapsulated:** *Streptococcus pneumoniae, Neisseria meningitides, H. influenzae*

**What is the most common bacteria in OPSS?**

*Streptococcus pneumoniae*

**What is the preventive treatment of OPSS?**

Vaccinations for pneumococcus, *H. influenzae,* and meningococcus
Prophylactic penicillin for all minor infections/illnesses and immediate medical care if febrile illness develops

**What is the best time to give immunizations to splenectomy patients?**

**Preoperatively,** if at all possible
If emergent, then *two weeks* postoperatively

**What lab tests are abnormal after splenectomy?**

WBC count increases by 50% over the baseline; marked **thrombocytosis** occurs; RBC smear is abnormal.

| | |
|---|---|
| **What are the findings on postsplenectomy RBC smear?** | Peripheral smear will show Pappenheimer bodies, Howell-Jolly bodies, and Heinz bodies. |
| **When and how should thrombocytosis be treated?** | When platelet count is >1 million, most surgeons will treat with **aspirin.** |
| **What is the most common cause of splenic vein thrombosis?** | Pancreatitis |
| **What opsonins does the spleen produce?** | Properdin, tuftsin (think: "PROfessionally TUF spleen") |
| **What is the most common cause of ISOLATED GASTRIC varices?** | Splenic vein thrombosis (usually from pancreatitis) |
| **What is the treatment of gastric varices caused by splenic vein thrombosis?** | Splenectomy |
| **Which patients develop hyposplenism?** | Patients with ulcerative colitis |
| **What vaccinations should every patient with a splenectomy receive?** | Pneumococcus Meningococcus *Haemophilus influenzae* type B |
| **Define hypersplenism.** | Hyperfunctioning spleen Documented loss of blood elements (WBC, Hct, platelets) Large spleen (splenomegaly) Hyperactive bone marrow (trying to keep up with loss of blood elements) |
| **Define splenomegaly.** | Enlarged spleen |
| **What is ITP?** | Autoimmune (antiplatelet antibodies IgG in >90% of patients) platelet destruction leading to troublesome bleeding and purpura |

| | |
|---|---|
| **What is the most common cause of failure to correct thrombocytopenia after splenectomy for ITP?** | Missed accessory spleen |
| **What are the "I's" of ITP?** | **I**mmune etiology (**I**gG antiplatelets ABs)<br>**I**mmunosuppressive treatment (initially treated with steroids)<br>**I**mmune globulin<br>**I**mprovement with splenectomy (75% of patients have improved platelet counts after splenectomy) |
| **What is the treatment of choice for TTP?** | Plasmapheresis (splenectomy reserved as a last resort) |
| **What is the most common physical finding of portal hypertension?** | Splenomegaly |

---

# Chapter 61

# Surgically Correctable HTN

| | |
|---|---|
| **What is it?** | Hypertension caused by conditions that are amenable to surgical correction |
| **What percentage of patients with HTN have a surgically correctable cause?** | Approximately 7% |
| **What diseases that cause HTN are surgically correctable?** | Think "CAN I CHURP?":<br>**C**ushing's syndrome<br>**A**ortic coarctation<br>**N**euroblastoma/neoplasia<br><br>**I**ncreased intracranial pressure<br><br>**C**onn's syndrome (primary hyperaldosteronism)<br>**H**yperparathyroidism/hyperthyroidism |

Unilateral renal parenchymal disease
Renal artery stenosis
Pheochromocytoma

| | |
|---|---|
| **What is the formula for pressure?** | Pressure = flow × resistance or P = F × R (think: **P**ower **FoR**ward); thus, an increase in flow, resistance, or both results in an increase in pressure |

# Chapter 62

# Soft Tissue Sarcomas and Lymphomas

## SOFT TISSUE SARCOMAS

| | |
|---|---|
| **What are they?** | Soft tissue tumors, derived from mesoderm |
| **Sarcoma means what in GREEK?** | Fish flesh |
| **Sarcomas are more common in upper or lower extremities?** | 50% of sarcomas are in the extremities and are 3.5 times **more** common in the **lower** extremity (thigh). |
| **How common are they?** | They comprise 0.6% of malignant tumors. |
| **What is the median age at diagnosis?** | 55 |
| **What are the risk factors?** | "R.A.L.E.S.": Radiation AIDS (Immunosuppression) Lymphedema Exposure to chemicals Syndromes (e.g., Gardner's/Le-Fraumeni) |

**Name the following types of malignant sarcoma:**

| | |
|---|---|
| Fat | Liposarcoma |
| Smooth muscle | Leiomyosarcoma |
| Myofibroblast | Malignant fibrous histiocytoma |
| Striated muscle | Rhabdomyosarcoma |
| Vascular endothelium | Angiosarcoma |
| Fibroblast | Fibrosarcoma |
| Lymph vessel | Lymphangiosarcoma |
| Peripheral nerve | Malignant neurilemmoma or schwannoma |
| AIDS | Kaposi's sarcoma |
| Lymphedema | Lymphangiosarcoma |

**What are the signs/symptoms?**
Soft tissue mass; pain from compression of adjacent structures, often noticed after minor trauma to area of mass

**How do most sarcomas metastasize?**
Hematogenously (i.e., via blood)

**What is the most common location and route of metastasis?**
**Lungs** via hematogenous route

**What tests should be done in the preoperative work-up?**
CXR, ± chest CT, LFTs

**What are the three most common malignant sarcomas in adults?**
Fibrous histiocytoma (25%), liposarcoma (20%), leiomyosarcoma (15%)

**What are the two most common in children?**
Rhabdomyosarcoma (about 50%), fibrosarcoma (20%)

| | |
|---|---|
| **What is the most common type to metastasize to the lymph nodes?** | Malignant fibrous histiocytoma |
| **What is the most common sarcoma of the retroperitoneum?** | Liposarcoma |
| **How do sarcomas locally invade?** | Usually along anatomic planes such as fascia, vessels, etc. |
| **How is the diagnosis made?** | Imaging work-up—MRI is superior to CT at distinguishing the tumor from adjacent structures<br>Mass less than 3 cm: excisional biopsy<br>**Mass more than 3 cm:** incisional biopsy or **core biopsy** |
| **Define excisional biopsy.** | Biopsy by removing the **entire** mass |
| **Define incisional biopsy.** | Biopsy by removing a **piece** of the mass |
| **What is the orientation of incision for incisional biopsy of a suspected extremity sarcoma?** | **Longitudinal,** not transverse, so that the incision can be incorporated in a future resection if biopsy for sarcoma is positive |
| **Define core biopsy.** | A large-bore needle that takes a core of tissue (like an earth core sample) |
| **Define the following American Joint Committee for Cancer Staging (AJCC) Sarcoma Stages:** | |
| Stage I | Well differentiated (**grade**), any size, no nodes, no metastases |
| Stage II | Moderately differentiated (**grade**), any size, no nodes, no metastases |
| Stage III | Poorly differentiated or undifferentiated (**grade**), any size tumor, no nodes, no metastases |
| Stage IV | Positive nodes or distant metastases |

| | |
|---|---|
| **What is a pseudocapsule and what is its importance?** | It is the outer layer of a sarcoma that represents compressed malignant cells. Microscopic extensions of tumor cells invade through the pseudocapsule into adjacent structures. Thus, definitive therapy must include a wide margin of resection to account for this phenomenon and not just be "shelled-out" like a benign growth. |
| **What is the most important factor in the prognosis?** | **Histologic grade** of the primary lesion |
| **What is the treatment?** | Surgical resection and radiation (with or without chemotherapy) |
| **What surgical margins are obtained?** | 2 cm |
| **What is the "limb-sparing" surgery for extremity sarcoma?** | Avoidance of amputation with local resection and chemoradiation |
| **What is the treatment of pulmonary metastasis?** | Surgical resection for isolated lesions |
| **What tests should be done in the follow-up?** | Physical examination, CXR, repeat CT/ MRI of the area of resection to look for recurrence |
| **What syndrome of lymphangiosarcoma arises in chronic lymphedema after axillary dissection for breast cancer?** | Stewart-Treves syndrome |
| **What syndrome is associated with breast cancer and soft tissue sarcoma?** | Le-Fraumeni syndrome (p53 tumor suppressor gene mutation) |

## LYMPHOMA

| | |
|---|---|
| **How is the diagnosis made?** | Cervical or axillary node excisional biopsy |
| **What cell type is associated with the histology of Hodgkin's disease?** | Reed-Sternberg cells |

| | |
|---|---|
| **What are the four histopathologic types of Hodgkin's disease?** | 1. Nodular sclerosing (most common; about 50% of cases)<br>2. Mixed cellularity<br>3. Lymphocyte predominant (best prognosis)<br>4. Lymphocyte depleted |
| **What are the indications for a "staging laparotomy" in Hodgkin's disease?** | Controversial; rarely performed for the low stages because they are treated differently than advanced stages<br>Most experts rely on CT scans and do not perform laparotomy. |
| **What is a staging laparotomy for Hodgkin's lymphoma?** | A laparotomy to distinguish between advanced and low-stage disease to define proper therapy. It includes:<br>1. **Splenectomy**<br>2. Iliac crest bone aspiration<br>3. Biopsies of splenic hilar, celiac, mesenteric, porta hepatis, para-aortic, and iliac **lymph nodes**<br>4. **Liver biopsy**<br>5. **Oophoropexy:** if the patient is a woman of childbearing years, the ovaries are marked with metallic clips and then tacked behind the uterus for protection from the radiation field. |
| **Define the stages (Ann Arbor) of Hodgkin's disease:** | |
| **Stage I** | Single lymph node region (think: stage 1 = 1 region) |
| **Stage II** | Two or more lymph node regions on **the same side of the diaphragm** (think: stage 2 = >2 regions) |
| **Stage III** | Involvement on **both** sides of the diaphragm |
| **Stage IV** | Diffuse and/or disseminated involvement |
| **What is stage A Hodgkin's?** | Asymptomatic (think: **A**symptomatic = stage **A**) |

| | |
|---|---|
| **What is stage B Hodgkin's?** | Symptomatic: weight loss, fever, night sweats, etc. (think: stage **B** = **B**ad) |
| **What is the "E" on the staging?** | Extralymphatic site involvement (**E** = **E**xtralymphatic) |
| **What treatments are used for low versus advanced stage Hodgkin's lymphoma?** | Low stage: radiotherapy<br>Advanced stage: chemotherapy |
| **What percentage of patients with Hodgkin's disease can be cured?** | Approximately 80% |

## GI LYMPHOMA

| | |
|---|---|
| **What is it?** | Non-Hodgkin's lymphoma arising in the GI tract |
| **What is the risk factor for gastric lymphoma?** | Helicobacter *pylori* |
| **What are the signs/symptoms?** | Abdominal pain, obstruction, GI hemorrhage, GI tract perforation, fatigue |
| **What is the treatment for gastric lymphoma?** | **Controversial:** chemoradiation vs. surgical resection |
| **What is the treatment of intestinal lymphoma?** | Surgical resection with removal of draining lymph nodes and chemotherapy |
| **What is the most common site of primary GI tract lymphoma?** | The stomach (66%) |

# Chapter 63     **Skin Lesions**

| | |
|---|---|
| **What are the most common skin cancers?** | 1. Basal cell carcinoma (75%)<br>2. Squamous cell carcinoma (20%)<br>3. Melanoma (4%) |
| **What is the most common skin cancer that causes death?** | Melanoma |
| **What is malignant melanoma?** | A redundancy! All melanomas are considered malignant. |

## SQUAMOUS CELL CARCINOMA

| | |
|---|---|
| **What is it?** | Carcinoma arising from epidermal cells |
| **What are the most common sites?** | Head, neck, and hands |
| **What are the risk factors?** | Sun exposure, pale skin, chronic inflammatory process, immunosuppression, xeroderma pigmentosum, arsenic |
| **What is a precursor skin lesion?** | Actinic keratosis |
| **What are the signs/ symptoms?** | Raised, slightly pigmented skin lesion; ulceration/exudate; chronic scab; itching |
| **How is the diagnosis made?** | Small lesion—excisional biopsy<br>Large lesions—incisional biopsy |
| **What is the treatment?** | Small lesion (<1 cm): excise with 0.5 cm margin<br>Large lesion >1 cm: resect with 1 to 2 cm margins of normal tissue (large lesions may require skin graft/flap) |

| | |
|---|---|
| **What is the dreaded sign of metastasis?** | Palpable lymph nodes (remove involved lymph nodes) |
| **What is Marjolin's ulcer?** | Squamous cell carcinoma that arises in an area of chronic inflammation (e.g., chronic fistula, burn wound, osteomyelitis) |
| **What is the prognosis?** | Excellent if totally excised (95% cure rate); most patients with positive lymph-node metastasis eventually die from metastatic disease |
| **What is the treatment for solitary metastasis?** | Surgical resection |

## BASAL CELL CARCINOMA

| | |
|---|---|
| **What is it?** | Carcinoma arising in the germinating basal cell layer of epithelial cells |
| **What are the risk factors?** | Sun exposure, fair skin, radiation, chronic dermatitis, xeroderma pigmentosum |
| **What are the most common sites?** | Head, neck, and hands |
| **What are the signs/ symptoms?** | Slow-growing skin mass (chronic, scaly); scab; ulceration, with or without pigmentation, often described as "pearl"-like |
| **How is the diagnosis made?** | Excisional or incisional biopsy |
| **What is the treatment?** | Resection with 5-mm margins (2-mm margin in cosmetically sensitive areas) |
| **What is the risk of metastasis?** | Very low (recur locally) |

## MISCELLANEOUS SKIN LESIONS

| | |
|---|---|
| **What is an epidermal inclusion cyst?** | EIC = A benign subcutaneous cyst filled with epidermal cells (should be removed surgically) filled with waxy material; no clinical difference from a sebaceous cyst |

| | |
|---|---|
| **What is a sebaceous cyst?** | A benign subcutaneous cyst filled with sebum (waxy, paste-like substance) from a blocked sweat gland (should be removed with a small area of skin that includes the blocked gland); may become infected; much less common than EIC |
| **What is actinic keratosis?** | A premalignant skin lesion from sun exposure; seen as a scaly skin lesion (surgical removal eliminates the 20% risk of cancer transformation) |
| **What is seborrheic keratosis?** | Benign pigmented lesion in the elderly; observe or treat by excision (especially if there is any question of melanoma), curettage, or topical agents |
| **How to remember actinic keratosis vs. seborrheic keratosis malignant potential?** | Actinic keratosis = AK = asset kicker = premalignant<br>Seborrheic keratosis = SK = soft kicker = benign |
| **What is Bowen's disease of the skin?** | Squamous carcinoma in situ (should be removed or destroyed, thereby removing the problem) |
| **What is "Mohs" surgery?** | Mohs technique or surgery: repeats thin excision until margins are clear by microscopic review (named after Dr. Mohs)—used to minimize collateral skin excision (e.g., on the face) |

# Chapter 64      Melanoma

| | |
|---|---|
| **What is it?** | Neoplastic disorder produced by malignant transformation of the melanocyte; melanocytes are derived from neural crest cells |

**Which patients are at greatest risk?**

White patients with blonde/red hair, fair skin, freckling, a history of blistering sunburns, blue/green eyes, actinic keratosis

Male > female

**What are the most common sites (3)?**

1. Skin
2. Eyes
3. Anus

Think: **SEA** = **S**kin, **E**yes, **A**nus

**What is the most common site in African Americans?**

Palms of the hands, soles of the feet (acral lentiginous melanoma)

**What characteristics are suggestive of melanoma?**

Usually a pigmented lesion with an irregular border, irregular surface, or irregular coloration

Other clues: darkening of a pigmented lesion, development of pigmented satellite lesions, irregular margins or surface elevations, notching, recent or rapid enlargement, erosion or ulceration of surface, pruritus

**What are the "A, B, C, D's" of melanoma?**

**A**symmetry
**B**order irregularity
**C**olor variation
**D**iameter >6 mm and **D**ark lesion

**What are the associated risk factors?**

Severe sunburn before age 18, giant congenital nevi, family history, race (white), ultraviolet radiation (sun), multiple dysplastic nevi

**How does location differ in men and women?**

Men get more lesions on the trunk; women get more on the extremities.

**Which locations are unusual?**

Noncutaneous regions, such as mucous membranes of the vulva/vagina, anorectum, esophagus, and choroidal layer of the eye

**What is the most common site of melanoma in men?**

Back (one-third)

| | |
|---|---|
| **What is the most common site of melanoma in women?** | Legs (one-third) |
| **What are the four major histologic types?** | 1. Superficial spreading<br>2. Lentigo maligna<br>3. Acral lentiginous<br>4. Nodular |

**Define the following terms:**

**Superficial spreading melanoma**

Occurs in both sun-exposed and nonexposed areas

Superficial spread is the most common type (75% of melanomas).

**Lentigo maligna melanoma**

Malignant cells that are superficial, found usually in elderly patients on the head or neck

Called "Hutchinson's freckle" if noninvasive

Least aggressive type; very good prognosis

Accounts for <10% of melanomas

**Acral lentiginous melanoma**

Occurs on the palms, soles, subungual areas, and mucous membranes

Accounts for ≈ 5% of melanomas (most common melanoma in African-American patients ≈ 50%)

**Nodular melanoma**

Vertical growth predominates

Lesions are usually dark

Most aggressive type; worst prognosis

Accounts for ≈ 15% of melanomas

**Amelanotic melanoma**

Melanoma from melanocytes but with obvious lack of pigment

**What is the most common type of melanoma?**

Superficial spreading (>70%) (think: **SUPER**ficial = **SUPER**ior)

**What type of melanoma arises in Hutchinson's freckle?**

Lentigo maligna melanoma

| | |
|---|---|
| **What is Hutchinson's freckle?** | Lentigo melanoma in the radial growth phase without vertical extension (non-invasive); usually occurs on the faces of elderly women |

## STAGING

**What is Clark's classification (microstaging of tumor):**

| | |
|---|---|
| **I?** | Tumor confined to the epidermis; recurrence rate of 0% to 5% |
| **II?** | Tumor invading the papillary dermis; 5-year recurrence rate of 5% |
| **III?** | Tumor cells up to the junction of the papillary and reticular dermis; 5-year recurrence rate of 33% |
| **IV?** | Invasion into the reticular dermis; 5-year recurrence rate of approximately 66% |
| **V?** | Invasion into subcutaneous fat; 5-year recurrence rate of approximately 75% |

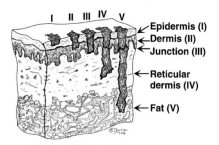

| | |
|---|---|
| **How can Clark's stages be remembered?** | Think "**E**very **P**igmented **J**unction **R**equires **F**ormalin": **E**pidermis (I) **P**apillary dermis (II) **J**unction of papillary/reticular dermis (III) **R**eticular dermis (IV) **F**at (V) |

| | |
|---|---|
| **What is the Breslow classification (microstaging of tumor)?** | Staging by actually measuring the depth of the lesion:<br>Less than 0.76 mm thickness has more than 90% cure with excision.<br>More than 4.0 mm has at least an 80% risk of local recurrence or metastasis in 5 years. |
| **How can Breslow versus Clarke's classifications be remembered?** | Think: Bres**low** = **low** = depth by measurement |
| **Which tumor staging is more accurate in predicting survival?** | The Breslow classification (a more consistent measure of tumor thickness) |

**What are the American Joint Committee on Cancer (AJCC) stages simplified:**

| | |
|---|---|
| **I?** | Less than 1.5 mm depth |
| **II?** | More than 1.5 mm depth |
| **III?** | Positive nodes (regional nodal basin) |
| **IV?** | Metastases (including NONregional nodal basin) |
| **What are the common sites of metastasis?** | Nodes local<br>Distant skin recurrence, lung, liver, bone, heart, and brain<br>Melanoma has a specific attraction for small bowel mucosa and distant cutaneous sites.<br>Brain metastases are a common cause of death. |
| **What are the metastatic routes?** | Both lymphatic and hematogenous |
| **How is the diagnosis made?** | Excisional biopsy (complete removal leaving only normal tissue) or incisioned biopsy for very large lesions (Early diagnosis is crucial.) |

**What is the role of shave biopsy?**

No role

**What is the "sentinel node" biopsy?**

Inject Lymphazurin® blue dye, colloid with a radiolabel, or both around the melanoma; the first LN in the draining chain is identified as the "sentinel lymph node" and reflects the metastatic status of the group of lymph nodes.

**When is elective lymph node dissection recommended?**

Controversial—possible advantage in melanomas 1 to 2 mm in depth but jury still out. Sentinel node biopsy if >1 mm is getting very common. Remember, lymph node dissection is fraught with morbidity (e.g., lymphedema).

**What is the recommended size of the surgical margin for depth of invasion:**
    **Melanoma in situ?**

0.5 cm margin

    **1 mm thick?**

1 cm margin

    **1–4 mm thick?**

2 cm margin

    **>4 mm thick?**

2–3 cm margin

**What is the treatment for digital melanoma?**

Amputation

**What is the treatment of palpable lymph node metastasis?**

Lymphadenectomy

**What factors determine the prognosis?**

Depth of invasion and metastasis are the most important factors. (Superficial spreading and lentigo maligna have a better prognosis because they have a longer horizontal phase of growth and are thus diagnosed at an earlier stage. Nodular has the worst prognosis because it grows predominantly vertically and metastasizes earlier.)

| | |
|---|---|
| **What is the workup to survey for metastasis in the patient with melanoma?** | Physical exam, LFTs, CXR (bone scan/CT/MRI reserved for symptoms) |
| **What is the treatment of intestinal metastasis?** | Surgical resection to prevent bleeding/obstruction |
| **Which malignancy is most likely to metastasize to the bowel?** | Melanoma |
| **What is the surgical treatment of nodal metastasis?** | Lymphadenectomy |
| **What is FDA-approved adjuvant therapy?** | Interferon-alfa-2B |
| **What is the treatment of unresectable brain metastasis?** | Radiation |
| **What is the treatment of isolated adrenal metastasis?** | Surgical resection |
| **What is the treatment of isolated lung metastasis?** | Surgical resection |
| **What is the most common symptom of anal melanoma?** | Bleeding |
| **What is the treatment of anal melanoma?** | APR or wide excision (no survival benefit from APR, but better local control) |
| **What other experimental therapy is available for metastatic disease?** | 1. Monoclonal antibodies<br>2. Chemotherapy (e.g., dacarbazine)<br>3. Vaccinations |
| **What is the median survival with distant metastasis?** | $\approx 6$ months |

# Chapter 65

# Surgical Intensive Care

## INTENSIVE CARE UNIT (ICU) BASICS

**How is an ICU note written?**

The note is by **systems:**
Neurologic (e.g., GCS, MAE, pain control)
Pulmonary (e.g., vent settings)
CVS (e.g., pressors, Swan numbers)
GI (gastrointestinal)
Heme (CBC)
FEN (e.g., Chem 10, nutrition)
Renal (e.g., urine output, BUN, Cr)
ID (e.g., Tmax, WBC, antibiotics)
Assessment
Plan
(**FEN** = **F**luids, **E**lectrolytes, **N**utrition); physical exam included in each section

**What is the best way to report urine output in the ICU?**

24 hrs/last shift/last 3 hourly rate = "urine output has been 2 liters over last 24 hrs, 350 last shift, and 45, 35, 40 cc over the last 3 hours"

**What are the possible causes of fever in the ICU?**

Central line infection
Pneumonia/atelectasis
UTI, urosepsis
Intra-abdominal abscess
Sinusitis
DVT
Thrombophlebitis
Drug fever
Fungal infection, meningitis, wound infection
Endocarditis

**What is the most common bacteria in ICU pneumonia?**

Gram-negative rods

| | |
|---|---|
| **What is the acronym for the basic ICU care check list (Dr. Vincent)?** | **F.A.S.T.  H.U.G.:**<br><br>**F**eeding<br>**A**nalgesia<br>**S**edation<br>**T**hromboembolic prophylaxis<br><br>**H**ead-of-bed elevation (pneumonia prevention)<br>**U**lcer prevention<br>**G**lucose control |

## INTENSIVE CARE UNIT FORMULAS AND TERMS YOU SHOULD KNOW

| | |
|---|---|
| **What is CO?** | **C**ardiac **O**utput: HR (heart rate) × SV (stroke volume) |
| **What is the normal CO?** | Between 4 and 8 L/min |
| **What factors increase CO?** | Increased contractility, heart rate, and preload; decreased afterload |
| **What is CI?** | **C**ardiac **I**ndex: CO/BSA (body surface area) |
| **What is the normal CI?** | Between 2.5 and 3.5 $L/min/M_2$ |
| **What is SV?** | **S**troke **V**olume: the amount of blood pumped out of the ventricle each beat; simply, end diastolic volume minus the end systolic volume **or** CO/HR |
| **What is the normal SV?** | Between 60 and 100 cc |
| **What is CVP?** | **C**entral **V**enous **P**ressure: indirect measurement of intravascular volume status |
| **What is the normal CVP?** | Between 4 and 11 |
| **What is PCWP?** | **P**ulmonary **C**apillary **W**edge **P**ressure: indirectly measures left atrial pressure, which is an estimate of intravascular volume (LV filling pressure) |

| | |
|---|---|
| **What is the normal PCWP?** | Between 5 and 15 |
| **What is anion gap?** | $Na^+ - (Cl^- + HCO_3^-)$ |
| **What are the normal values for anion gap?** | Between 10 and 14 |
| **Why do you get an increased anion gap?** | The unmeasured acids are unmeasured anions in the equation that are part of the "counterbalance" to the sodium cation. |
| **What are the causes of increased anion gap acidosis in surgical patients?** | Think **"S.A.L.U.D.":** **S**tarvation **A**lcohol (ethanol/methanol) **L**actic acidosis **U**remia (renal failure) **D**KA |
| **Define MODS.** | **M**ultiple **O**rgan **D**ysfunction **S**yndrome |
| **What is SVR?** | **S**ystemic **V**ascular **R**esistance: MAP − CVP / CO × 80 (remember, P = F × R, **P**ower **FoR**ward; and calculating resistance: **R = P/F**) |
| **What is SVRI?** | **S**ystemic **V**ascular **R**esistance **I**ndex: SVR/BSA |
| **What is the normal SVRI?** | Between 1500 and 2400 |
| **What is MAP?** | **M**ean **A**rterial **P**ressure: diastolic blood pressure **+ 1/3 (systolic−diastolic pressure)** *Note:* Not the mean between diastolic and systolic blood pressure because diastole lasts longer than systole |
| **What is PVR?** | **P**ulmonary **V**ascular **R**esistance: PA(MEAN) − PCWP / CO × 80 (PA is pulmonary artery pressure and LA is left atrial or PCWP pressure) |
| **What is the normal PVR value?** | 100 ± 50 |
| **What is the formula for arterial oxygen content?** | Hemoglobin × $O_2$ saturation ($SaO_2$) |

**What is the formula for oxygen delivery?**

$CO \times (\text{hemoglobin} \times SaO_2)$

**What factors can increase oxygen delivery?**

Increased CO by increasing SV, HR, or both; increased $O_2$ content by increasing the hemoglobin content, $SaO_2$, or both

**What is mixed venous oxygen saturation?**

$SvO_2$; simply, the $O_2$ saturation of the blood in the right ventricle or pulmonary artery; an indirect measure of peripheral oxygen supply and demand

**Which lab values help assess adequate oxygen delivery?**

$SvO_2$ (low with inadequate delivery), lactic acid (elevated with inadequate delivery), pH (acidosis with inadequate delivery), base deficit

**What is FENA?**

**F**ractional **E**xcretion of Sodium (**Na$^+$**): $(U_{Na^+} \times P_{cr} / P_{Na^+} \times U_{cr}) \times 100$

**What is the memory aid for calculating FENA?**

Think: **"You need pee"** = You (**U**rine) **need** (**Na$^+$**) **pee** (**P**lasma); therefore, $U_{Na^+} \times P_{cr}$; and for the denominator switch everything, or $P_{Na^+} \times U_{cr}$

**What is the prerenal FENA value?**

$<1.0$; renal failure from decreased renal blood flow (e.g., cardiogenic, hypovolemia, arterial obstruction, etc.)

**How long does Lasix® effect last?**

6 hours = **LASIX** = **LA**sts **SIX** hours

**What is the formula for flow/pressure/resistance?**

Remember **P**ower **F**o**R**ward: **P**ressure = **F**low $\times$ **R**esistance

**What is the "10 for 0.08 rule" of acid-base?**

For every increase of $PaCO_2$ by 10 mm Hg, the pH falls by 0.08.

**What is the "40, 50, 60 for 70, 80, 90 rule" for $O_2$ sats?**

A $PaO_2$ of **40, 50, 60** corresponds roughly to an $O_2$ sat of **70, 80, 90**, respectively.

**One liter of $O_2$ via nasal cannula raises $FiO_2$ by how much?**

Approximately 3% to 4%

| | |
|---|---|
| **What is pure respiratory acidosis?** | Low pH (acidosis), increased $PaCO_2$, normal bicarbonate |
| **What is pure respiratory alkalosis?** | High pH (alkalosis), decreased $PaCO_2$, normal bicarbonate |
| **What is pure metabolic acidosis?** | Low pH, low bicarbonate, normal $PaCO_2$ |
| **What is pure metabolic alkalosis?** | High pH, high bicarbonate, normal $PaCO_2$ |

**List how the body compensates for each of the following:**

| | |
|---|---|
| **Respiratory acidosis** | Increased bicarbonate |
| **Respiratory alkalosis** | Decreased bicarbonate |
| **Metabolic acidosis** | Decreased $PaCO_2$ |
| **Metabolic alkalosis** | Increased $PaCO_2$ |
| **What does MOF stand for?** | **M**ultiple **O**rgan **F**ailure |
| **What does SIRS stand for?** | **S**ystemic **I**nflammatory **R**esponse **S**yndrome |

## SICU DRUGS

DOPAMINE

**What is the site of action and effect at the following levels:**

| | |
|---|---|
| **Low dose (1–3 µg/kg/ min)?** | ++ dopa agonist; **renal vasodilation** (A.K.A. "renal dose dopamine") |
| **Intermediate dose (4–10 µg/kg/min)?** | + alpha$_1$, ++ beta$_1$; positive inotropy and some vasoconstriction |
| **High dose (> µg/kg/min)?** | +++ alpha$_1$ agonist; marked afterload increase from arteriolar vasoconstriction |
| **Has "renal dose" dopamine been shown to decrease renal failure?** | NO |

## DOBUTAMINE

| | |
|---|---|
| **What is the site of action?** | $+++$ beta$_1$ agonist, $++$ beta$_2$ |
| **What is the effect?** | ↑ inotropy; ↑ chronotropy, **decrease in systemic vascular resistance** |

## ISOPROTERENOL

| | |
|---|---|
| **What is the site of action?** | $+++$ beta$_1$ and beta$_2$ agonist |
| **What is the effect?** | ↑ inotropy; ↑ chronotropy; ($+$ vasodilation of skeletal and mesenteric vascular beds) |

## EPINEPHRINE (EPI)

| | |
|---|---|
| **What is the site of action?** | $++$ alpha$_1$, alpha$_2$, $++++$ beta$_1$, and beta$_2$ agonist |
| **What is the effect?** | ↑ inotropy; ↑ chronotropy |
| **What is the effect at high doses?** | Vasoconstriction |

## NOREPINEPHRINE (NE)

| | |
|---|---|
| **What is the site of action?** | $+++$ alpha$_1$, alpha$_2$, $+++$ beta$_1$, and beta$_1$ agonist |
| **What is the effect?** | ↑ inotropy; ↑ chronotropy; $++$ increase in blood pressure |
| **What is the effect at high doses?** | Severe vasoconstriction |

## NITROGLYCERINE (NTG)

| | |
|---|---|
| **What is the site of action?** | $+++$ venodilation; $+$ arteriolar dilation |
| **What is the effect?** | Increased venous capacitance, decreased preload, coronary arteriole vasodilation |

## SODIUM NITROPRUSSIDE (SNP)

| | |
|---|---|
| **What is the site of action?** | $+++$ venodilation; $+++$ arteriolar dilation |

| | |
|---|---|
| **What is the effect?** | Decreased preload and afterload (allowing blood pressure titration) |
| **What is the major toxicity of SNP?** | **Cyanide** toxicity |

## INTENSIVE CARE PHYSIOLOGY

**Define the following terms:**

| | |
|---|---|
| **Preload** | Load on the heart muscle that stretches it to end-diastolic volume (end-diastolic pressure) = intravascular volume |
| **Afterload** | Load or resistance the heart must pump against = vascular tone = SVR |
| **Contractility** | Force of heart muscle contraction |
| **Compliance** | Distensibility of heart by the preload |
| **What is the Frank-Starling curve?** | Cardiac output increases with increasing preload up to a point. |
| **What is the clinical significance of the steep slope of the Starling curve relating end-diastolic volume to cardiac output?** | It demonstrates the importance of preload in determining cardiac output. |
| **What factors influence the oxygen content of whole blood?** | Oxygen content is composed largely of that oxygen bound to hemoglobin, and is thus determined by the hemoglobin concentration and the arterial oxygen saturation; the partial pressure of oxygen dissolved in plasma plays a minor role. |
| **What factors influence mixed venous oxygen saturation?** | Oxygen **delivery** (hemoglobin concentration, arterial oxygen saturation, cardiac output) and oxygen **extraction** by the peripheral tissues |
| **What lab test for tissue ischemia is based on the shift from aerobic to anaerobic metabolism?** | Serum lactic acid levels |

**Define the following terms:**
**Dead space**

That part of the inspired air that will not participate in gas exchange (e.g., the gas in the large airways/ET tube not in contact with capillaries)
Think: space = air

**Shunt fraction**

That fraction of pulmonary venous blood that did not participate in gas exchange
Think: shunt = blood

**What causes increased dead space?**

Overventilation (emphysema, excessive PEEP) or underperfusion (pulmonary embolus, low cardiac output, pulmonary artery vasoconstriction)

**At high shunt fractions, what is the effect of increasing $FiO_2$ on arterial $PO_2$?**

At high shunt fractions (>50%), changes in $FiO_2$ have almost no effect on arterial $PO_2$ because the blood that does "see" the $O_2$ is already at maximal $O_2$ absorption and, thus, increasing the $FiO_2$ has no effect ($FiO_2$ can be minimized to prevent oxygen toxicity).

**Define ARDS.**

**A**cute **R**espiratory **D**istress **S**yndrome (previously known as **A**dult **R**espiratory **D**istress **S**yndrome) = noncardiac pulmonary edema

**What is the ARDS diagnostic triad?**

"C.X.R.":
**C**apillary wedge pressure <18
**X**-ray of chest with bilateral infiltrates
**R**atio of $PaO_2$ to $FiO_2$ <200

**What does the classic chest x-ray look like with ARDS?**

Bilateral fluffy infiltrates

**How can you remember the $PaO_2$ to $FiO_2$, or PF, ratio?**

Think: "**PuF**f" ratio: PF ratio = $PaO_2$–$FiO_2$ ratio

**At what concentration does $O_2$ toxicity occur?**

$FiO_2$ of >60% × 48 hours; thus, try to keep $FiO_2$ below 60% at all times

**What is the ONLY ventilatory parameter that has been shown to decrease mortality in ARDS patients?**

Low tidal volumes ($\leq 6$ cc/kg) and low plateau pressures <30

**What are the main causes of carbon dioxide retention?**

Hypoventilation, increased dead space ventilation, and increased carbon dioxide production (as in hypermetabolic states)

**Why are carbohydrates minimized in the diet/TPN of patients having difficulty with hypercapnia?**

The respiratory quotient (RQ) is the ratio of $CO_2$ production to $O_2$ consumption and is highest for carbohydrates (1.0) and lowest for fats (0.7).

## HEMODYNAMIC MONITORING

**Why are indwelling arterial lines used for blood pressure monitoring in critically ill patients?**

Because of the need for frequent measurements, the inaccuracy of frequently repeated cuff measurements, the inaccuracy of cuff measurements in hypotension, and the need for frequent arterial blood sampling/labs

**Which pressures/values are obtained from a Swan-Ganz catheter?**

CVP, PA pressures, PCWP, CO, PVR, SVR, mixed venous $O_2$ saturation

**Identify the Swan-Ganz waveforms.**

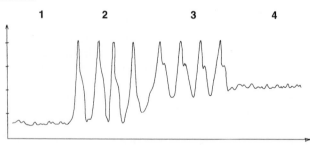

1. CVP/right atrium
2. Right ventricle
3. Pulmonary artery
4. Wedge

**What does the abbreviation PCWP stand for?**

**P**ulmonary **C**apillary **W**edge **P**ressure

**Give other names for PCWP.**

Wedge or wedge pressure, pulmonary artery occlusion pressure (PAOP)

**What is it?**

Pulmonary capillary pressure after balloon occlusion of the pulmonary artery, which is equal to left atrial pressure because there are no valves in the pulmonary system.

Left atrial pressure is essentially equal to left ventricular end diastolic pressure (LVEDP): left heart preload, and, thus, intravascular volume status.

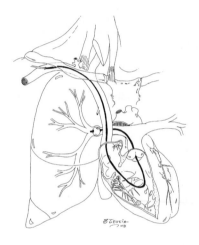

**What is the primary use of the PCWP?**

As an indirect measure of preload = intravascular volume

**Has the usage of a Swan-Ganz catheter been shown to decrease mortality in ICU patients?**

NO

**At what point in the respiratory cycle is PCWP most accurate?**

Positive pressure
Ventilated patient—at end expiration
Nonventilated patient—at peak inspiration
Think: "Peaks and valleys":
**P**eaks—**P**atient breathing on his own = **P**eak of inspiration
**V**alleys—**V**entilated patient = **V**alley of expiration

**In which clinical situations is PCWP not an accurate estimate of preload?**

Pulmonary disease, such as ARDS; pulmonary hypertension; valvular heart disease; ischemic heart disease with a noncompliant ventricle; high levels of PEEP; tamponade; PTX

**How does thermodilution determine the cardiac output (CO)?**

The temperature of a proximal saline injection or heater probe is determined at a point distal (pulmonary artery) to its origin. The temperature difference determines amount of blood flow and, thus, CO.

## MECHANICAL VENTILATION

**Define ventilation.**

Air through the lungs; monitored by $PCO_2$

**Define oxygenation.**

Oxygen delivery to the alveoli; monitored by $O_2$ sats and $PO_2$

**What can increase ventilation to decrease $PCO_2$?**

Increased respiratory rate (RR), increased tidal volume (minute ventilation)

**What is minute ventilation?**

Volume of gas ventilated through the lungs (RR $\times$ tidal volume)

**Define tidal volume.**

Volume delivered with each breath; should be 6 to 8 cc/kg on the ventilator

**Are ventilation and oxygenation related?**

Basically no; you can have an $O_2$ sat of 100% and a $PCO_2$ of 150. $O_2$ sats do not tell you anything about the $PCO_2$ (key point!).

**What can increase $PO_2$ (oxygenation) in the ventilated patient?**

Increased $FiO_2$
Increased PEEP

**What can decrease $PCO_2$ in the ventilated patient?**

Increased RR
Increased tidal volume (i.e., increase minute ventilation)

**Define the following modes:**

**IMV**

Intermittent Mandatory Ventilation: mode with intermittent mandatory ventilations at a predetermined rate; patients can also breathe on their own above the mandatory rate **without** help from the ventilator

**SIMV**

Synchronous **IMV:** mode of IMV that delivers the mandatory breath synchronously with patient's initiated effort; if no breath is initiated, the ventilator delivers the predetermined mandatory breath

**A-C**

Assist-Control Ventilation: mode in which the ventilator delivers a breath when the patient initiates a breath, or the ventilator "assists" the patient to breathe; if the patient does not initiate a breath, the ventilator takes "control" and delivers a breath at a predetermined rate
In contrast to IMV, all breaths are by the ventilator.

**CPAP**

Continuous Positive Airway Pressure: positive pressure delivered **continuously** (during expiration and inspiration) by ventilator, but no volume breaths (patient breathes on own)

**Pressure support**

Pressure is delivered only **with an initiated breath.** Pressure support decreases the work of breathing by overcoming the resistance in the ventilator circuit.

**What are the effects of positive pressure ventilation in a patient with hypovolemia or low lung compliance?**

Venous return and cardiac output are decreased.

**Define PEEP.**

Positive End Expiration Pressure: positive pressure maintained at the end of a breath; keeps alveoli open

| | |
|---|---|
| **What is "physiologic PEEP"?** | PEEP of 5 cm $H_2O$; thought to approximate normal pressure in normal nonintubated people caused by the closed glottis |
| **What are the side effects of increasing levels of PEEP?** | Barotrauma (injury to airway = pneumothorax), decreased CO from decreased preload |

**What are the typical initial ventilator settings:**

| | |
|---|---|
| Mode? | Intermittent mandatory ventilation |
| Tidal volume? | 6–8 ml/kg |
| Ventilator rate? | 10 breaths/min |
| $FiO_2$? | 100% and wean down |
| PEEP? | 5 cm $H_2O$<br>From these parameters, change according to blood-gas analysis |

| | |
|---|---|
| **What is a normal I:E (inspiratory to expiratory time)?** | 1:2 |
| **When would you use an inverse I:E ratio (e.g., 2:1, 3:1, etc.)?** | To allow for longer inspiration in patients with poor compliance, to allow for "alveolar recruitment" |
| **When would you use a prolonged I:E ratio (e.g., 1:4)?** | COPD to allow time for complete exhalation (prevents "breath stacking") |
| **What clinical situations cause increased airway resistance?** | Airway or endotracheal tube obstruction, bronchospasm, ARDS, mucus plug, CHF (pulmonary edema) |
| **What are the presumed advantages of PEEP?** | Prevention of alveolar collapse and atelectasis, improved gas exchange, increased pulmonary compliance, decreased shunt fraction |
| **What are the possible disadvantages of PEEP?** | Decreased cardiac output, especially in the setting of hypovolemia; decreased gas exchange; ↓ compliance with high levels of PEEP, fluid retention, increased intracranial pressure, barotrauma |

**What parameters must be evaluated in deciding if a patient is ready to be extubated?**

Patient alert and able to protect airway, gas exchange ($PaO_2$ >70, $PaCO_2$ <50), tidal volume (>5 cc/kg), minute ventilation (<10 L/min), negative inspiratory pressure (< −20 cm $H_2O$ or more negative), $FiO_2 \le 40\%$, PEEP 5, PH > 7.25, RR < 35, Tobin index < 105

**What is the Tobin index?**

**R**ate: **T**idal volume ratio. A Tobin index < 105 is associated with successful extubation (think: **R**espiratory **T**herapist = **RT** = **R**ate: **T**idal volume)

**What is a possible source of fever in a patient with an NG or nasal endotracheal tube?**

Sinusitis (diagnosed by sinus films/CT)

**What is the 35−45 rule of blood gas values?**

Normal values:
pH = 7.**35**−7.**45**
$PCO_2$ = **35**−**45**

**Which medications can be delivered via an endotracheal tube?**

Think **"N.A.V.E.L.":**
**N**arcan
**A**tropine
**V**asopressin
**E**pinephrine
**L**idocaine

**What conditions should you think of with ↑ peak airway pressure and decreased urine output?**

1. Tension pneumothorax
2. Abdominal compartment syndrome

---

# Chapter 66

# Vascular Surgery

**What is atherosclerosis?**

A diffuse disease process in arteries; atheromas containing cholesterol and lipid form within the intima and inner media, often accompanied by ulcerations and smooth muscle hyperplasia

**What is the common theory of how atherosclerosis is initiated?**

Endothelial injury → platelets adhere → growth factors released → smooth muscle hyperplasia/plaque deposition

**What are the risk factors for atherosclerosis?**

Hypertension, **smoking,** diabetes mellitus, family history, hyper-cholesterolemia, high LDL, obesity, and sedentary lifestyle

**What are the common sites of plaque formation in arteries?**

Branch points (carotid bifurcation), tethered sites (superficial femoral artery [SFA] in Hunter's canal in the leg)

**What must be present for a successful arterial bypass operation?**

1. Inflow (e.g., patent aorta)
2. Outflow (e.g., open distal popliteal artery)
3. Run off (e.g., patent trifurcation vessels down to the foot)

**What is the major principle of safe vascular surgery?**

Get **proximal** and **distal** control of the vessel to be worked on!

**What does it mean to "POTTS" a vessel?**

Place a vessel loop twice around a vessel so that if you put tension on the vessel loop, it will occlude the vessel.

**What is the suture needle orientation through graft versus diseased artery in a graft to artery anastomosis?**

Needle "in to out" of the lumen in diseased artery to help **tack down the plaque** and the needle "out-to-in" on the graft

**What are the layers of an artery?**

1. Intima
2. Media
3. Adventitia

**Which arteries supply the blood vessel itself?**

Vasovasorum

**What is a true aneurysm?**

Dilation (> 2× nL diameter) of all three layers of a vessel

**What is a false (pseudo)aneurysm?**

Dilation of artery not involving all three layers (e.g., hematoma with fibrous covering)

Often connects with vessel lumen and blood swirls inside the false aneurysm

**What is "ENDOVASCULAR" repair?**

Placement of a catheter in artery and then deployment of a graft intraluminally

## PERIPHERAL VASCULAR DISEASE

**Define the arterial anatomy.**

1. Aorta
2. Internal iliac (hypogastric)
3. External iliac
4. Common femoral artery
5. Profundi femoral artery
6. Superficial femoral artery (SFA)
7. Popliteal artery
8. Trifurcation
9. Anterior tibial artery
10. Peroneal artery
11. Posterior tibial artery
12. Dorsalis pedis artery

**How can you remember the orientation of the lower exterior arteries below the knee on A-gram?**

Use the acronym "**L.A.M.P.**":
**L**ateral **A**nterior tibial
**M**edial **P**osterior tibial

**What is peripheral vascular disease (PVD)?**

Occlusive atherosclerotic disease in the lower extremities

**What is the most common site of arterial atherosclerotic occlusion in the lower extremities?**

Occlusion of the SFA in Hunter's canal

**What are the symptoms of PVD?**

Intermittent claudication, rest pain, erectile dysfunction, sensorimotor impairment, tissue loss

**What is intermittent claudication?**

Pain, cramping, or both of the lower extremity, usually the calf muscle, after walking a specific distance; then the pain/cramping resolves after stopping for a specific amount of time while standing; this pattern is reproducible

**What is rest pain?**

Pain in the foot, usually over the distal metatarsals; this pain arises at rest (classically at night, awakening the patient)

**What classically resolves rest pain?**

Hanging the foot over the side of the bed or standing; gravity affords some extra flow to the ischemic areas

**How can vascular causes of claudication be differentiated from nonvascular causes, such as neurogenic claudication or arthritis?**

History (in the vast majority of patients) and noninvasive tests; remember, vascular claudication appears after a specific distance and resolves after a specific time of rest while standing (not so with most other forms of claudication)

**What is the differential diagnosis of lower extremity claudication?**

Neurogenic (e.g., nerve entrapment/discs), arthritis, coarctation of the aorta, popliteal artery syndrome, chronic compartment syndrome, neuromas, anemia, diabetic neuropathy pain

**What are the signs of PVD?**   Absent pulses, bruits, muscular atrophy, decreased hair growth, thick toenails, tissue necrosis/ulcers/infection

**What is the site of a PVD ulcer vs. a venous stasis ulcer?**   PVD arterial insufficiency ulcer—usually on the toes/foot
Venous stasis ulcer—medial malleolus (ankle)

**What is the ABI?**   The **A**nkle to **B**rachial **I**ndex (**ABI**); simply, the ratio of the systolic blood pressure at the ankle to the systolic blood pressure at the arm (brachial artery) A:B; ankle pressure taken with Doppler; the ABI is noninvasive

**What ABIs are associated with normals, claudicators, and rest pain?**   Normal ABI— $\geq 1.0$
Claudicator ABI— $<0.6$
Rest pain ABI— $<0.4$

**Who gets false ABI readings?**   Patients with calcified arteries, especially those with diabetes

**What are PVRs?**   **P**ulse **V**olume **R**ecordings; pulse wave forms are recorded from lower extremities representing volume of blood per heart beat at sequential sites down leg
A large wave form means good collateral blood flow.
(Noninvasive using pressure cuffs)

**Prior to surgery for chronic PVD, what diagnostic test will every patient receive?**   **A-gram** (arteriogram: dye in vessel and x-rays) maps disease and allows for best treatment option (i.e., angioplasty vs. surgical bypass vs. endarterectomy)
Gold standard for diagnosing PVD

**What is the bedside management of a patient with PVD?**   1. Sheep skin (easy on the heels)
2. Foot cradle (keeps sheets/blankets off the feet)
3. Skin lotion to avoid further cracks in the skin that can go on to form a fissure and then an ulcer

**What are the indications for surgical treatment in PVD?**

Use the acronym **"S.T.I.R."**:

**S**evere claudication refractory to conservative treatment that affects quality of life/livelihood (e.g., can't work because of the claudication)

**T**issue necrosis

**I**nfection

**R**est pain

**What is the treatment of claudication?**

For the vast majority, conservative treatment, including exercise, smoking cessation, treatment of HTN, diet, aspirin, with or without Trental (pentoxifylline)

**How can you remember the medical conservative treatment for claudication?**

Use the acronym **P.A.C.E.**:

**P**entoxifylline

**A**spirin

**C**essation of smoking

**E**xercise

**How does aspirin work?**

Inhibits platelets (inhibits cyclooxygenase and platelet aggregation)

**How does Trental® (pentoxifylline) work?**

Results in increased RBC deformity and flexibility (think: pento**X**ifylline = RBC fle**X**ibility)

**What is the risk of limb loss with claudication?**

Five percent limb loss at 5 years (think: 5 in 5), 10% at 10 years (think: 10 in 10)

**What is the risk of limb loss with rest pain?**

More than 50% of patients will have amputation of the limb at some point.

**In the patient with PVD, what is the main postoperative concern?**

Cardiac status, because most patients with PVD have coronary artery disease; about 20% have an AAA

MI is the most common cause of postoperative death after a PVD operation.

**What is Leriche's syndrome?**

Impotence, buttock claudication, and leg muscle atrophy from occlusive disease of the iliacs/distal aorta

Think: **"C.I.A."**:

Claudication
Impotence
Atrophy
(think: CIA spy Leriche)

**What are the treatment options for severe PVD?**

1. Surgical graft bypass
2. Angioplasty—balloon dilation
3. Endarterectomy—remove diseased intima and media
4. Surgical patch angioplasty (place patch over stenosis)

**What is a FEM-POP bypass?**

Bypass SFA occlusion with a graft from the femoral artery to the popliteal artery

Graft

**What is a FEM-DISTAL bypass?**

Bypass from the femoral artery to a distal artery (peroneal artery, anterior tibial artery, or posterior tibial artery)

Graft

**What graft material has the longest patency rate?**

Autologous vein graft

**What is an "in situ" vein graft?**

Saphenous vein is more or less left in place, all branches are ligated, and the vein valves are broken with a small hook or cut out. A vein can also be used if reversed so that the valves do not cause a problem.

**What type of graft is used for above-the-knee FEM-POP bypass?**

Either vein or Gortex® graft; vein still has better patency

**What type of graft is used for below-the-knee FEM-POP or FEM-DISTAL bypass?**

Must use vein graft; prosthetic grafts have a prohibitive thrombosis rate

**What is DRY gangrene?**

Dry necrosis of tissue without signs of infection ("mummified tissue")

**What is WET gangrene?**

Moist necrotic tissue with signs of infection

**What is blue toe syndrome?**

Intermittent painful blue toes (or fingers) due to microemboli from a proximal arterial plaque

## LOWER EXTREMITY AMPUTATIONS

**What are the indications?**

Irreversible tissue ischemia (no hope for revascularization bypass) and necrotic tissue, severe infection, severe pain with no bypassable vessels, or if patient is not interested in a bypass procedure

**Identify the level of the following amputations:**

1. Above-the-knee amputation (AKA)
2. Below-the-knee amputation (BKA)
3. Symes amputation
4. Transmetatarsal amputation
5. Toe amputation

**What is a Ray amputation?**

Removal of toe and head of metatarsal

## ACUTE ARTERIAL OCCLUSION

**What is it?**

Acute occlusion of an artery, usually by embolization; other causes include acute thrombosis of an atheromatous lesion, vascular trauma

**What are the classic signs/ symptoms of acute arterial occlusion?**

The "six P's": **P**ain, **P**aralysis, **P**allor, **P**aresthesia, **P**olar (some say poikilothermia—you pick), **P**ulselessness (you **must** know these!)

**What is the classic timing of pain with acute arterial occlusion from an embolus?**

Acute onset; the patient can classically tell you exactly when and where it happened

**What is the immediate preoperative management?**

1. Anticoagulate with IV heparin (bolus followed by constant infusion)
2. A-gram

**What are the sources of emboli?**

1. Heart—85% (e.g., clot from AFib, clot forming on dead muscle after MI, endocarditis, myxoma)
2. Aneurysms
3. Atheromatous plaque (atheroembolism)

**What is the most common cause of embolus from the heart?**

AFib

**What is the most common site of arterial occlusion by an embolus?**

Common femoral artery (SFA is the most common site of arterial occlusion from atherosclerosis)

**What diagnostic studies are in order?**

1. A-gram
2. ECG (looking for MI, AFib)
3. Echocardiogram ($\pm$) looking for clot, MI, valve vegetation

**What is the treatment?**

Surgical embolectomy via cutdown and Fogarty balloon (bypass is reserved for embolectomy failure)

**What is a Fogarty?**

Fogarty balloon catheter—catheter with a balloon tip that can be inflated with saline; used for embolectomy

**How do you use a Fogarty catheter?**

Insinuate the catheter with the balloon deflated past the embolus and then inflate the balloon and pull the catheter out; the balloon brings the embolus with it

**How many mm in diameter is a 12 French Fogarty catheter?**

Simple; to get mm from French measurements, divide the French number by pi, or 3.14; thus, a 12 French catheter is $12/3 = 4$ mm in diameter

| | |
|---|---|
| **What must you look for postoperatively after reperfusion of a limb?** | Compartment syndrome, hyperkalemia, renal failure from myoglobinuria, MI |
| **What is compartment syndrome?** | The leg (calf) is separated into compartments by very unyielding fascia; **tissue swelling** from reperfusion can increase the intracompartmental pressure, resulting in decreased capillary flow, ischemia, and myonecrosis; myonecrosis may occur after the intracompartment pressure reaches only 30 mm Hg. |
| **What are the signs/ symptoms of compartment syndrome?** | Classic signs include pain, especially after passive flexing/extension of the foot, paralysis, paresthesias, and pallor; **pulses are present** in most cases because systolic pressure is much higher than the minimal 30 mm Hg needed for the syndrome! |
| **Can a patient have a pulse and compartment syndrome?** | YES! |
| **How is the diagnosis made?** | History/suspicion, compartment pressure measurement |
| **What is the treatment of compartment syndrome?** | Treatment includes opening compartments via bilateral calf-incision fasciotomies of all four compartments in the calf. |

## ABDOMINAL AORTIC ANEURYSMS

| | |
|---|---|
| **What is it also known as?** | AAA, or "triple A" |
| **What is it?** | An abnormal dilation of the abdominal aorta ($>1.5-2\times$ normal), forming a true aneurysm |

| | |
|---|---|
| **What is the male to female ratio?** | M:F = approximately 6:1 |
| **By far, who is at the highest risk?** | White males |
| **What is the common etiology?** | Believed to be **atherosclerotic** in 95% of cases; 5% inflammatory |
| **What is the most common site?** | Infrarenal (95%) |
| **What is the incidence?** | Five percent of all adults older than 60 years of age |
| **What percentage of patients with AAA have a peripheral arterial aneurysm?** | 20% |
| **What are the risk factors?** | **Atherosclerosis,** hypertension, smoking, male gender, advanced age, connective tissue disease |
| **What are the symptoms?** | Most AAAs are **asymptomatic** and discovered during routine abdominal exam by primary care physicians; in the remainder, symptoms range from vague epigastric discomfort to back and abdominal pain. |
| **Classically, what does testicular pain and an AAA signify?** | Retroperitoneal rupture with ureteral stretch and referred pain to the testicle |

| | |
|---|---|
| **What are the risk factors for rupture?** | Increasing aneurysm diameter, COPD, HTN, recent rapid expansion, large diameter, hypertension, symptomatic |
| **What are the signs of rupture?** | Classic triad of ruptured AAA:<br>1. **Abdominal pain**<br>2. **Pulsatile abdominal mass**<br>3. **Hypotension** |
| **By how much each year do AAAs grow?** | Approximately 3 mm/year on average (larger AAAs grow faster than smaller AAAs) |
| **Why do larger AAAs rupture more often and grow faster than smaller AAAs?** | Probably because of Laplace's law (wall tension = pressure × diameter) |
| **What is the risk of rupture per year based on AAA diameter size?** | Less than 5 cm = 4%<br>Between 5 and 7 cm = 7%<br>More than 7 cm = 20% |
| **Where does the aorta bifurcate?** | At the level of the **umbilicus;** therefore, when palpating for an AAA, palpate above the umbilicus and below the xiphoid process |
| **What is the differential diagnosis?** | Acute pancreatitis, aortic dissection, mesenteric ischemia, MI, perforated ulcer, diverticulosis, renal colic, etc. |
| **What are the diagnostic tests?** | Use U/S to follow AAA clinically; other tests involve contrast CT and A-gram; A-gram will assess lumen patency and iliac/renal involvement. |
| **What is the limitation of A-gram?** | AAAs often have large mural thrombi, which result in a falsely reduced diameter because only the patent lumen is visualized. |
| **What are the signs of AAA on AXR?** | Calcification in the aneurysm wall, best seen on lateral projection (A.K.A. eggshell calcifications) |

**What are the indications for surgical repair of AAA?**

**AAA more than 5.5 cm** in diameter, if the patient is not an overwhelming high risk for surgery; also, rupture of the AAA, any size AAA with rapid growth, symptoms/embolization of plaque

**What is the treatment?**

1. Prosthetic graft placement, with rewrapping of the native aneurysm adventitia around the prosthetic graft after the thrombus is removed; when rupture is strongly suspected, **proceed to immediate laparotomy; there is no time for diagnostic tests!**

2. Endovascular repair

**What is endovascular repair?**

Endovascular repair is a repair of the AAA by femoral catheter placed stents

**Why wrap the graft in the native aorta?**

To reduce the incidence of enterograft fistula formation

**What type of repair should be performed with AAA and iliacs severely occluded or iliac aneurysm(s)?**

Aortobi-iliac or aortobifemoral graft replacement (bifurcated graft)

**What is the treatment if the patient has abdominal pain, pulsatile abdominal mass, and hypotension?**

Take the patient to the **O.R.** for emergent AAA repair

**What is the treatment if the patient has known AAA and new onset of abdominal pain or back pain?**

CT scan
1. Leak → straight to OR
2. No leak → repair during next elective slot

**What is the mortality rate associated with the following types of AAA treatment:**
  **Elective?**

Good; less than 4% operative mortality

  **Ruptured?**

≈ 50% operative mortality

**What is the leading cause of postoperative death in a patient undergoing elective AAA treatment?**

Myocardial infarction (MI)

**What are the other etiologies of AAA?**

Inflammatory (connective tissue diseases), mycotic (a misnomer because most result from bacteria, not fungi)

**What is the mean normal abdominal aortic diameter?**

2 cm

**What are the possible operative complications?**

MI, atheroembolism, declamping hypotension, acute renal failure (especially if aneurysm involves the renal arteries), ureteral injury, hemorrhage

**Why is colonic ischemia a concern in the repair of AAAs?**

Often the IMA is sacrificed during surgery; if the collaterals are not adequate, the patient will have colonic ischemia.

**What are the signs of colonic ischemia?**

Heme-positive stool, or bright red blood per rectum (BRBPR), diarrhea, abdominal pain

**What is the study of choice to diagnose colonic ischemia?**

Colonoscopy

**When is colonic ischemia seen postoperatively?**

Usually in the first week

**What is the treatment of necrotic sigmoid colon from colonic ischemia?**

1. Resection of necrotic colon
2. Hartmann's pouch or mucus fistula
3. End colostomy

**What is the possible long-term complication that often presents with both upper and lower GI bleeding?**

Aortoenteric fistula (fistula between aorta and duodenum)

**What are the other possible postoperative complications?**

Erectile dysfunction (sympathetic plexus injury), retrograde ejaculation, aortovenous fistula (to IVC), graft infection, **anterior spinal syndrome**

**What is the anterior spinal syndrome?**

Classically:
1. Paraplegia
2. Loss of bladder/bowel control
3. Loss of pain/temperature sensation below level of involvement
4. **Sparing of proprioception**

**Which artery is involved in anterior spinal cord syndrome?**

Artery of **Adamkiewicz**—supplies the anterior spinal cord

**What are the most common bacteria involved in aortic graft infections?**

1. *Staphylococcus aureus*
2. *Staphylococcus epidermidis* (usually late)

**How is a graft infection and an aortoenteric fistula treated?**

Perform an **extra-anatomic bypass** with resection of the graft

**What is an extra-anatomic bypass graft?**

Axillofemoral bypass graft—**graft not in a normal vascular path;** usually, the graft goes from the axillary artery to the femoral artery and then from one femoral artery to the other (fem-fem bypass)

| | |
|---|---|
| **What is an endovascular repair?** | Placement of a stent proximal and distal to an AAA through a distant percutaneous access (usually through the groin); less invasive; long-term results pending |

## CLASSIC INTRAOP QUESTIONS DURING AAA REPAIR

| | |
|---|---|
| **Which vein crosses the neck of the AAA proximally?** | The renal vein (left) |
| **What part of the small bowel crosses in front of the AAA?** | The duodenum |
| **Which large vein runs to the left of the AAA?** | IMV |
| **Which artery comes off the middle of the AAA and runs to the left?** | IMA |
| **Which vein runs behind the RIGHT common iliac artery?** | The **LEFT** common iliac vein |
| **Which renal vein is longer?** | Left |

# MESENTERIC ISCHEMIA

## CHRONIC MESENTERIC ISCHEMIA

| | |
|---|---|
| **What is it?** | Chronic intestinal ischemia from long-term occlusion of the intestinal arteries; most commonly results from atherosclerosis; usually in two or more arteries because of the extensive collaterals |
| **What are the symptoms?** | Weight loss, postprandial abdominal pain, anxiety/fear of food because of postprandial pain, ± heme occult, ± diarrhea/vomiting |
| **What is "intestinal angina"?** | Postprandial pain from gut ischemia |
| **What are the signs?** | Abdominal bruit is commonly heard. |
| **How is the diagnosis made?** | A-gram, duplex, MRA |
| **What supplies blood to the gut?** | 1. Celiac axis vessels<br>2. SMA<br>3. IMA |
| **What is the classic finding on A-gram?** | Two of the three mesenteric arteries are occluded, and there is atherosclerotic narrowing of the third patent artery. |
| **What are the treatment options?** | Bypass, endarterectomy, angioplasty, stenting |

## ACUTE MESENTERIC ISCHEMIA

| | |
|---|---|
| **What is it?** | Acute onset of intestinal ischemia |
| **What are the causes?** | 1. **Emboli** to a mesenteric vessel from the heart<br>2. **Acute thrombosis** of long-standing atherosclerosis of mesenteric artery |
| **What are the causes of emboli from the heart?** | **AFib,** MI, cardiomyopathy, valve disease/endocarditis, mechanical heart valve |

| | |
|---|---|
| **What drug has been associated with acute intestinal ischemia?** | Digitalis |
| **To which intestinal artery do emboli preferentially go?** | Superior mesenteric artery (SMA) |
| **What are the signs/ symptoms of acute mesenteric ischemia?** | Severe pain—classically **"pain out of proportion to physical exam,"** no peritoneal signs until necrosis, vomiting/ diarrhea/hyperdefecation, ± heme stools |
| **What is the classic triad of acute mesenteric ischemia?** | 1. Acute onset of pain<br>2. Vomiting, diarrhea, or both<br>3. History of AFib or heart disease |
| **What is the gold standard diagnostic test?** | Mesenteric A-gram |
| **What is the treatment of a mesenteric embolus?** | Perform Fogarty catheter embolectomy, resect obviously necrotic intestine, and leave marginal looking bowel until a second look laparotomy is performed 24 to 72 hours postoperatively. |
| **What is the treatment of acute thrombosis?** | **Papaverine** vasodilator via A-gram catheter until **patient is in the OR;** then, most surgeons would perform a supraceliac aorta graft to the involved intestinal artery or endarterectomy; intestinal resection/second look as needed |

## MEDIAN ARCUATE LIGAMENT SYNDROME

| | |
|---|---|
| **What is it?** | Mesenteric ischemia resulting from narrowing of the celiac axis vessels by extrinsic compression by the median arcuate ligament |
| **What is the median arcuate ligament?** | Diaphragm hiatus fibers |
| **What are the symptoms?** | Postprandial pain, weight loss |

| | |
|---|---|
| **What are the signs?** | Abdominal bruit in almost all patients |
| **How is the diagnosis made?** | A-gram |
| **What is the treatment?** | Release arcuate ligament surgically |

## CAROTID VASCULAR DISEASE

### ANATOMY

**Identify the following structures:**

1. Internal carotid artery
2. External carotid artery
3. Carotid "bulb"
4. Superior thyroid artery
5. Common carotid artery

Shaded area: common site of plaque formation

| | |
|---|---|
| **What are the signs/ symptoms?** | Amaurosis fugax, TIA, RIND, CVA |
| **Define the following terms:** | |
| **Amaurosis fugax** | Temporary monocular blindness ("curtain coming down"): seen with microemboli to retina; example of TIA |
| **TIA** | **T**ransient **I**schemic **A**ttack: focal neurologic deficit with resolution of all symptoms within 24 hours |
| **RIND** | **R**eversible **I**schemic **N**eurologic **D**eficit: transient neurologic impairment (without any lasting sequelae) lasting 24 to 72 hours |

| | |
|---|---|
| **CVA** | **C**erebro**V**ascular **A**ccident (stroke): neurologic deficit with permanent brain damage |
| **What is the risk of a CVA in patients with TIA?** | About 10% a year |
| **What is the noninvasive method of evaluating carotid disease?** | **Carotid ultrasound/Doppler:** gives general location and degree of stenosis |
| **What is the gold standard invasive method of evaluating carotid disease?** | A-gram |
| **What is the surgical treatment of carotid stenosis?** | Carotid endarterectomy (CEA): the removal of the diseased intima and media of the carotid artery, often performed with a shunt in place |
| **What are the indications for CEA in the ASYMPTOMATIC patient?** | Carotid artery stenosis >60% (greatest benefit is probably in patients with >80% stenosis) |
| **What are the indications for CEA in the SYMPTOMATIC (CVA, TIA, RIND) patient?** | Carotid stenosis >50% |
| **Before performing a CEA in the symptomatic patient, what study other than the A-gram should be performed?** | Head CT |
| **In bilateral high-grade carotid stenosis, on which side should the CEA be performed in the asymptomatic, right-handed patient?** | Left CEA first, to protect the dominant hemisphere and speech center |
| **What is the dreaded complication after a CEA?** | Stroke (CVA) |

| | |
|---|---|
| **What are the possible postoperative complications after a CEA?** | CVA, MI, hematoma, wound infection, hemorrhage, hypotension/hypertension, thrombosis, vagus nerve injury (change in voice), hypoglossal nerve injury (tongue deviation toward side of injury— "wheel-barrow" effect), intracranial hemorrhage |
| **What is the mortality rate after CEA?** | About 1% |
| **What is the perioperative stroke rate after CEA?** | Between 1% (asymptomatic patient) and 5% (symptomatic patient) |
| **What is the postoperative medication?** | Aspirin (inhibits platelets by inhibiting cyclo-oxygenase) |
| **What is the most common cause of death during the early postoperative period after a CEA?** | MI |
| **Define "Hollenhorst plaque"?** | Microemboli to retinal arterioles seen as bright defects |

## CLASSIC CEA INTRAOP QUESTIONS

| | |
|---|---|
| **What thin muscle is cut right under the skin in the neck?** | Platysma muscle |
| **What are the extracranial branches of the internal carotid artery?** | None |
| **Which vein crosses the carotid bifurcation?** | The facial vein |
| **What is the first branch of the external carotid?** | The superior thyroidal artery |
| **Which muscle crosses the common carotid proximally?** | Omohyoid muscle |
| **Which muscle crosses the carotid artery distally?** | Digastric muscle (think: **D**igastric = **D**istal) |

**Which nerve crosses approximately 1 cm distal to the carotid bifurcation?**

Hypoglossal nerve; cut it and you get a tongue deviating toward the side of the injury (the "wheelbarrow effect")

**Which nerve crosses the internal carotid near the ear?**

Facial nerve (marginal branch)

**What is in the carotid sheath?**

1. Carotid artery
2. Internal jugular vein
3. **Vagus** nerve (lies posteriorly in 98% of patients and anterior in 2%)
4. Deep cervical lymph nodes

## SUBCLAVIAN STEAL SYNDROME

**What is it?**

Arm fatigue and vertebrobasilar insufficiency from obstruction of the left subclavian artery or innominate proximal to the vertebral artery branch point; ipsilateral arm movement causes increased blood flow demand, which is met by retrograde flow from the vertebral artery, thereby "stealing" from the vertebrobasilar arteries

| | |
|---|---|
| **Which artery is most commonly occluded?** | Left subclavian |
| **What are the signs/ symptoms?** | Upper extremity claudication and signs of vertebrobasilar insufficiency: syncopal attacks, vertigo, confusion, dysarthria, blindness, or ataxia |
| **What are the signs?** | Upper extremity blood pressure discrepancy, bruit (above the clavicle) |
| **What is the treatment?** | Surgical bypass or endovascular stent |

## RENAL ARTERY STENOSIS

| | |
|---|---|
| **What is it?** | Stenosis of renal artery, resulting in decreased perfusion of the juxtaglomerular apparatus and subsequent activation of the renin-angiotensin-aldosterone system (i.e., hypertension from renal artery stenosis) |
| **What is the incidence?** | ~ 10% to 15% of the U.S. population has HTN; of these, approximately 4% have potentially correctable renovascular HTN<br>Also note that 30% of malignant HTN has a renovascular etiology |
| **What is the etiology of the stenosis?** | ~ Two-thirds result from atherosclerosis (men > women), ~ one-third result from fibromuscular dysplasia (women > men, average age 40 years, and 50% with bilateral disease)<br>*Note:* another rare cause is hypoplasia of the renal artery |
| **What is the classic profile of a patient with renal artery stenosis from fibromuscular dysplasia?** | A young woman with hypertension |
| **What are the associated risks/clues?** | Family history, early onset of HTN, HTN refractory to medical treatment |

| | |
|---|---|
| **What are the signs/ symptoms?** | Most patients are asymptomatic but may have headache, **diastolic** HTN, flank bruits (present in 50%), and decreased renal function. |
| **What are the diagnostic tests?** | |
| **A-gram** | Maps artery and extent of stenosis; gold standard |
| **IVP** | 80% of patients have delayed nephrogram phase (i.e., delayed filling of contrast) |
| **Renal vein renin ratio (RVRR)** | If sampling of renal vein renin levels shows ratio between the two kidneys $\geq 1.5$, then diagnostic for a unilateral stenosis |
| **Captopril provocation test** | Will show a drop in BP |
| **Are renin levels in serum ALWAYS elevated?** | No; systemic renin levels may also be measured but are only increased in malignant HTN, as the increased intravascular volume dilutes the elevated renin level in most patients. |
| **What is the invasive nonsurgical treatment?** | Percutaneous renal transluminal angioplasty (PRTA)/stenting<br>Much better results with fibromuscular dysplasia but also good for isolated short-segment atherosclerotic lesions away from the ostium of the renal artery<br>With FM dysplasia: 85% to 100% success rate using PRTA and 5% restenosis rate<br>With atherosclerosis: 40% to 90% success using PRTA and about one-fourth restenosis |
| **What is the surgical treatment?** | Resection, bypass, vein/graft interposition, or endarterectomy |

| | |
|---|---|
| **What antihypertensive medication is CONTRAINDICATED in patients with hypertension from renovascular stenosis?** | ACE inhibitors (result in renal insufficiency) |

## SPLENIC ARTERY ANEURYSM

| | |
|---|---|
| **What is it?** | Aneurysm of the splenic artery |
| **What are the causes?** | Women—medial dysplasia<br>Men—atherosclerosis |
| **How is the diagnosis made?** | Usually by abdominal pain → U/S or CT, in the OR after rupture, or incidentally **by eggshell calcifications seen on AXR** |
| **What is the risk factor for rupture?** | Pregnancy |
| **What are the indications for splenic artery aneurysm removal?** | Pregnancy, > 2 cm in diameter, symptoms, and in women of childbearing age |
| **What is the treatment for splenic aneurysm?** | Resection or percutaneous catheter embolization in high-risk (e.g., portal hypertension) patients |

## POPLITEAL ARTERY ANEURYSM

| | |
|---|---|
| **What is it?** | Aneurysm of the popliteal artery caused by atherosclerosis and, rarely, bacterial infection |
| **How is the diagnosis made?** | Usually by physical exam → A-gram, U/S |
| **Why examine the contralateral popliteal artery?** | Half of all patients with a popliteal artery aneurysm have a popliteal artery aneurysm in the contralateral popliteal artery |
| **What are the indications for elective surgical repair of a popliteal aneurysm?** | 1. ≥ 2 cm in diameter<br>2. Intraluminal thrombus<br>3. Artery deformation |

**Why examine the rest of the arterial tree (especially the abdominal aorta)?**

**Three-fourths of all patients with popliteal aneurysms have additional aneurysms elsewhere;** more than half of these are located in the abdominal aorta/iliacs.

**What size of the following aneurysms are indications for surgical repair:**

    **Thoracic aorta?**      >7 cm

    **Abdominal aorta?**      >5.5 cm

    **Iliac artery?**      >4 cm

    **Femoral artery?**      >2.5 cm

    **Popliteal artery?**      >2 cm

## MISCELLANEOUS

**Define the following terms:**

    **"Milk leg"**

A.K.A. phlegmasia alba dolens (alba = white): often seen in pregnant women with occlusion of iliac vein resulting from extrinsic compression by the uterus (thus, the leg is "white" because of subcutaneous edema)

    **Phlegmasia cerulea dolens**

In comparison, phlegmasia cerulea dolens is secondary to severe venous outflow obstruction and results in a cyanotic leg. The extensive venous thrombosis results in arterial inflow impairment.

    **Raynaud's phenomenon**

Vasospasm of digital arteries with color changes of the digits; usually initiated by cold/emotion
White (spasm), then blue (cyanosis), then red (hyperemia)

**Takayasu's arteritis**

Arteritis of the aorta and aortic branches, resulting in stenosis/occlusion/ aneurysms
Seen mostly in women

**Buerger's disease**

A.K.A. thromboangiitis obliterans: occlusion of the small vessels of the hands and feet; seen in **young men who smoke;** often results in digital gangrene → amputations

**What is the treatment for Buerger's disease?**

Smoking **cessation,** +/− sympathectomy

**What is blue toe syndrome?**

Microembolization from proximal atherosclerotic disease of the aorta resulting in blue, painful, ischemic toes

**What is a "paradoxical embolus"?**

Venous embolus gains access to the left heart after going through an intracardiac defect, most commonly a patent foramen ovale, and then lodges in a peripheral artery.

**What size iliac aneurysm should be repaired?**

> 4 cm diameter

# Section III

## Subspecialty Surgery

# Chapter 67

## Pediatric Surgery

**What is the motto of pediatric surgery?**

"Children are NOT little adults!"

**What is a simple way to distract a pediatric patient when examining the abdomen for tenderness?**

Listen to the abdomen with the stethoscope and then push down on the abdomen with the stethoscope to check for tenderness.

## PEDIATRIC IV FLUIDS AND NUTRITION

**What is the estimated blood volume of infants and children?**

About 8% of body weight or approximately **80 cc/kg**

**What is the maintenance IV fluid for children?**

D5 1/4 NS + 20 mEq KCl

**Why 1/4 NS?**

Children (especially those younger than 4 years of age) cannot concentrate their urine and cannot clear excess sodium.

**How are maintenance fluid rates calculated in children?**

4, 2, 1 per hour:
**4 cc/kg for the first 10 kg of body weight**
**2 cc/kg for the second 10 kg of body weight**
**1 cc/kg for every kilogram over the first 20** (e.g., the rate for a child weighing 25 kg is $4 \times 10 = 40$ plus $2 \times 10 = 20$ plus $1 \times 5 = 5$, for an IVF rate of 65 cc/hr)

| | |
|---|---|
| **What is the minimal urine output for children?** | From 1 to 2 mL/kg/hr |
| **What is the best way to present urine output measurements on rounds?** | Urine output total per shift THEN cc/kg/hr |
| **What is the major difference between adult and pediatric nutritional needs?** | Premature infants/infants/children need more calories and protein/kg/day. |

**What are the caloric requirements by age for the following patients:**

| | |
|---|---|
| **Premature infants?** | 80 Kcal/kg/day and then go up |
| **Children younger than 1 year?** | Approximately 100 Kcal/kg/day (90–120) |
| **Children aged 1 to 7?** | Approximately 85 Kcal/kg/day (75–90) |
| **Children aged 7 to 12?** | Approximately 70 Kcal/kg/day (60–75) |
| **Youths aged 12 to 18** | Approximately 40 Kcal/kg/day (30–60) |

**What are the protein requirements by age for the following patients:**

| | |
|---|---|
| **Children younger than 1 year?** | 3 g/kg/day (2–3.5) |
| **Children aged 1 to 7?** | 2 g/kg/day (2–2.5) |
| **Children aged 7 to 12?** | 2 g/kg/day |
| **Youths aged 12 to 18?** | 1.5 grams/kg/day |
| **How many calories are in breast milk?** | 20 Kcal/30 cc (same as most formulas) |

## PEDIATRIC BLOOD VOLUMES

Give blood volume per
kilogram:
    Newborn infant?        85 cc

    Infant 1–3 months of age?    75 cc

    Child?        70 cc

## FETAL CIRCULATION

What is the number of    1 (usually)
umbilical veins?

What is the number of    2
umbilical arteries?

Which umbilical vessel    Umbilical vein
carries oxygenated blood?

The oxygenated blood travels    Ductus venosus
through the liver to the IVC
through which structure?

Oxygenated blood passes    Foramen ovale
from the right atrium to the
left atrium through which
structure?

Unsaturated blood goes    Ductus arteriosum
from the right ventricle
to the descending aorta
through which structure?

**Define the overall fetal circulation.**

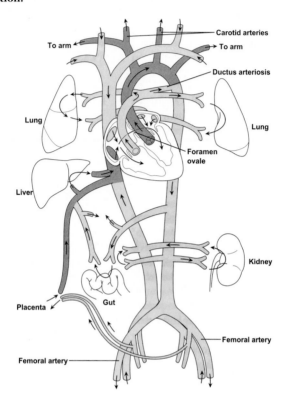

**What are the ADULT structures of the following fetal structures:**

| | |
|---|---|
| **Ductus venosus?** | Ligamentum venosum |
| **Umbilical vein?** | Ligamentum teres |
| **Umbilical artery?** | Medial umbilical ligament |
| **Ductus arteriosus?** | Ligamentum arteriosum |
| **Urachus?** | Median umbilical ligament |

| | |
|---|---|
| **Tongue remnant of thyroid's descent?** | Foramen cecum |
| **Persistent remnant of vitelline duct?** | Meckel's diverticulum |

## ECMO

| | |
|---|---|
| **What is ECMO?** | **E**xtra**C**orporeal **M**embrane **O**xygenation chronic cardiopulmonary bypass—for complete respiratory support |
| **What are the types of ECMO?** | Venovenous: Blood from vein → oxygenated → back to vein<br>Venoarterial: Blood from vein (IJ) → oxygenated → back to artery (carotid) |
| **What are the indications?** | Severe hypoxia, usually from congenital diaphragmatic hernia, meconium aspiration, persistent pulmonary hypertension, sepsis |
| **What are the contraindications?** | Weight <2 kg, IVH (intraventricular hemorrhage in brain contraindicated because of heparin in line) |

## NECK

| | |
|---|---|
| **What is the major differential diagnosis of a pediatric neck mass?** | Thyroglossal duct cyst (midline), branchial cleft cyst (lateral), lymphadenopathy, abscess, cystic hygroma, hemangioma, teratoma/dermoid cyst, thyroid nodule, lymphoma/leukemia (also parathyroid tumors, neuroblastoma, histiocytosis X, rhabdomyosarcoma, salivary gland tumors, neurofibroma) |

### THYROGLOSSAL DUCT CYST

| | |
|---|---|
| **What is it?** | Remnant of the diverticulum formed by migration of thyroid tissue; normal development involves migration of thyroid tissue from the foramen cecum at the base of the tongue through the hyoid bone to its final position around the tracheal cartilage |

**What is the average age at diagnosis?**

Usually presents around 5 years of age

**How is the diagnosis made?**

Ultrasound

**What are the complications?**

Enlargement, infection, and fistula formation between oropharynx or salivary gland; aberrant thyroid tissue may masquerade as thyroglossal duct cyst, and if it is not cystic, deserves a thyroid scan

**What is the anatomic location?**

Almost always in the **midline**

**How can one remember the position of the thyroglossal duct cyst?**

Think: thyroGLOSSAL = TONGUE midline sticking out

| | |
|---|---|
| **What is the treatment?** | Antibiotics if infection is present, then excision, which must include the midportion of the hyoid bone and entire tract to foramen cecum (**Sistrunk** procedure) |

## BRANCHIAL CLEFT ANOMALIES

| | |
|---|---|
| **What is it?** | Remnant of the primitive branchial clefts in which epithelium forms a sinus tract between the pharynx (second cleft), or the external auditory canal (first cleft), and the skin of the anterior neck; if the sinus ends blindly, a cyst may form |
| **What is the common presentation?** | Infection because of communication between pharynx and external ear canal |
| **What is the anatomic position?** | Second cleft anomaly—**lateral to the midline** along anterior border of the sternocleidomastoid, anywhere from angle of jaw to clavicle<br><br>First cleft anomaly—less common than second cleft anomalies; tend to be located higher under the mandible |
| **What is the most common cleft remnant?** | Second; thus, these are found most often laterally versus thyroglossal cysts, which are found centrally (think: **s**econd = **s**uperior) |
| **What is the treatment?** | Antibiotics if infection is present, then surgical excision of cyst and tract once inflammation is resolved |
| **What is the major anatomic difference between thyroglossal cyst and branchial cleft cyst?** | Thyroglossal cyst = **midline**<br>Branchial cleft cyst = **lateral**<br>(think: br**A**nchial = l**A**teral) |

## STRIDOR

| | |
|---|---|
| **What is stridor?** | A harsh, high-pitched sound heard on breathing caused by obstruction of the trachea or larynx |

| | |
|---|---|
| **What are the signs/ symptoms?** | Dyspnea, cyanosis, difficulty with feedings |
| **What is the differential diagnosis?** | Laryngomalacia—leading cause of stridor in infants; results from inadequate development of supporting laryngeal structures; usually self-limited and treatment is expectant unless respiratory compromise is present<br><br>Tracheobronchomalacia—similar to laryngomalacia, but involves the entire trachea<br><br>Vascular rings and slings—abnormal development or placement of thoracic large vessels resulting in obstruction of trachea/bronchus |
| **What are the symptoms of vascular rings?** | Stridor, dyspnea on exertion, or dysphagia |
| **How is the diagnosis of vascular rings made?** | Barium swallow revealing typical configuration of esophageal compression<br><br>Echo/arteriogram |
| **What is the treatment of vascular rings?** | Surgical division of the ring, if the patient is symptomatic |

## CYSTIC HYGROMA

| | |
|---|---|
| **What is it?** | Congenital abnormality of lymph sac resulting in lymphangioma |
| **What is the anatomic location?** | Occurs in sites of primitive lymphatic lakes and can occur virtually anywhere in the body, most commonly in the floor of mouth, under the jaw, or in the neck, axilla, or thorax |
| **What is the treatment?** | Early total surgical removal because they tend to enlarge; sclerosis may be needed if the lesion is unresectable |

| | |
|---|---|
| **What are the possible complications?** | Enlargement in critical regions, such as the floor of the mouth or paratracheal region, may cause airway obstruction; also, they tend to insinuate onto major structures (although not malignant), making excision difficult and hazardous |

## ASPIRATED FOREIGN BODY (FB)

| | |
|---|---|
| **Which bronchus do FBs go into more commonly (left or right)?** | Younger than age 4—50/50<br>Age 4 and older—most go into right bronchus because it develops into a straight shot (less of an angle) |
| **What is the most commonly aspirated object?** | Peanut |
| **What is the associated risk with peanut aspiration?** | Lipoid pneumonia |
| **How can an FB result in "air trapping and hyperinflation"?** | By forming a "ball valve" (i.e., air in, no air out) as seen on CXR as a hyperinflated lung on expiratory film |
| **How can you tell on A-P CXR if a coin is in the esophagus or the trachea?** | Coin in **esophagus** results in the coin lying "en face" with face of the coin viewed as a **round object** because of compression by anterior and posterior structures<br>If coin is in the **trachea,** it is viewed as a **side projection** due to the U-shaped cartilage with membrane posteriorly |
| **What is the treatment of tracheal or esophageal FB?** | Remove FB with **rigid** bronchoscope or **rigid** esophagoscope |

## CHEST

| | |
|---|---|
| **What is the differential diagnosis of a lung mass?** | Bronchial adenoma (carcinoid is most common), pulmonary sequestration, pulmonary blastoma, rhabdomyosarcoma, chondroma, hamartoma, leiomyoma, mucus gland adenoma, metastasis |

| | |
|---|---|
| **What is the differential diagnosis of mediastinal tumor/mass?** | 1. Neurogenic tumor (ganglioneuromas, neurofibromas)<br>2. Teratoma<br>3. Lymphoma<br>4. Thymoma<br>(T's: teratoma, terrible lymphoma, thymoma, thyroid tumor)<br>Rare: pheochromocytoma, hemangioma, rhabdomyosarcoma, osteochondroma |

## PECTUS DEFORMITY

| | |
|---|---|
| **What heart abnormality is associated with pectus abnormality?** | Mitral valve prolapse (many patients receive preoperative echocardiogram) |

## PECTUS EXCAVATUM

| | |
|---|---|
| **What is it?** | Chest wall deformity with sternum caving inward (think: ex**CAV**atum = **CAVE**) |

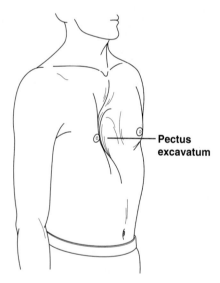

Pectus excavatum

| | |
|---|---|
| **What is the cause?** | Abnormal, unequal overgrowth of rib cartilage |
| **What are the signs/ symptoms?** | Often asymptomatic; mental distress, dyspnea on exertion, chest pain |

| | |
|---|---|
| **What is the treatment?** | Open perichondrium, remove abnormal cartilage, place substernal strut; new cartilage grows back in the perichondrium in normal position; remove strut 6 months later |
| **What is the NUSS procedure?** | Placement of metal strut to elevate sternum **without** removing cartilage |

## PECTUS CARINATUM

| | |
|---|---|
| **What is it?** | Chest wall deformity with sternum outward (pectus = chest, carinatum = pigeon); much less common than pectus excavatum |

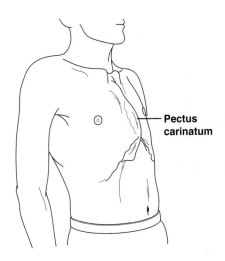

Pectus carinatum

| | |
|---|---|
| **What is the cause?** | Abnormal, unequal overgrowth of rib cartilage |
| **What is the treatment?** | Open perichondrium and remove abnormal cartilage. Place substernal strut. New cartilage grows into normal position. Remove strut 6 months later. |

## ESOPHAGEAL ATRESIA WITHOUT TRACHEOESOPHAGEAL (TE) FISTULA

| | |
|---|---|
| **What is it?** | Blind-ending esophagus from atresia |
| **What are the signs?** | Excessive oral secretions and inability to keep food down |
| **How is the diagnosis made?** | Inability to pass NG tube; plain x-ray shows tube coiled in upper esophagus and no gas in abdomen |
| **What is the primary treatment?** | Suction blind pouch, IVFs, (gastrostomy to drain stomach if prolonged preoperative esophageal stretching is planned) |
| **What is the definitive treatment?** | Surgical with 1° anastomosis, often with preoperative stretching of blind pouch (other options include colonic or jejunal interposition graft or gastric tube formation if esophageal gap is long) |

## ESOPHAGEAL ATRESIA WITH TRACHEOESOPHAGEAL (TE) FISTULA

| | |
|---|---|
| **What is it?** | Esophageal atresia occurring with a fistula to the trachea; occurs in more than 90% of cases of esophageal atresia |
| **What is the incidence?** | One in 1500 to 3000 births |
| **Define the following types of fistulas/atresias:** | |
| Type A | Esophageal atresia without TE fistula (8%) |

**Type B**                    Proximal esophageal atresia with proximal
                              TE fistula (1%)

**Type C**                    Proximal esophageal atresia with distal
                              TE fistula (85%); most common type

**Type D**                    Proximal esophageal atresia with both
                              proximal and distal TE fistulas (2%) (think:
                              **D** = **D**ouble connection to trachea)

**Type E**                    "H-type" TE fistula without esophageal
                              atresia (4%)

| | |
|---|---|
| **How do you remember which type is most common?** | Simple: the most **C**ommon type is type **C**. |
| **What are the symptoms?** | Excessive secretions caused by an accumulation of saliva (may not occur with type E) |
| **What are the signs?** | Obvious respiratory compromise, aspiration pneumonia, postprandial regurgitation, gastric distention as air enters the stomach directly from the trachea |
| **How is the diagnosis made?** | Failure to pass an NG tube (although this will not be seen with type E); plain film demonstrates tube coiled in the upper esophagus; "pouchogram" (contrast in esophageal pouch); gas on AXR (tracheoesophageal fistula) |
| **What is the initial treatment?** | Directed toward minimizing complications from aspiration: <br> 1. Suction blind pouch (NPO/TPN) <br> 2. Upright position of child <br> 3. Prophylactic antibiotics (Amp/gent) |
| **What is the definitive treatment?** | Surgical correction via a thoracotomy, usually through the right chest with division of fistula and end-to-end esophageal anastomosis, if possible |

**What can be done to lengthen the proximal esophageal pouch?**

Delayed repair: with or without G-tube and daily **stretching** of proximal pouch

**Which type should be fixed via a right neck incision?**

"H-Type" (type E) is high in the thorax and can most often be approached via a right neck incision.

**What is the work up of a patient with a TE fistula?**

To evaluate the TE fistula and **associated anomalies:** CXR, AXR, U/S of kidneys, cardiac echo (rest of work-up directed by physical exam)

**What are the associated anomalies?**

**VACTERL** cluster (present in about 10% of cases):

**V**ertebral or vascular, **A**norectal, **C**ardiac, **TE** fistula, **E**sophageal atresia
**R**adial limb and renal abnormalities, **L**umbar and limb
Previously known as **VATER**:
**V**ertebral, **A**nus, **TE** fistula, **R**adial

**What is the significance of a "gasless" abdomen on AXR?**

No air to the stomach and, thus, no tracheoesophageal fistula

## CONGENITAL DIAPHRAGMATIC HERNIA

**What is it?**

Failure of complete formation of the diaphragm, leading to a defect through which abdominal organs are herniated

**What is the incidence?**

One in 2100 live births; males are more commonly affected

**What are the types of hernias?**

Bochdalek and Morgagni

**What are the associated positions?**

Bochdalek—posterolateral with L > R
Morgagni—anterior parasternal hernia, relatively uncommon

**How to remember the position of the Bochdalek hernia?**

Think BOCH DA LEK = "BACK TO THE LEFT"

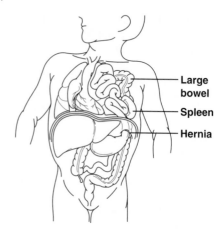

**What are the signs?**

Respiratory distress, dyspnea, tachypnea, retractions, and cyanosis; bowel sounds in the chest; rarely, maximal heart sounds on the right; ipsilateral chest dullness to percussion

**What are the effects on the lungs?**

1. Pulmonary hypoplasia
2. Pulmonary hypertension

**What inhaled agent is often used?**

Inhaled nitric oxide (pulmonary vasodilator), which decreases the shunt and decreases pulmonary hypertension

**What is the treatment?**

NG tube, ET tube, stabilization, and if patient is stable, surgical repair; if patient is unstable: nitric oxide +/− ECMO then to the OR when feasible

## PULMONARY SEQUESTRATION

**What is it?**

Abnormal benign lung tissue with separate blood supply that **DOES NOT** communicate with the normal tracheobronchial airway

**Define the following terms:**
**Interlobar**

Sequestration in the normal lung tissue covered by normal visceral pleura

| | |
|---|---|
| **Extralobar** | Sequestration not in the normal lung covered by its own pleura |
| **What are the signs/ symptoms?** | Asymptomatic, recurrent pneumonia |
| **How is the diagnosis made?** | CXR, chest CT, A-gram, U/S with Doppler flow to ascertain blood supply |
| **What is the treatment of each type:** | |
| **Extralobar?** | Surgical resection |
| **Intralobar?** | Lobectomy |
| **What is the major risk during operation for sequestration?** | Anomalous blood supply from below the diaphragm (can be cut and retracted into the abdomen and result in exsanguination!); always document blood supply by A-gram or U/S with Doppler flow |

## ABDOMEN

| | |
|---|---|
| **What is the differential diagnosis of pediatric upper GI bleeding?** | Gastritis, esophagitis, gastric ulcer, duodenal ulcer, esophageal varices, foreign body, epistaxis, coagulopathy, vascular malformation, duplication cyst |
| **What is the differential diagnosis of pediatric lower GI bleeding?** | Upper GI bleeding, anal fissures, NEC (premature infants), midgut volvulus (usually children younger than 1 year), strangulated hernia, intussusception, Meckel's diverticulum, infectious diarrhea, polyps, IBD, hemolytic uremic syndrome, Henoch-Schönlein purpura, vascular malformation, coagulopathy |
| **What is the differential diagnosis of neonatal bowel obstruction?** | Malrotation with volvulus, intestinal atresia, duodenal web, annular pancreas, imperforate anus, Hirschsprung's disease, NEC, intussusception (rare), Meckel's diverticulum, incarcerated hernia, meconium ileus, meconium plug, maternal narcotic abuse (ileus), maternal hypermagnesemia (ileus), sepsis (ileus) |

| | |
|---|---|
| **What is the differential diagnosis of infant constipation?** | Hirschsprung's disease, CF (cystic fibrosis), anteriorly displaced anus, polyps |

## INGUINAL HERNIA

| | |
|---|---|
| **What is the most commonly performed procedure by U.S. pediatric surgeons?** | Indirect inguinal hernia repair |
| **What is the most common inguinal hernia in children?** | Indirect |
| **What is an indirect inguinal hernia?** | Hernia lateral to Hesselbach's triangle into the internal inguinal ring and down the inguinal canal (think: through the abdominal wall indirectly into the internal ring and out through the external inguinal ring) |
| **What is Hesselbach's triangle?** | A triangle formed by:<br>1. Epigastric vessels<br>2. Inguinal ligament<br>3. Lateral border of the rectus sheath |
| **What type of hernia goes through Hesselbach's triangle?** | A direct hernia from a weak abdominal floor; rare in children (0.5% of all inguinal hernias) |
| **What is the incidence of indirect inguinal hernia in all children?** | Approximately 3% |
| **What is the incidence in premature infants?** | Up to 30% |
| **What is the male to female ratio?** | 6:1 |
| **What are the risk factors for an indirect inguinal hernia?** | Male gender, ascites, V-P shunt, prematurity, family history, meconium ileus, abdominal wall defect elsewhere, hypo/epispadias, connective tissue disease, bladder exstrophy, undescended testicle, CF |

| | |
|---|---|
| **Which side is affected more commonly?** | **Right** (about 60%) |
| **What percentage are bilateral?** | Approximately 15% |
| **What percentage have a family history of indirect hernias?** | Approximately 10% |
| **What are the signs/ symptoms?** | Groin bulge, scrotal mass, thickened cord, silk glove sign |
| **What is the silk glove sign?** | The hernia sac rolls under the finger like the finger of a silk glove. |
| **Why should it be repaired?** | Risk of incarcerated/strangulated bowel or ovary; will not go away on its own |
| **How is a pediatric inguinal hernia repaired?** | High ligation of hernia sac (no repair of the abdominal wall floor, which is a big difference between the procedure in children and adults; high refers to high position on the sac neck next to the peritoneal cavity) |
| **Which infants need overnight apnea monitoring/ observation?** | Premature infants; infants younger than 3 months of age |
| **What is the risk of recurrence after high ligation of an indirect pediatric hernia?** | Approximately 1% |
| **Describe the steps in the repair of an indirect inguinal hernia from skin to skin.** | Cut skin, then fat, then Scarpa's fascia, then external oblique fascia through the external inguinal ring; find hernia sac anteriomedially and bluntly separate from the other cord structures; ligate sac high at the neck at the internal inguinal ring; resect sac and allow sac stump to retract into the peritoneal cavity; close external oblique; close Scarpa's fascia; close skin. |

**Define the following terms:**

**Cryptorchidism**

Failure of the testicle to descend into the scrotum

**Hydrocele**

Fluid-filled sac (i.e., fluid in a patent processus vaginalis or in the tunica vaginalis around the testicle)

**Communicating hydrocele**

Hydrocele that communicates with the peritoneal cavity and thus fills and drains peritoneal fluid or gets bigger, then smaller

**Noncommunicating hydrocele**

Hydrocele that does not communicate with the peritoneal cavity; stays about the same size

**Can a hernia be ruled out if an inguinal mass transilluminates?**

NO; baby bowel is very thin and will often transilluminate.

## CLASSIC INTRAOPERATIVE QUESTIONS DURING REPAIR OF AN INDIRECT INGUINAL HERNIA

**From what abdominal muscle layer is the cremaster muscle derived?**

Internal oblique muscle

**From what abdominal muscle layer is the inguinal ligament (A.K.A. Poupart's ligament) derived?**

External oblique

**What nerve travels with the spermatic cord?**

Ilioinguinal nerve

**What is in the spermatic cord (5 structures)?**

1. Cremasteric muscle fibers
2. Vas deferens
3. Testicular artery
4. Testicular pampiniform venous plexus
5. With or without hernia sac

**What is the hernia sac made of?**

Basically peritoneum or a patent processus vaginalis

| | |
|---|---|
| **What is the name of the fossa between the testicle and epididymis?** | Fossa of Geraldi |
| **What attaches the testicle to the scrotum?** | The gubernaculum |
| **How can the opposite side be assessed for a hernia intraoperatively?** | Many surgeons operatively explore the opposite side when they repair the affected side. A laparoscope is placed into the abdomen via the hernia sac and the opposite side internal inguinal ring is examined. |
| **Name the remnant of the processus vaginalis around the testicle.** | Tunica vaginalis |
| **What is a Littre's inguinal hernia?** | Hernia with a Meckel's diverticulum in the hernia sac |
| **What may a yellow/orange tissue that is not fat be on the spermatic cord/testicle?** | Adrenal rest |
| **What is the most common organ in an inguinal hernia sac in boys?** | Small intestine |
| **What is the most common organ in an inguinal hernia sac in girls?** | Ovary/fallopian tube |
| **What lies in the inguinal canal in girls instead of the vas?** | Round ligament |
| **Where in the inguinal canal does the hernia sac lie in relation to the other structures?** | Anteriomedially |

| | |
|---|---|
| **What is a "cord lipoma"?** | Preperitoneal fat on the cord structures (pushed in by the hernia sac); not a real lipoma<br>Should be removed surgically, if feasible |
| **Within the spermatic cord, do the vessels or the vas lie medially?** | The vas is medial to the testicular vessels. |
| **What is a small outpouching of testicular tissue off of the testicle?** | Testicular appendage (A.K.A. the appendix testes); should be removed with electrocautery |
| **What is a "blue dot sign"?** | A blue dot on the scrotal skin from a twisted testicular appendage |
| **How is a transected vas treated?** | Repair with primary anastomosis |
| **How do you treat a transected ilioinguinal nerve?** | Should not be repaired; many surgeons ligate it to inhibit neuroma formation |
| **What happens if you cut the ilioinguinal nerve?** | Loss of sensation to the medial aspect of the inner thigh and scrotum/labia; loss of cremasteric reflex |

## UMBILICAL HERNIA

| | |
|---|---|
| **What is it?** | Fascial defect at the umbilical ring |
| **What are the risk factors?** | 1. Black or African American infant<br>2. Premature infant |
| **What are the indications for surgical repair?** | 1. >1.5 cm defect<br>2. Bowel incarceration<br>3. >4 years of age |

## GERD

| | |
|---|---|
| **What is it?** | **G**astro **E**sophageal **R**eflux **D**isease |
| **What are the causes?** | LES malfunction/malposition, hiatal hernia, gastric outlet obstruction, partial bowel obstruction, common in cerebral palsy |

| | |
|---|---|
| **What are the signs/ symptoms?** | Spitting up, emesis, URTI, pneumonia, laryngospasm from aspiration of gastric contents into the tracheobronchial tree, failure to thrive |
| **How is the diagnosis made?** | 24 hour Ph probe, bronchoscopy, UGI (manometry, EGD, U/S) |
| **What cytologic aspirate finding on bronchoscopy can diagnose aspiration of gastric contents?** | Lipid-laden macrophages (from phagocytosis of fat) |
| **What is the medical/ conservative treatment?** | H$_2$ blockers <br> Small meals/rice cereal <br> Elevation of head |
| **What are the indications for surgery?** | "S.A.F.E.": <br> **S**tricture <br> **A**spiration, pneumonia/asthma <br> **F**ailure to thrive <br> **E**sophagitis |
| **What is the surgical treatment?** | **Nissen** 360° fundoplication, with or without G tube |

## CONGENITAL PYLORC STENOSIS

| | |
|---|---|
| **What is it?** | Hypertrophy of smooth muscle of pylorus, resulting in obstruction of outflow |

| | |
|---|---|
| **What are the associated risks?** | Family history, firstborn males are affected most commonly, decreased incidence in African American population |
| **What is the incidence?** | One in 750 births, male to female ratio = 4:1 |
| **What is the average age at onset?** | Usually from 2 weeks after birth to about 2 months (2 to 2) |
| **What are the symptoms?** | Increasing frequency of regurgitation, leading to eventual nonbilious projectile vomiting |
| **Why is the vomiting nonbilious?** | The obstruction is proximal to the ampulla of Vater. |
| **What are the signs?** | Abdominal mass or "olive" in epigastric region (85%), hypokalemic hypochloremic metabolic alkalosis, icterus (10%), visible gastric peristalsis, paradoxic aciduria, hematemesis (<10%) |
| **What is the differential diagnosis?** | Pylorospasm, milk allergy, increased ICP, hiatal hernia, GERD, adrenal insufficiency, uremia, malrotation, duodenal atresia, annular pancreas, duodenal web |
| **How is the diagnosis made?** | Usually by history and physical exam alone<br>U/S—demonstrates elongated (>15 mm) pyloric channel and thickened muscle wall (>3.5 mm)<br>If U/S is nondiagnostic, then barium swallow—shows "string sign" or "double railroad track sign" |
| **What is the initial treatment?** | Hydration and correction of alkalosis with D10 NS plus 20 mEq of KCl; *Note:* the infant's liver glycogen stores are very small; therefore, use D10; Cl⁻ and hydration will correct the alkalosis. |

| | |
|---|---|
| **What is the definitive treatment?** | Surgical, via Fredet-Ramstedt pyloromyotomy (division of circular muscle fibers without entering the lumen/mucosa) |
| **What are the postoperative complications?** | Unrecognized incision through the duodenal mucosa, bleeding, wound infection, aspiration pneumonia |
| **What is the appropriate postoperative feeding?** | Between 6 and 12 hours postoperative feeding with Pedialyte, advanced to full-strength formula over 24 hours |
| **Which vein crosses the pylorus?** | Vein of Mayo |

## DUODENAL ATRESIA

| | |
|---|---|
| **What is it?** | Complete obstruction or stenosis of duodenum caused by an ischemic insult during development or failure of recanalization |
| **What is the anatomic location?** | 85% are distal to the ampulla of Vater, 15% are proximal to the ampulla of Vater (these present with nonbilious vomiting). |
| **What are the signs?** | Bilious vomiting (if distal to the ampulla), epigastric distention |
| **What is the differential diagnosis?** | Malrotation with Ladd's bands, annular pancreas |
| **How is the diagnosis made?** | Plain abdominal film revealing "double bubble," with one air bubble in the stomach and the other in the duodenum |
| **What is the treatment?** | Duodenoduodenostomy or duodenojejunostomy |
| **What are the associated abnormalities?** | Between 50% and 70% have cardiac, renal, or other gastrointestinal defects; 30% have trisomy 21 |

## MECONIUM ILEUS

| | |
|---|---|
| **What is it?** | Intestinal obstruction from solid meconium concretions |
| **What is the incidence?** | Occurs in about 15% of infants with CF |
| **What percentage of patients with meconium ileus have CF?** | More than 95% |
| **What are the signs/symptoms?** | Bilious vomiting, abdominal distention, failure to pass meconium, Neuhauser's sign, peritoneal calcifications |
| **What is Neuhauser's sign?** | A.K.A. "soap bubble" sign: ground glass appearance in the RLQ on AXR from viscous meconium mixing with air |
| **How is the diagnosis made?** | Family history of CF, plain abdominal films showing significant dilation of similar-sized bowel loops, but few if any air-fluid levels, BE may demonstrate "microcolon" and inspissated meconium pellets in the terminal ileum |
| **What is the treatment?** | 70% nonoperative clearance of meconium using Gastrografin enema, +/− acetylcysteine, which is hypertonic and therefore draws fluid into lumen, separating meconium pellets from bowel wall (60% success rate) |
| **What should you remove during all operative cases?** | Appendix |
| **What is the surgical treatment?** | If enema is unsuccessful, then enterotomy with intraoperative catheter irrigation using acetylcysteine (Mucomyst®) |
| **What is the long-term medical treatment?** | Pancreatic enzyme replacement |

| | |
|---|---|
| **What is cystic fibrosis (CF)?** | Inherited disorder of epithelial $Cl^-$ transport defect affecting sweat glands, airways, and GI tract (pancreas, intestine); diagnosed by sweat test (elevated levels of NaCl >60 mEq/liter) and genetic testing |
| **What is DIOS?** | **D**istal **I**ntestinal **O**bstruction **S**yndrome: intestinal obstruction in older patients with CF from inspissated luminal contents |

## MECONIUM PERITONITIS

| | |
|---|---|
| **What is it?** | A sign of **intrauterine** bowel perforation; sterile meconium leads to an intense local inflammatory reaction with eventual formation of calcifications |
| **What are the signs?** | Calcifications on plain films |

## MECONIUM PLUG SYNDROME

| | |
|---|---|
| **What is it?** | Colonic obstruction from unknown factors that dehydrate meconium, forming a "plug" |
| **What is it also known as?** | Neonatal small left colon syndrome |
| **What are the signs/ symptoms?** | Abdominal distention and **failure to pass meconium within first 24 hours of life;** plain films demonstrate many loops of distended bowel and air-fluid levels |
| **What is the nonoperative treatment?** | Contrast enema is both diagnostic and therapeutic; it demonstrates "microcolon" to the point of dilated colon (usually in transverse colon) and reveals copious intraluminal material. |
| **What is the major differential diagnosis?** | Hirschsprung's disease |
| **Is meconium plug highly associated with CF?** | No; less than 5% of patients have CF, in contrast to meconium ileus, in which nearly all have CF (95%) |

## ANORECTAL MALFORMATIONS

| | |
|---|---|
| **What are they?** | Malformations of the distal GI tract in the general categories of anal atresia, imperforate anus, and rectal atresia |

### IMPERFORATE ANUS

| | |
|---|---|
| **What is it?** | Congenital absence of normal anus (complete absence or fistula) |
| **Define a "high" imperforate anus.** | Rectum patent to level above puborectalis sling |
| **Define "low" imperforate anus.** | Rectum patent to below puborectalis sling |
| **Which type is much more common in women?** | Low |
| **What are the associated anomalies?** | **V**ertebral abnormalities, **A**nal abnormalities, **C**ardiac, **TE** fistulas, **E**sophageal Atresia, **R**adial/**R**enal abnormalities, **L**umbar abnormalities (**VACTERL**; most commonly TE fistula) |
| **What are the signs/ symptoms?** | No anus, fistula to anal skin or bladder, UTI, fistula to vagina or urethra, bowel obstruction, distended abdomen, hyperchloremic acidosis |
| **How is the diagnosis made?** | Physical exam, the classic Cross table "invertogram" plain x-ray to see level of rectal gas (not very accurate), perineal ultrasound |
| **What is the treatment of the following conditions:** | |
|     **Low imperforate anus with anal fistula?** | Dilatation of anal fistula and subsequent anoplasty |
|     **High imperforate anus?** | Diverting colostomy and mucus fistula; neoanus is usually made at 1 year of age |

## HIRSCHSPRUNG'S DISEASE

| | |
|---|---|
| **What is it also known as?** | Aganglionic megacolon |
| **What is it?** | Neurogenic form of intestinal obstruction in which obstruction results from inadequate relaxation and peristalsis; absence of normal ganglion cells of the rectum and colon |
| **What are the associated risks?** | Family history; 5% chance of having a second child with the affliction |
| **What is the male to female ratio?** | 4:1 |
| **What is the anatomic location?** | Aganglionosis begins at the anorectal line and involves rectosigmoid in 80% of cases (10% have involvement to splenic flexure, and 10% have involvement of entire colon). |
| **What are the signs/ symptoms?** | Abdominal distention and bilious vomiting; more than 95% present with failure to pass meconium in the first 24 hours; can also present later with constipation, diarrhea, and decreased growth |
| **What is the classic history?** | Failure to pass meconium in the first 24 hours of life |
| **What is the differential diagnosis?** | Meconium plug syndrome, meconium ileus, sepsis with adynamic ileus, colonic neuronal dysplasia, hypothyroidism, maternal narcotic abuse, maternal hypermagnesemia (tocolysis) |
| **What imaging studies should be ordered?** | **AXR:** reveals dilated colon <br> **Unprepared barium enema:** reveals constricted aganglionic segment with dilated proximal segment, but this picture may not develop for 3 to 6 weeks; BE will also demonstrate retention of barium for 24 to 48 hours (normal evacuation = 10 to 18 hours) |

**What is needed for definitive diagnosis?**

**Rectal biopsy:** for definitive diagnosis, submucosal suction biopsy is adequate in 90% of cases; otherwise, full-thickness biopsy should be performed to evaluate Auerbach's plexus

**What is the "colonic transition zone"?**

The transition (taper) from aganglionic small colon into the large dilated normal colon seen on BE

**What is the initial treatment?**

In neonates, a colostomy proximal to the transition zone prior to correction, to allow for pelvic growth and dilated bowel to return to normal size

**What is a "leveling" colostomy?**

The colostomy performed for Hirschsprung's disease at the level of normally innervated ganglion cells as ascertained on frozen section intraoperatively

**Describe the following procedures:**
  **Swenson**

Primary anastomosis between the anal canal and healthy bowel (rectum removed)

**Duhamel**

The anterior, aganglionic region of the rectum is preserved and anastomosed to a posterior portion of healthy bowel; a functional rectal pouch is thereby created (think: **duha** = **dual** barrels side by side)

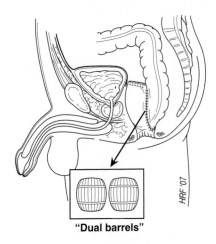

**"Dual barrels"**

**Soave**

(A.K.A. endorectal pull-through); this procedure involves bringing proximal normal colon through the aganglionic rectum, which has been stripped of its mucosa but otherwise present (think: **soave** = **save** the rectum, lose the mucosa)

| | |
|---|---|
| **What is the new trend in surgery for Hirschsprung's disease?** | No colostomy; remove aganglionic colon (as confirmed on frozen section) and perform pull-through anastomosis at the same time (Boley modification) |
| **What is the prognosis?** | Overall survival rate >90%; >96% of patients continent; postoperative symptoms improve with age |

## MALROTATION AND MIDGUT VOLVULUS

| | |
|---|---|
| **What is it?** | Failure of the normal bowel rotation, with resultant abnormal intestinal attachments and anatomic positions |
| **Where is the cecum?** | With malrotation, the cecum usually ends up in the RUQ |
| **What are Ladd's bands?** | Fibrous bands that extend from the abnormally placed cecum in the RUQ, often crossing over the duodenum and causing obstruction |

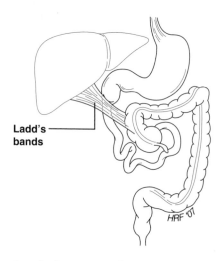

Ladd's bands

HRF '01

| | |
|---|---|
| **What is the usual age at onset?** | One-third are present by 1 week of age, three-fourths by 1 month of age, and 90% by 1 year of age. |

| | |
|---|---|
| **What is the usual presentation?** | Sudden onset of bilious vomiting (**bilious vomiting in an infant is malrotation until proven otherwise!**) |
| **Why is the vomiting bilious?** | The "twist" is distal to the ampulla of Vater |
| **How is the diagnosis made?** | Upper GI contrast study showing cut off in duodenum; BE showing abnormal position of cecum in the upper abdomen |
| **What are the possible complications?** | Volvulus with midgut infarction, leading to death or necessitating massive enterectomy (**rapid diagnosis is essential!**) |
| **What is the treatment?** | IV antibiotics and fluid resuscitation with LR, followed by emergent laparotomy with Ladd's procedure; second-look laparotomy if bowel is severely ischemic in 24 hours to determine if remaining bowel is viable |
| **What is the Ladd's procedure?** | 1. **Counterclockwise** reduction of mid-gut volvulus<br>2. Splitting of Ladd's bands<br>3. Division of peritoneal attachments to the cecum, ascending colon<br>4. Appendectomy |
| **In what direction is the volvulus reduced—clockwise or counterclockwise?** | Rotation of the bowel in a counterclockwise direction |
| **Where is the cecum after reduction?** | In the LLQ |
| **What is the cause of bilious vomiting in an infant until proven otherwise?** | Malrotation with midgut volvulus |

## OMPHALOCELE

| | |
|---|---|
| **What is it?** | Defect of abdominal wall at umbilical ring; sac **covers** extruded viscera |

| | |
|---|---|
| **How is it diagnosed prenatally?** | It may be seen on **fetal** U/S after 13 weeks' gestation, with elevated maternal AFP. |
| **What comprises the "sac"?** | Peritoneum and amnion |
| **What organ is often found protruding from an omphalocele, but is almost never found with a gastroschisis?** | The liver |
| **What is the incidence?** | Approximately 1 in 5000 births |
| **How is the diagnosis made?** | Prenatal U/S |
| **What are the possible complications?** | Malrotation of the gut, anomalies |
| **What is the treatment?** | 1. NG tube for decompression<br>2. IV fluids<br>3. Prophylactic antibiotics<br>4. Surgical repair of the defect |
| **What is the treatment of a small defect (>2 cm)?** | Closure of abdominal wall |
| **What is the treatment of a medium defect (2–10 cm)?** | Removal of outer membrane and placement of a silicone patch to form a "silo," temporarily housing abdominal contents; the silo is then slowly decreased in size over 4 to 7 days, as the abdomen accommodates the viscera; then the defect is closed |

**What is the treatment of "giant" defects (>10 cm)?**

Skin flaps or treatment with Betadine® spray, mercurochrome, or silver sulfadiazine (Silvadene®) over the defect; this allows an eschar to form, which epithelializes over time, allowing opportunity for future repair months to years later

**What are the associated abnormalities?**

50% of cases occur with often severe abnormalities of the GI tract, cardiovascular system, GU tract, musculoskeletal system, CNS, and chromosomes.

| | |
|---|---|
| **Of what "pentalogy" is omphalocele a part?** | Pentalogy of Cantrell |
| **What is the pentalogy of Cantrell?** | **"D COPS":**<br>**D**iaphragmatic defect (hernia)<br>**C**ardiac abnormality<br>**O**mphalocele<br>**P**ericardium malformation/absence<br>**S**ternal cleft |

## GASTROSCHISIS

| | |
|---|---|
| **What is it?** | Defect of abdominal wall; sac does not cover extruded viscera |
| **How is it diagnosed prenatally?** | Possible at fetal ultrasound after 13 weeks' gestation, elevated maternal AFP |
| **Where is the defect?** | Lateral to the umbilicus (think: g**A**strochisis = l**A**teral) |
| **On what side of the umbilicus is the defect found most commonly?** | The right |
| **What is the usual size of the defect?** | Between 2 and 4 cm |
| **What are the possible complications?** | Thick edematous peritoneum from exposure to amnionic fluid; malrotation of the gut<br>Other complications include hypothermia; hypovolemia from third-spacing; sepsis; and metabolic acidosis from hypovolemia and poor perfusion, NEC, prolonged ileus |
| **How is the diagnosis made?** | Prenatal U/S |
| **What is the treatment?** | Primary—NG tube decompression, IV fluids (D10 LR), and IV antibiotics<br>Definitive—surgical reduction of viscera and abdominal closure; may require staged closure with silo |

| | |
|---|---|
| **What is a "silo"?** | Silastic silo is a temporary housing for external abdominal contents; silo is slowly tightened over time |
| **What is the prognosis?** | More than 90% survival rate |
| **What are the associated anomalies?** | Unlike omphalocele, relatively uncommon except for intestinal atresia, which occurs in 10% to 15% of cases |
| **How do you remember that omphalocele is associated with abnormailties in 50% of cases?** | Think: **O**mphalocele = "**O**h no, lots of abnormalities" |
| **What are the major differences compared with omphalocele?** | No membrane coverings<br>Uncommon associated abnormalities<br>Lateral to umbilicus not on umbilicus |
| **How can you remember the position of omphalocele vs. gastroschisis?** | Think: **OM**phalocele = **ON** the umbilicus |

## POWER REVIEW OF OMPHALOCELE AND GASTROSCHISIS

| | |
|---|---|
| **What are the differences between omphalocele and gastroschisis in terms of the following characteristics:** | |
| **Anomalies?** | Common in omphalocele (50%), uncommon in gastroschisis |
| **Peritoneal/amnion covering (sac)?** | Always with omphalocele, never with gastroschisis |
| **Position of umbilical cord?** | On the sac with omphalocele, from skin to the left of the gastroschisis defect |
| **Thick bowel?** | Common with gastroschisis, rare with omphalocele (unless sac ruptures) |
| **Protrusion of liver?** | Common with omphalocele, almost never with gastroschisis |
| **Large defect?** | Omphalocele |

## APPENDICITIS

| | |
|---|---|
| **What is it?** | Obstruction of the appendiceal lumen (fecalith, lymphoid hyperplasia), producing a closed loop with resultant inflammation that can lead to necrosis and perforation |
| **What is its claim to fame?** | Most common surgical disease requiring emergency surgery in children |
| **What is the affected age?** | Very rare before 3 years of age |
| **What is the usual presentation?** | Onset of referred or **periumbilical pain** followed by **anorexia,** nausea, and vomiting; *Note:* unlike gastroenteritis, **pain precedes vomiting;** pain then migrates to the **RLQ,** where it becomes more intense and localized from local peritoneal irritation<br>If the patient is hungry and can eat, seriously question the diagnosis of appendicitis. |
| **How is the diagnosis made?** | History and physical exam |
| **What are the signs/ symptoms?** | Signs of peritoneal irritation may be present—guarding, muscle spasm, rebound tenderness, obturator and Psoas signs; low-grade fever rising to high grade if perforation occurs |
| **What is the differential diagnosis?** | Intussusception, volvulus, Meckel's diverticulum, Crohn's disease, ovarian torsion, cyst, tumor, perforated ulcer, pancreatitis, PID, ruptured ectopic pregnancy, mesenteric lymphadenitis |
| **What is the common bacterial cause of mesenteric lymphadenitis?** | *Yersinia enterocolitica* |
| **What are the associated lab findings?** | Increased WBC ($>$10,000 per mm$^3$ in $>$90% of cases, with a left shift in most) |

**What is the role of urinalysis?**

To evaluate for possible pyelonephritis or renal calculus, but mild hematuria and pyuria are common in appendicitis because of ureteral inflammation

**What is the "hamburger" sign?**

Ask patients with suspected appendicitis if they would like a hamburger or favorite food; if they can eat, seriously question the diagnosis.

**What radiographic studies may be performed?**

Often none; CXR to rule out RML or RLL pneumonia; abdominal films are usually nonspecific, but calcified fecalith is present in 5% of cases; U/S to evaluate for ovarian/gynecologic pathology

**What is the treatment?**

**Nonperforated**—prompt appendectomy and cefoxitin to avoid perforation
**Perforated**—triple antibiotics, fluid resuscitation, and prompt appendectomy; all pus is drained and cultures obtained, with postoperative antibiotics continued for 5 to 7 days, ± drain

**How long should antibiotics be administered if nonperforated?**

24 hours

**How long if perforated?**

Usually 5 to 7 days or until WBCs are normal and patient is afebrile

**If a normal appendix is found upon exploration, what must be examined/ ruled out?**

Meckel's diverticulum, Crohn's disease, intussusception, gynecologic disease

**What is the approximate risk of perforation?**

~ 25% after 24 hours from onset of symptoms
~ 50% by 36 hours
~ 75% by 48 hours

## INTUSSUSCEPTION

| | |
|---|---|
| **What is it?** | Obstruction caused by bowel telescoping into the lumen of adjacent distal bowel; may result when peristalsis carries a "leadpoint" downstream |
| **What is its claim to fame?** | Most common cause of small bowel obstruction in toddlers (<2 years old) |
| **What is the usual age at presentation?** | Disease of infancy; 60% present from 4 to 12 months of age, 80% by 2 years of age |
| **What is the most common site?** | Terminal ileum involving ileocecal valve and extending into ascending colon |
| **What is the most common cause?** | Hypertrophic Peyer's patches, which act as a lead point; many patients have prior viral illness |
| **What are the signs/ symptoms?** | Alternating lethargy and irritability (colic), bilious vomiting, "currant jelly" stools, RLQ mass on plain abdominal film, empty RLQ on palpation (Dance's sign) |
| **What is the intussuscipiens?** | The recipient segment of bowel (think: **recipiens** = intussus**cipiens**) |
| **What is the intussusceptum?** | The leading point or bowel that enters the intussuscipiens |
| **Identify locations 1 and 2 on the following illustration:** | 1. Intussuscipiens<br>2. Intussusceptum |

**How can the spelling of intussusception be remembered?**

Intussusception—two "s's," followed by one "s." Think: the United States ship the U.S. = the U.S.S. U.S. (analogous to the ship the U.S.S. Constitution)

**What is the treatment?**

**Air** or barium enema; 85% reduce with hydrostatic pressure (i.e., barium = meter elevation air = maximum of 120 mm Hg); if unsuccessful, then laparotomy and reduction by "milking" the ileum from the colon should be performed

**What are the causes of intussusception in older patients?**

Meckel's diverticulum, polyps, and tumors, all of which act as a lead point

## MECKEL'S DIVERTICULUM

**What is it?**

Remnant of the omphalomesenteric duct/vitelline duct, which connects the yolk sac with the primitive midgut in the embryo

**What is the usual location?**

Between 45 and 90 cm proximal to the ileocecal valve on the antimesenteric border of the bowel

**What is the major differential diagnosis?**

Appendicitis

**Is it a true diverticulum?**

Yes; all layers of the intestine are found in the wall.

**What is the incidence?**

2% of the population at autopsy, but more than 90% of these are asymptomatic

**What is the gender ratio?**

Two to three times more common in males

**What is the usual age at onset of symptoms?**

Most frequently in the first 2 years of life, but can occur at any age

| | |
|---|---|
| **What are the possible complications?** | **Intestinal hemorrhage** (painless)— 50% |
| | Accounts for 50% of all lower GI bleeding in patients younger than 2 years; bleeding results from ectopic gastric mucosa secreting acid → ulcer → bleeding |
| | **Intestinal obstruction**—25% |
| | Most common complication in adults; includes volvulus and intussusception |
| | **Inflammation** (± perforation)—20% |
| **What percentage of cases have heterotopic tissue?** | More than 50%; usually gastric mucosa (85%), but duodenal, pancreatic, and colonic mucosa have been described |
| **What is the most common ectopic tissue in a Meckel's diverticulum?** | Gastric mucosa |
| **What other pediatric disease entity can also present with GI bleeding secondary to ectopic gastric mucosa?** | Enteric duplications |
| **What is the most common cause of lower GI bleeding in children?** | Meckel's diverticulum with ectopic gastric mucosa |
| **What is the "rule of 2s"?** | **2% are symptomatic.** Found about **2** feet from ileocecal valve Found in **2%** of the population Most symptoms occur before age **2**. One of **2** will have ectopic tissue. Most diverticula are about **2** inches long. Male:female ratio = **2**:1 |
| **What is a Meckel's scan?** | Scan for ectopic gastric mucosa in Meckel's diverticulum; uses **technetium** Tc 99m **pertechnetate** IV, which is preferentially taken up by gastric mucosa |

## NECROTIZING ENTEROCOLITIS

| | |
|---|---|
| **What is it also known as?** | NEC |
| **What is it?** | Necrosis of intestinal mucosa often with bleeding; may progress to transmural intestinal necrosis, shock/sepsis, and death |
| **What are the predisposing conditions?** | **PREMATURITY** Stress: shock, hypoxia, RDS, apneic episodes, sepsis, exchange transfusions, PDA and cyanotic heart disease, hyperosmolar feedings, polycythemia, indomethacin |
| **What is the pathophysiologic mechanism?** | Probable splanchnic vasoconstriction with decreased perfusion, mucosal injury, and probable bacterial invasion |
| **What is its claim to fame?** | Most common cause of emergent laparotomy in the neonate |
| **What are the signs/ symptoms?** | Abdominal distention, vomiting, heme positive or gross rectal bleeding, fever or hypothermia, jaundice, abdominal wall erythema (consistent with perforation and abscess formation) |
| **What are the radiographic findings?** | Fixed, dilated intestinal loops; pneumatosis intestinalis (air in the bowel wall); free air; and portal vein air (sign of advanced disease) |
| **What are the lab findings?** | Low hematocrit, glucose, and platelets |
| **What is the treatment?** | Most are managed medically: 1. Cessation of feedings 2. OG tube 3. IV fluids 4. IV antibiotics 5. Ventilator support, as needed |

| | |
|---|---|
| **What are the surgical indications?** | Free air in abdomen revealing perforation, and positive peritoneal tap revealing transmural bowel necrosis |
| **Operation?** | 1. Resect<br>2. Stoma |
| **What is an option for bowel perforation in <1000 gram NEC patients?** | Placement of percutaneous drain (without laparotomy!) |
| **Is portal vein gas or pneumatosis intestinalis alone an indication for operation with NEC?** | No |
| **What are the indications for peritoneal tap?** | Severe thrombocytopenia, distended abdomen, abdominal wall erythema, unexplained clinical downturn |
| **What are the possible complications?** | Bowel necrosis, gram-negative sepsis, DIC, wound infection, cholestasis, short bowel syndrome, strictures, SBO |
| **What is the prognosis?** | >80% overall survival rate |

## BILIARY TRACT

| | |
|---|---|
| **What is "physiologic jaundice"?** | Hyperbilirubinemia in the first 2 weeks of life from inadequate conjugation of bilirubin |
| **What enzyme is responsible for conjugation of bilirubin?** | Glucuronyl transferase |
| **How is hyperbilirubinemia from "physiologic jaundice" treated?** | UV light |
| **What is Gilbert's syndrome?** | Partial deficiency of glucuronosyl-transferase, leading to intermittent asymptomatic jaundice in the second or third decade of life |

| | |
|---|---|
| **What is Crigler-Najjar syndrome?** | Rare genetic absence of glucuronosyl-transferase activity, causing unconjugated hyperbilirubinemia, jaundice, and death from kernicterus (usually within the first year) |

## BILIARY ATRESIA

| | |
|---|---|
| **What is it?** | Obliteration of extrahepatic biliary tree |
| **What is the incidence?** | One in 16,000 births |
| **What are the signs/ symptoms?** | Persistent jaundice (normal physiologic jaundice resolves in <2 weeks), hepatomegaly, splenomegaly, ascites and other signs of portal hypertension, acholic stools, biliuria |
| **What are the lab findings?** | Mixed jaundice is always present (i.e., both direct and indirect bilirubin increased), with an elevated serum alkaline phosphatase level. |
| **What is the classic "rule of 5s" of indirect bilirubinemia?** | Bizarre: with progressive hyperbilirubinemia, jaundice progresses by levels of 5 from the head to toes: 5 mg/dL = jaundice of head, 10 mg/dL = jaundice of trunk, 15 mg/dL = jaundice of leg/feet |
| **What is the differential diagnosis?** | Neonatal hepatitis (TORCH); biliary hypoplasia |
| **How is the diagnosis made?** | 1. U/S to rule out choledochal cyst and to examine extrahepatic bile ducts and gallbladder<br>2. HIDA scan—shows no excretion into the GI tract (with phenobarbital preparation)<br>3. Operative cholangiogram and liver biopsy |
| **What is the treatment?** | Early laparotomy by 2 months of age with a modified form of the Kasai hepatoportoenterostomy |

**How does a Kasai work?**

The anastomosis of the porta hepatis and the small bowel allows drainage of bile via many microscopic bile ducts in the fibrous structure of the porta hepatis.

**What if the Kasai fails?**

Revise or liver transplantation

**What are the possible postoperative complications?**

Cholangitis (manifested as decreased bile secretion, fever, leukocytosis, and recurrence of jaundice), progressive cirrhosis (manifested as portal hypertension with bleeding varices, ascites, hypoalbuminemia, hypothrombinemia, and fat-soluble vitamin K, A, D, E deficiencies)

**What are the associated abnormalities?**

Between 25% and 30% have other anomalies, including annular pancreas, duodenal atresia, malrotation, polysplenic syndrome, situs inversus, and preduodenal portal vein; 15% have congenital heart defects.

## CHOLEDOCHAL CYST

**What is it?**

Cystic enlargement of bile ducts; most commonly arises in extrahepatic ducts, but can also arise in intrahepatic ducts

**What is the usual presentation?**

50% present with intermittent jaundice, RUQ mass, and abdominal pain; may also present with pancreatitis.

**What are the possible complications?**

Cholelithiasis, cirrhosis, carcinoma, and portal HTN

**What are the anatomic variants:**
    **I?**

Dilation of common hepatic and common bile duct, with cystic duct entering the cyst; most common type (90%)

Type I

**II?**                     Lateral saccular cystic dilation

Type II

**III?**                    Choledochocele represented by an
                           intraduodenal cyst

Type III

**IV?**                     Multiple extrahepatic cysts, intrahepatic
                           cysts, or both

Type IV

**V?**

Single or multiple intrahepatic cysts

**Type V**

**How is the diagnosis made?**

U/S

**What is the treatment?**

Operative cholangiogram to clarify pathologic process and delineate the pancreatic duct, followed by complete resection of the cyst and a Roux-en-Y hepatojejunostomy

**What condition are these patients at increased risk of developing?**

**Cholangiocarcinoma** often arises in the cyst; therefore, treat by complete prophylactic resection of the cyst.

CHOLELITHIASIS

**What is it?**

The formation of gallstones

**What are the common causes in children?**

The etiology differs somewhat from that of adults; the most common cause is cholesterol stones, but there is an increased percentage of pigmented stones from hemolytic disorders.

**What is the differential diagnosis?**

Hereditary spherocytosis, thalassemia, pyruvate kinase deficiency, sickle-cell disease, cystic fibrosis, long-term parenteral nutrition, idiopathic

**What are the associated risks?**

Use of oral contraceptives, teenage, positive family history

**What is the treatment?**

Cholecystectomy is recommended for all children with gallstones.

## ANNULAR PANCREAS

| | |
|---|---|
| **What is an annular pancreas?** | Congenital pancreatic abnormality with complete encirclement of the duodenum by the pancreas |
| **What are the symptoms of annular pancreas?** | Duodenal obstruction |
| **What is the treatment of annular pancreas?** | Duodenoduodenostomy bypass of obstruction (do not resect the pancreas!) |

## TUMORS

| | |
|---|---|
| **What is the differential diagnosis of pediatric abdominal mass?** | Wilms' tumor, neuroblastoma, hernia, intussusception, malrotation with volvulus, mesenteric cyst, duplication cyst, liver tumor (hepatoblastoma/hemangioma), rhabdomyosarcoma, teratoma |

## WILMS' TUMOR

| | |
|---|---|
| **What is it?** | Embryonal tumor of **renal** origin |
| **What is the incidence?** | Very rare: 500 new cases in the United States per year |
| **What is the average age at diagnosis?** | Usually between 2 and 4 years of age |
| **What are the symptoms?** | Usually asymptomatic except for abdominal mass; 20% of patients present with minimal blunt trauma to mass |
| **What are the signs?** | Abdominal mass (most do not cross the midline); hematuria (10–15%); HTN in 20% of cases, related to compression of juxtaglomerular apparatus; signs of Beckwith-Wiedemann syndrome |
| **What are the diagnostic radiologic tests?** | Abdominal and chest CT |
| **Define the stages:** | |
| **Stage I** | Limited to kidney and completely resected |

| | |
|---|---|
| **Stage II** | Extends beyond kidney, but completely resected; capsule invasion and perirenal tissues may be involved |
| **Stage III** | Residual nonhematogenous tumor after resection |
| **Stage IV** | Hematogenous metastases (lung, distal lymph nodes, and brain) |
| **Stage V** | Bilateral renal involvement |
| **What are the best indicators of survival?** | Stage and histologic subtype of tumor; 85% of patients have favorable histology (FH); 15% have unfavorable histology (UH); overall survival for FH is 85% for all stages |
| **What is the treatment?** | Radical resection of affected kidney with evaluation for staging, followed by chemotherapy (low stages) and radiation (higher stages) |
| **What is the neoadjuvant treatment?** | Large tumors may be shrunk with chemotherapy/XRT to allow for surgical resection. |
| **What are the associated abnormalities?** | **Aniridia,** hemihypertrophy, Beckwith-Wiedemann syndrome, neurofibromatosis, horseshoe kidney |
| **What is the Beckwith-Wiedemann syndrome?** | **Syndrome of:** 1. Umbilical defect 2. Macroglossia (big tongue) 3. Gigantism 4. Visceromegaly (big organs) (think: **W**ilms' = Beckwith-**W**iedemann) |

## NEUROBLASTOMA

| | |
|---|---|
| **What is it?** | Embryonal tumor of neural crest origin |
| **What are the anatomic locations?** | **Adrenal medulla**—50% Paraaortic abdominal paraspinal ganglia—25% |

Posterior mediastinum—20%
Neck—3%
Pelvis—3%

**With which type of tumor does a patient with Horner's syndrome present?**

Neck, superior mediastinal tumors

**What is the incidence?**

One in 7,000 to 10,000 live births; most common solid malignant tumor of infancy; most common solid tumor in children outside the CNS

**What is the average age at diagnosis?**

Approximately 50% are diagnosed by 2 years of age
Approximately 90% are diagnosed by 8 years of age

**What are the symptoms?**

Vary by tumor location—anemia, failure to thrive, weight loss, and poor nutritional status with advanced disease

**What are the signs?**

Asymptomatic abdominal mass (palpable in 50% of cases), respiratory distress (mediastinal tumors), Horner's syndrome (upper chest or neck tumors), proptosis (with orbital metastases), subcutaneous tumor nodules, HTN (20–35%)

**CABS?**

24-hour urine to measure VMA, HVA, and metanephrines (elevated in >85%); neuron-specific enolase, N-*myc* oncogene, DNA ploidy

**What are the diagnostic radiologic tests?**

CT, MRI, I-MIBG, somatostatin receptor scan

**What is the classic abdominal plain x-ray finding?**

Calcifications (approximately 50%)

**How do you access bone marrow involvement?**

Bone marrow aspirate

**What is the difference in position of tumors in neuroblastoma versus Wilms' tumors?**

Neuroblastoma may cross the midline, but Wilms' tumors do so only rarely.

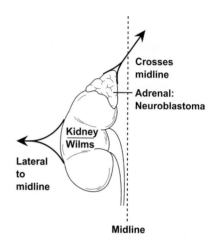

**What is the treatment?**

Depends on staging

**Define the stages:**

**Stage I**

Tumor is confined to organ of origin.

**Stage II**

Tumor extends beyond organ of origin **but not** across the midline.

**Stage III**

Tumor extends **across the midline.**

**Stage IV**

Metastatic disease

**Stage IVS**

Infants: Localized primary tumor does not cross the midline, but **remote disease** is confined to the liver, subcutaneous/skin, and bone marrow.

**What is the treatment of each stage:**

**Stage I?**

Surgical resection

**Stage II?**

Resection and chemotherapy +/− XRT

**Stage III?**

Resection and chemotherapy/XRT

**Stage IV?**

Chemotherapy/XRT → resection

**What is the survival rate of each stage:**

| | |
|---|---|
| **Stage I?** | Approximately 90% |
| **Stage II?** | Approximately 80% |
| **Stage III?** | Approximately 40% |
| **Stage IV?** | Approximately 15% |
| **Stage IVS?** | Survival rate is more than 80%! *Note:* these tumors are basically stage I or II with metastasis to liver, subcutaneous tissue, or bone marrow; most of these patients, if younger than 1 year of age, have a spontaneous cure. (think: stage **IVS** = **S**pecial condition) |

**What are the laboratory prognosticators?**

Aneuploidy is favorable! The lower the number of N-*myc* oncogene copies, the better the prognosis.

**Which oncogene is associated with neuroblastoma?**

N-*myc* oncogene
Think: **N**-*myc* = **N**euroblastoma

## RHABDOMYOSARCOMA

**What is it?**

Highly malignant **striated muscle** sarcoma

**What is its claim to fame?**

Most common sarcoma in children

**What is the age distribution?**

Bimodal:
1. 2–5 years
2. 15–19 years

**What are the most common sites?**

1. Head and neck (40%)
2. GU tract (20%)
3. Extremities (20%)

**What are the signs/ symptoms?**

Mass

**How is the diagnosis made?**

Tissue biopsy, CT, MRI, bone marrow

| | |
|---|---|
| **What is the treatment:** | |
| **Resectable?** | Surgical excision +/− chemotherapy and radiation therapy |
| **Unresectable?** | Neoadjuvant chemo/XRT then surgical excision |

## HEPATOBLASTOMA

| | |
|---|---|
| **What is it?** | Malignant tumor of the liver (derived from embryonic liver cells) |
| **What is the average age at diagnosis?** | Presents in the first 3 years of life |
| **What is the male to female ratio?** | 2:1 |
| **How is the diagnosis made?** | Physical exam—abdominal distention; **RUQ mass that moves with respiration** Elevated serum $\alpha$-fetoprotein and ferritin (can be used as tumor markers) CT scan of abdomen, which often predicts resectability |
| **What percentage will have an elevated $\alpha$-fetoprotein level?** | Approximately 90% |
| **What is the treatment?** | Resection by lobectomy or trisegmentectomy is the treatment of choice (plus postoperative chemotherapy); large tumors may require preoperative chemotherapy and **subsequent** hepatic resection. |
| **What is the overall survival rate?** | Approximately 50% |
| **What is the major difference in age presentation between hepatoma and hepatoblastoma?** | Hepatoblastoma presents at younger than 3 years of age; hepatoma presents at older than 3 years of age and in adolescents. |

## PEDIATRIC TRAUMA

| | |
|---|---|
| **What is the leading cause of death in pediatric patients?** | Trauma |
| **How are the vast majority of splenic and liver injuries treated in children?** | Observation (i.e., nonoperatively) |
| **What is a common simulator of peritoneal signs in the blunt pediatric trauma victim?** | Gastric distention (place an NG tube) |
| **How do you estimate normal systolic blood pressure (SBP) in a child?** | 80 plus 2 multiplied by age (e.g., a 5-year-old child should have an SBP of about 90) |
| **What is the 20–20–10 rule for fluid resuscitation of the unstable pediatric trauma patient?** | Fluid resuscitation in the unstable pediatric patient: first give a **20** cc/kg LR bolus followed by a second bolus of **20** cc/kg LR bolus if needed. If the patient is still unstable after the second LR bolus, then administer a **10** cc/kg bolus of **blood** |
| **What CT scan findings suggest small bowel injury?** | Free fluid with **no** evidence of liver or spleen injury, free air, contrast leak, bowel thickening, mesentery streaking |
| **What is the treatment for duodenal hematoma?** | Observation with NGT and TPN |

## OTHER PEDIATRIC SURGERY QUESTIONS

| | |
|---|---|
| **What is bilious vomiting in an infant?** | Malrotation, until proven otherwise! (About 90% of patients with malrotation present before the first year of life.) |
| **What does TORCHES stand for?** | Nonbacterial fetal and neonatal infections: **TO**xoplasmosis, **R**ubella, **C**ytomegalovirus (CMV), **H**erpes, **S**yphilis |
| **What is the common pediatric sedative?** | Chloral hydrate |

**What are the contraindications to circumcision?**

Hypospadias, etc., because the foreskin might be needed for future repair of the abnormality

**When should an umbilical hernia be repaired?**

After 4 years of age; otherwise observe, because most close spontaneously; repair before school age if it persists

**What is the cancer risk in the cryptorchid testicle?**

More than ten times the normal testicular cancer rate

**When should orchidopexy be performed?**

All patients with undescended testicle undergo orchidopexy after 1 year of age

**What are the signs of child abuse?**

Cigarette burns, rope burns, scald to posterior thighs and buttocks, multiple fractures/old fractures, genital trauma, delay in accessing health care system

**What is the treatment of child abuse?**

**Admit the patient** to the hospital.

**What is Dance's sign?**

Empty RLQ in patients with ileocecal intussusception

**What is the treatment of hemangioma?**

Observation, because most regress spontaneously

**What are the indications for operation in hemangiomas?**

Severe thrombocytopenia, congestive heart failure, functional impairment (vision, breathing)

**What are treatment options for hemangiomas?**

Steroids, radiation, surgical resection, angiographic embolization

**What is the most common benign liver tumor in children?**

Hemangioma

**What is Eagle-Barrett's syndrome?**

A.K.A. prune belly; congenital inadequate abdominal musculature (very lax and thin)

**What is the Pierre-Robin syndrome?**

Classic triad:
1. Big, protruding tongue (glossoptosis)
2. Small mandible (micrognathia)
3. Cleft palate

**What is the major concern with Pierre-Robin syndrome?**

Airway obstruction by the tongue!

**What are the most common cancers in children?**

1. Leukemia
2. CNS tumors
3. Lymphomas

**What is the most common solid neoplasm in infants?**

Neuroblastoma

**What is the most common solid tumor in children?**

CNS tumors

**What syndrome must you consider in the patient with abdominal pain, hematuria, history of joint pain, and a purpuric rash?**

Henoch-Schönlein syndrome; patient may also have melena (50%) or at least guaiac-positive stools (75%)

**What is Apley's law?**

The further a chronically recurrent abdominal pain is from the umbilicus, the greater is the likelihood of an organic cause for the pain.

**What is the most common cause of SBO in children?**

Hernias

**What is a patent urachus?**

Persistence of the urachus, a communication between the bladder and umbilicus; presents with urine out of the umbilicus and recurrent UTIs

**What is a "Replogle tube"?**

10 French sump pump NG tube for babies (originally designed by Dr. Replogle for suction of the esophageal blind pouch of esophageal atresia)

**What are "A's and B's"?**

**A**pnea and **B**radycardia episodes in babies

| | |
|---|---|
| **What is the "Double Bubble" sign on AXR?** | Gastric bubble and **duodenal bubble** on AXR; seen with duodenal obstruction (web, annular pancreas, malrotation with volvulus, duodenal atresia, etc.) |
| **What is Poland's syndrome?** | Absence of pectoralis major muscle<br>Absence of pectoralis minor muscle<br>Often associated with ipsilateral hand malformation<br>Nipple/breast/right-breast hypoplasia |
| **What is the treatment of ATYPICAL mycobacterial lymph node infection?** | Surgical removal of the node |
| **What is the most common cause of rectal bleeding in infants?** | Anal fissure |
| **What chromosomal abnormality is associated with duodenal web/atresia/stenosis?** | Trisomy 21 |
| **Which foreign body past the pylorus must be surgically removed?** | Batteries! |

## POWER REVIEW

| | |
|---|---|
| **What is the usual age at presentation of the following conditions:** | |
| **Pyloric stenosis?** | From 2 weeks to 2 months of age |
| **Intussusception?** | From 4 months to 2 years of age (>80%) |
| **Wilms' tumor?** | Between 1 and 4 years of age |
| **Malrotation?** | Birth to 1 year of age (>85%) |

| | |
|---|---|
| **Neuroblastoma?** | Approximately 50% present by 2 years of age, and more than 80% present by 8 years of age |
| **Hepatoblastoma?** | Younger than 3 years of age |
| **Appendicitis?** | Older than 3 years of age (but must be considered at *any* age!) |

---

# Chapter 68          Plastic Surgery

**Define the following terms:**

| | |
|---|---|
| **Blepharoplasty** | Eyelid surgery—removing excess skin/fat |
| **Face lift** | Removal of excess facial skin via hairline/chin/ear incisions |
| **FTSG** | **F**ull **T**hickness **S**kin **G**raft |
| **Langer's lines** | The natural skin lines of minimal tension (e.g., lines across the forehead), incisions perpendicular to Langer's lines result in larger scars than incision parallel to the lines |

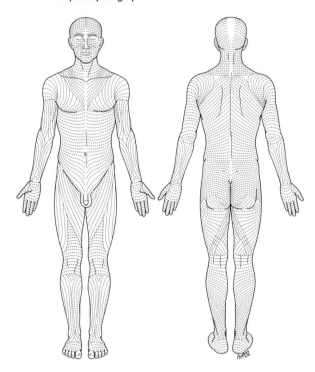

| | |
|---|---|
| **Mammoplasty** | Breast surgery (reduction/augmentation) |
| **Polydactyly** | Extra fingers |
| **Rhinoplasty** | Nose surgery, after trauma or cosmetic |
| **STSG** | **S**plit **T**hickness **S**kin **G**raft |
| **Syndactyly** | Webbed fingers |

## WOUND HEALING

| | |
|---|---|
| **What are the phases of wound healing?** | 1. Inflammation<br>2. Epithelialization<br>3. Fibroplasia<br>4. Contraction |
| **What is a memory aid for the phases of wound healing?** | "**In E**very **F**resh **C**ut" = **I.E.F.C.:**<br>**I**nflammation<br>**E**pithelialization |

Fibroplasia
Contraction

**What are the actions of the following phases:**

**Inflammation?**

Vasoconstriction followed by vasodilation, capillary leak

**Epithelialization?**

Epithelial coverage of wound

**Fibroplasia?**

Fibroblasts and accumulation of collagen, elastin, and reticulin

**Wound contraction?**

Myofibroblasts contract wound

**What is the maximal contraction of a wound in mm/day?**

0.75 mm/day

## EPITHELIALIZATION

**What degree of bacterial contamination prevents epithelialization?**

More than 100,000 organisms/gm tissue ($10^5$)

**What structures does the epithelium grow in from superficial burns/wounds?**

Epithelial lining of sweat glands and hair follicles

**In full-thickness burns?**

From wound margins, grows in less than 1 cm from wound edge because no sweat glands or hair remains; this epithelium has no underlying dermis

**What malignant ulcer is associated with a long-standing scar/burn?**

Marjolin's ulcer (A.K.A. burn scar carcinoma)

## WOUND CONTRACTION

**What are myofibroblasts?**

Specialized fibroblasts that behave like smooth muscle cells to pull the wound edges together following granulation

**Which contracts more: an STSG or an FTSG?**

An STSG contracts up to 41% in surface area, whereas an FTSG contracts little, if at all.

| | |
|---|---|
| **What is granulation tissue?** | Within 4 to 6 days after an open wound, development of capillary beds and fibroblasts provides a healthy base for epithelial growth from wound edges; this tissue also resists bacterial infection. |
| **Name the local factors that impair wound healing.** | Hematoma, seroma, infection, tight sutures, tight wrap, movement/disturbance of the wound (i.e., poking it with a finger) |
| **What generalized conditions inhibit wound healing?** | Anemia<br>Malnutrition<br>Steroids<br>Cancer<br>Radiation<br>Hypoxia<br>Sepsis |
| **What helps wound healing in patients taking steroids?** | Vitamin A is thought to counteract the deleterious effect of steroids on wound healing. |
| **When does a wound gain more than 90% of its maximal tensile strength?** | After approximately 6 weeks |
| **Define the following terms:**<br>  **Laceration** | A jagged wound |
|   **Abrasion** | Superficial skin removal |
|   **Contusion** | Bruise without a break in the skin |
|   **Hypertrophic scar** | Hypertrophic scar within original wound margins |
|   **Keloid** | Proliferative scar tumor progressively enlarging scar beyond original wound margins |
| **Why not clean lacerations with Betadine®?** | Betadine® is harmful to and inhibits normal healthy tissue. |
| **What is the best way to clean out a laceration?** | $H_2O$ irrigation. Remember, "the solution to pollution is dilution." |

## SKIN GRAFTS

| | |
|---|---|
| **What is an STSG?** | Split thickness: includes the epidermis and a variable amount of the dermis |
| **How thick is it?** | Between 12/1000 and 18/1000 of an inch (Think: 12–18 = teenager) |
| **What is an FTSG?** | Full thickness: includes the entire epidermis and dermis |
| **What are the prerequisites for a skin graft to take?** | The bed must be vascularized; a graft to a bone or tendon will not take. Bacteria must be less than 100,000. Shearing motion and fluid beneath the graft must be minimized. |
| **What is a better bed for a skin graft: fascia or fat?** | Fascia (much better blood supply) |
| **How do you increase surface area of an STSG?** | Mesh it (also allows for blood/serum to be removed from underneath the graft) |
| **How does an STSG get nutrition for the first 24 hours?** | Imbibition |

## FLAPS

| | |
|---|---|
| **Where does a random skin flap get its blood supply?** | From the dermal-subdermal plexus |
| **Where does an axial skin flap get its blood supply?** | It is vascularized by direct cutaneous arteries. |
| **Name some axial flaps and their arterial supply.** | Forehead flap—superficial temporal artery; often used for intraoral lesions<br>Deltopectoral flap—second, third, and fourth anterior perforators of the internal mammary artery; often used for head and neck wounds<br>Groin flap—superficial circumflex iliac artery; allows coverage of hand and forearm wounds |

**What is the most common cause of flap loss?**

Venous thrombosis

**What is a simple advancement flap?**

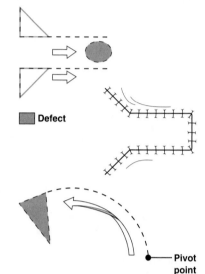

Defect

**What is a rotational flap?**

Pivot point

Defect

**What is a "free flap"?**

A flap separated from all vascular supply that requires microvascular anastomosis (microscope)

**What is a TRAM flap?**

**T**ransverse **R**ectus **A**bdominis **M**yocutaneous flap (see page 411)

**What is a "Z-plasty"?**

**What is a "V-Y advancement flap"?**

 Defect

# Chapter 69 — Hand Surgery

| | |
|---|---|
| **Who operates on hands?** | Plastic surgeons **and** orthopaedic surgeons |
| **What are the bones of the hand?** | Phalanges (fingers)<br>Metacarpal bones<br>Carpal bones |
| **What is the distal finger joint?** | Distal interphalangeal (DIP) joint |
| **What is the middle finger joint?** | Proximal interphalangeal (PIP) joint |
| **What is the proximal finger joint?** | Metacarpal phalangeal (MP) joint |
| **What are the "intrinsic" hand muscles?** | Lumbricals, interosseous muscle |
| **Where is "no man's land"?** | The zone extending from the distal palmar crease to just beyond the PIP joint. (Zone 2) |

Zone ② "No Man's Land"

**What is the significance of the "no man's land"?**

Flexor tendon injuries here have a poor prognosis; a hand expert needs to repair these injuries.

**What are the trauma zones of the hand?**

## SENSORY SUPPLY TO THE HAND

**What is the ulnar nerve distribution?**

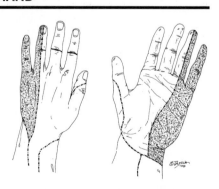

**What is the radial nerve distribution?**

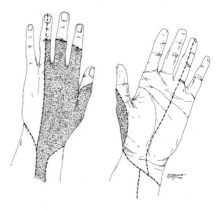

**What is the median nerve distribution?**

| | |
|---|---|
| **How can the radial nerve motor function be tested?** | 1. Wrist and MCP extension<br>2. Abduction and extension of thumb |
| **How can the ulnar nerve motor function be tested?** | 1. Spread fingers apart against resistance.<br>2. Check ability to cross index and middle fingers. |
| **How can the median nerve function be tested?** | 1. Touch the thumb to the pinky (distal median nerve).<br>2. Squeeze examiner's finger (proximal median nerve). |
| **How can the flexor digitorum *profundus* (FDP) apparatus be tested?** | Check isolated flexion of the finger DIP joint. |

**FDP**

| | |
|---|---|
| **How can the flexor digitorum *superficialis* (FDS) apparatus be tested?** | Check isolated flexion of the finger at the MP joint. |

**FDS**

| | |
|---|---|
| **Where do the digital arteries run?** | On medial and lateral sides of the digit |
| **What hand laceration should be left unsutured?** | Lacerations from human bites or animal bites |
| **Should a clamp ever be used to stop a laceration bleeder?** | **No;** use pressure and then tourniquet for definitive repair if bleeding does not cease because **nerves run with blood vessels!** |
| **What is a felon?** | Infection in **the tip** of the finger pad (think: felon = fingerprints = infection in pad); treat by incision and drainage |

**What is a paronychia?**
Infection on the **side** of the fingernail (nail fold); treat by incision and drainage

**What is tenosynovitis?**
Tendon sheath infection

**What are Kanavel's signs?**
Four signs of tenosynovitis:
1. Affected finger held in flexion
2. Pain over volar aspect of affected finger tendon sheath upon palpation
3. Swelling of affected finger (fusiform)
4. Pain on passive extension of affected finger

**Most common bacteria in tenosynovitis and paronychia?**
*Staphylococcus aureus*

**How are human and animal hand bites treated?**
Debridement/irrigation/administration of antibiotics; leave wound open

**What unique bacteria are found in human bites?**
*Eikenella corrodens*

**What unique bacteria are found in dog and cat bites?**
*Pasteurella multocida*

**What is the most common hand/wrist tumor?**
Ganglion cyst

**What is an extremely painful type of subungual tumor?**
Glomus tumor

**What is a "boxer's fracture"?**
Fracture of the fourth or fifth metacarpal

**What is a "drop finger" injury?**

**What is the classic deformity resulting from laceration of the extensor tendon over the DIP joint?**

Mallet finger

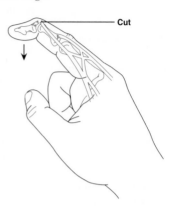

**What is the classic deformity resulting from laceration of the extensor tendon over the PIP joint?**

Boutonniere deformity

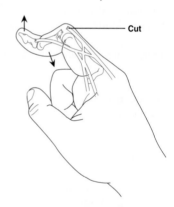

**Which fracture causes pain in the "anatomic snuffbox"?**

Scaphoid fracture; often not seen on x-ray at presentation, usually seen at a later date (2 weeks) on x-ray

Can result in avascular necrosis

Place in a cast if clinically suspected, regardless of x-ray findings.

**What is the "safe position" of hand splinting?**

**What is Dupuytren's contracture?**

Fibrosis of palmar fascia, causing contracture of and inability to extend digits

**What is Gamekeeper's thumb?**

Injury to the ulnar collateral ligament of the thumb

**How should a subungual (i.e., under the nail) hematoma be treated?**

Release pressure by burning a hole in the nail (use hand-held disposable battery-operated coagulation probe).

**What is a "Bible" cyst?**

Ganglion cyst—they used to be treated by a good whack from a Bible!

## CARPAL TUNNEL SYNDROME

**What is it?**

Compression of the median nerve in the carpal tunnel

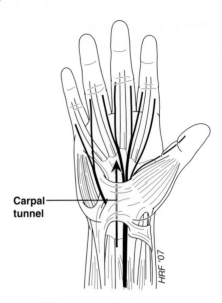

**Carpal tunnel**

HRF '07

| | |
|---|---|
| **What is the most common cause?** | Synovitis |
| **What are other causes?** | "MEDIAN TRAPS":<br>**M**edian artery (persistent)<br>**E**dema of pregnancy<br>**D**iabetes<br>**I**diopathic<br>**A**cromegaly<br>**N**eoplasm (e.g., ganglioneuroma)<br><br>**T**hyroid (myxedema)<br>**R**heumatoid arthritis<br>**A**myloid<br>**P**neumatic drill usage<br>**S**LE |
| **What are the symptoms?** | Pain and numbness in the median nerve distribution |
| **What are the signs?** | Tinel's sign (symptoms with percussion over median nerve), Phalen's test (symptoms with flexion of wrists), thenar atrophy |

| What is the work-up? | EMG, nerve conduction study |
| What is initial treatment? | Nonoperative + night wrist splint, vitamin B$_6$, NSAIDs, steroid injections |
| What are indications for surgery? | Refractory symptoms, thenar atrophy, thenar weakness |
| What surgery is performed? | Release transverse carpal ligament |

# Chapter 70

# Otolaryngology: Head and Neck Surgery

**Define:**

| Anosmia | Inability to **smell** |
| Otorrhea | Fluid discharge from ear |
| Dysphagia | Difficulty swallowing |
| Odynophagia | Painful swallowing |
| Globus | Sensation of a "lump in the throat" |
| Otalgia | Ear pain (often referred from throat) |
| Trismus | Difficulty opening mouth |

## ANATOMY

**Define the cranial nerves:**

| I | Olfactory nerve |
| II | Optic nerve |
| III | Oculomotor nerve |
| IV | Trochlear nerve |

| | |
|---|---|
| **V** | Trigeminal nerve |
| **VI** | Abducens nerve |
| **VII** | Facial nerve |
| **VIII** | Vestibulocochlear nerve |
| **IX** | Glossopharyngeal nerve |
| **X** | Vagus nerve |
| **XI** | Accessory nerve |
| **XII** | Hypoglossal nerve |

**Define motor/sensory actions of the following cranial nerves:**

| | |
|---|---|
| **I** | Smell |
| **II** | Sight (**sensory pupil reaction**) |
| **III** | Eyeball movement, pupil sphincter, ciliary muscle (**motor pupil reaction**) |
| **IV** | Superior oblique muscle movement |
| **V** | Sensory: face, teeth, sinuses, cornea<br>Motor: chewing (masseter muscle) |
| **VI** | Lateral rectus muscle (lateral gaze) |
| **VII** | Motor: facial muscles, lacrimal/ sublingual/submandibular glands<br>Sensory: anterior tongue/soft palate, taste |
| **VIII** | Hearing, positioning |
| **IX** | Motor: stylopharyngeus, parotid, pharynx<br>Sensory: posterior tongue, pharynx, middle ear |

| | |
|---|---|
| **X** | Motor: vocal cords, heart, bronchus, GI tract |
| | Sensory: bronchus, heart, GI tract, larynx, ear |
| **XI** | Motor: trapezius muscle, sternocleidomastoid muscle |
| **XII** | Motor: tongue, strap muscles (ansa cervicalis branch) |

**What are the three divisions of the trigeminal nerve (cranial nerve V)?**

1. Ophthalmic
2. Maxillary
3. Mandibular

**What happens when the hypoglossal nerve (cranial nerve XII) is cut?**

When the patient sticks out the tongue, it deviates to the same side as the injury (wheelbarrow effect).

**Name the duct of the submandibular gland.**

Wharton's duct

**Name the duct of the parotid gland.**

Stensen's duct

**What is the source of blood supply to the nose?**

1. Internal carotid artery: anterior and posterior ethmoidal arteries via ophthalmic artery
2. External carotid artery: superior labial artery (via facial artery) and sphenopalatine artery (via internal maxillary artery)

**Name the three bones that make up the posterior nasal septum.**

1. Ethmoid (perpendicular plate)
2. Vomer (Latin for plow)
3. Palatine (some also include maxillary crest)

**Name the seven bones of the bony eyeball orbit.**

1. Frontal
2. Zygoma
3. Maxillary
4. Lacrimal
5. Ethmoid
6. Palatine
7. Sphenoid

| | |
|---|---|
| **Which sinus is fully formed at birth?** | Ethmoid sinus |
| **Name the four strap muscles.** | "T.O.S.S.": <br> 1. **T**hyrohyoid <br> 2. **O**mohyoid <br> 3. **S**ternothyroid <br> 4. **S**ternohyoid |
| **Which muscle crosses the external and internal carotid arteries?** | Digastric muscle |
| **In a neck incision, what is the first muscle incised?** | Platysma |
| **Which nerve supplies the strap muscles?** | Ansa cervicalis (XII) |
| **What are the anterior and posterior neck triangles?** | Two regions of the neck divided by the sternocleidomastoid |

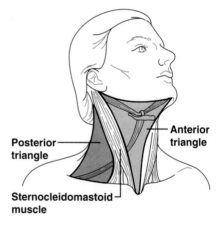

| | |
|---|---|
| **Which nerve runs with the carotid in the carotid sheath?** | Vagus |
| **Which nerve crosses the internal carotid artery at approximately 1 to 2 cm above the bifurcation?** | Hypoglossal nerve |

| | |
|---|---|
| **Name the three auditory ossicle bones.** | 1. Malleus (hammer)<br>2. Incus (anvil)<br>3. Stapes (stirrup) |
| **What comprises the middle ear?** | Eustachian tube, ossicle bones, tympanic membrane ("ear drum"), mastoid air cell |
| **What comprises the inner ear?** | Cochlea, semicircular canals, internal auditory canal |

## EAR

### OTITIS EXTERNA (SWIMMER'S EAR)

| | |
|---|---|
| **What is it?** | Generalized infection involving the external ear canal and often the tympanic membrane |
| **What is the usual cause?** | Prolonged water exposure and damaged squamous epithelium of the ear canal (i.e., swimming, hearing aid use) |
| **What are the typical pathogens?** | Most frequently *Pseudomonas;* may be *Proteus, Staphylococcus,* occasionally *Escherichia coli,* fungi (*Aspergillus, Candida*), or virus (herpes zoster or herpes simplex) |
| **What are the signs/ symptoms?** | Ear pain (otalgia); swelling of external ear, ear canal, or both; erythema; pain on manipulation of the auricle; debris in canal; otorrhea |
| **What is the treatment?** | Keep the ear dry; mild infections respond to cleaning and dilute acetic acid drops. Most infections require complete removal of all debris and topical antibiotics with or without hydrocortisone (antiinflammatory). |

### MALIGNANT OTITIS EXTERNA (MOE)

| | |
|---|---|
| **What is it?** | Fulminant **bacterial** otitis externa |
| **Is it malignant cancer?** | NO! |

| | |
|---|---|
| **Who is affected?** | Most common scenario: an elderly patient with poorly controlled diabetes (other forms of immunosuppression do not appear to predispose patients to MOE) |
| **What are the causative organisms?** | Usually *Pseudomonas aeruginosa* |
| **What is the classic feature?** | A nub of granulation tissue on the floor of the external ear canal at the bony-cartilaginous junction |
| **What are the other signs/symptoms?** | Severe ear pain, excessive purulent discharge, and usually **exposed bone** |
| **What are the diagnostic tests?** | 1. CT scan: shows erosion of bone, inflammation<br>2. Technetium-99 scan: temporal bone inflammatory process<br>3. Gallium-tagged white blood cell scan: to follow and document resolution |
| **What are the complications?** | Invasion of surrounding structures to produce a cellulitis, osteomyelitis of temporal bone, mastoiditis; later, a facial nerve palsy, meningitis, or brain abscess |
| **What is the treatment?** | Control of diabetes, meticulous local care with extensive debridement, hospitalization and IV antibiotics (anti-*Pseudomonas:* usually an aminoglycoside plus a penicillin) |

## TUMORS OF THE EXTERNAL EAR

| | |
|---|---|
| **What are the most common types?** | Squamous cell most common; occasionally, basal cell carcinoma or melanoma |
| **From what location do they usually arise?** | The auricle, but occasionally from the external canal |
| **What is the associated risk factor?** | Excessive sun exposure |

**What is the treatment of the following conditions:**

**Cancers of the auricle?**      Usually wedge excision

**Extension to the canal?**      May require excision of the external ear canal or partial temporal bone excision

**Middle ear involvement?**      Best treated by en bloc temporal bone resection and lymph node dissection

## TYMPANIC MEMBRANE (TM) PERFORATION

**What is the etiology?**      Usually the result of trauma (direct or indirect) or secondary to middle ear infection; often occurs secondary to slap to the side of the head (compression injury)

**What are the symptoms?**      Pain, conductive hearing loss, tinnitus

**What are the signs?**      Bleeding from the ear, clot in the meatus, visible tear in the TM

**What is the treatment?**      Keep dry; use systemic antibiotics if there is evidence of infection or contamination

**What is the prognosis?**      Most (90%) heal spontaneously, though larger perforations may require surgery (e.g., fat plug, temporalis fascia tympanoplasty).

## CHOLESTEATOMA

**What is it?**      An epidermal inclusion cyst of the middle ear or mastoid, containing desquamated keratin debris; may be acquired or congenital

**What are the causes?**      Negative middle ear pressure from eustachian tube dysfunction (primary acquired; typically in attic) or direct growth of epithelium through a TM perforation (secondary acquired)

| | |
|---|---|
| **What other condition is it often associated with?** | Chronic middle ear infection |
| **What is the usual history?** | Chronic ear infection with chronic, malodorous drainage |
| **What is the appearance?** | Grayish-white, shiny keratinous mass behind or involving the TM; often described as a "pearly" lesion |
| **What are the associated problems?** | Ossicular erosion, producing conductive hearing loss; also, local invasion resulting in: Vertigo/sensorineural hearing loss Facial paresis/paralysis CNS dysfunction/infection |
| **What is the treatment?** | Surgery (tympanoplasty/mastoidectomy) aimed at eradication of disease and reconstruction of the ossicular chain |

## BULLOUS MYRINGITIS

| | |
|---|---|
| **What is it?** | A vesicular infection of the TM and adjacent deep canal |
| **What are the causative agents?** | Unknown; viral should be suspected because of frequent association with viral URI (in some instances, *Mycoplasma pneumoniae* has been cultured) |
| **What are the symptoms?** | Acute, severe ear pain; low-grade fever; and bloody drainage |
| **What are the findings on otoscopic examination?** | Large, reddish blebs on the TM, wall of the meatus, or both |
| **Is hearing affected?** | Not usually; occasional reversible sensorineural loss |
| **What is the treatment?** | Oral antibiotics (erythromycin if *Mycoplasma* is suspected); topical analgesics may be used, with resolution of symptoms usually occurring in 36 hours |

## ACUTE SUPPURATIVE OTITIS MEDIA (OM)

**What is it?**

A bacterial infection of the middle ear, often following a viral URI; may be associated with a middle ear effusion

**What is the cause?**

Dysfunction of the eustachian tube that allows bacterial entry from nasopharynx; often associated with an occluded eustachian tube, although it is uncertain whether this is a cause or a result of the infection

**What are the predisposing factors?**

Young age, male gender, bottle feeding, crowded living conditions (i.e., day care), cleft palate, Down's syndrome, cystic fibrosis

**What is the etiology?**

1. *Streptococcus pneumoniae* (one-third of cases)
2. *Haemophilus influenzae*
3. *Moraxella catarrhalis*
4. *Staphylococcus*
5. β-hemolytic strep
6. *Pseudomonas aeruginosa*
7. Viral/no culture

**What is the etiology in infants younger than 6 months?**

1. *Staphylococcus aureus*
2. *E. coli*
3. *Klebsiella*

**What are the symptoms?**

Otalgia, fever, decreased hearing, infant pulls on ear, increased irritability; as many as 25% of patients are asymptomatic

**What are the signs?**

Early, redness of the TM; later, TM bulging with loss of the normal landmarks; finally, impaired TM mobility on pneumatic otoscopy

**If pain disappears instantly, what may have happened?**

TM perforation!

| | |
|---|---|
| **What are the complications?** | TM perforation, acute mastoiditis, meningitis, brain abscess, extradural abscess, labyrinthitis; if recurrent or chronic, OM may have adverse effects on speech and cognitive development as a result of decreased hearing |
| **What is the treatment?** | 10-day course of antibiotics; amoxicillin is the first-line agent; if the patient is allergic to PCN, trimethoprim-sulfamethoxazole or erythromycin should be administered |
| **What is the usual course?** | Symptoms usually resolve in 24 to 36 hours. |
| **What are the indications for myringotomy and PE tube placement?** | 1. Persistent middle ear effusion over 3 months<br>2. Debilitated or immunocompromised patient<br>3. More than three episodes over 6 months (especially if bilateral) |
| **What is a PE tube?** | **P**neumatic **E**qualization tube (tube placed across tympanic membrane) |
| **What is a Bezold's abscess?** | Abscess behind the superior attachment of the sternocleidomastoid muscle resulting from extension of a mastoid infection |
| **What are causes of chronic otitis media?** | Mixed, *S. aureus*, *P. aeruginosa* |
| **What are the signs/symptoms of chronic otitis media?** | Otorrhea and hearing loss |

## OTOSCLEROSIS

| | |
|---|---|
| **What is it?** | A genetic disease characterized by abnormal spongy and sclerotic bone formation in the temporal bone around the footplate of the stapes, thus preventing its normal movement |

| | |
|---|---|
| **What is the inheritance pattern?** | Autosomal dominant with incomplete one-third penetrance |
| **What are the symptoms?** | Painless, progressive hearing loss (may be unilateral or bilateral), tinnitus |
| **What is the usual age of onset?** | Second through fourth decade |
| **How is the diagnosis made?** | Normal TM with conductive hearing loss and no middle-ear effusion (though may be mixed or even sensorineural if bone of cochlea is affected) |
| **What is Schwartze's sign?** | Erythema around the stapes from hypervascularity of new bone formation |
| **What is the treatment?** | Frequently surgical (stapedectomy with placement of prosthesis), hearing aids, or observation; sodium fluoride may be used if a sensorineural component is present or for preoperative stabilization |

# MISCELLANEOUS

## FACIAL NERVE PARALYSIS

| | |
|---|---|
| **How is the defect localized?** | Supranuclear—paralysis of lower face only, forehead muscles are spared because of bilateral corticobulbar supply<br>Intratemporal bone—paralysis of upper and lower face, decreased tearing, altered taste, absent stapedius reflex<br>Distal to stylomastoid foramen—paralysis of facial muscles only |
| **What are the causes?** | Bell's palsy<br>Trauma<br>Cholesteatoma<br>Tumor (carcinoma, glomus jugulare)<br>Herpes zoster inflammation of geniculate ganglion (Ramsey-Hunt syndrome)<br>Peripheral lesions are usually parotid gland tumors |

| | |
|---|---|
| **What is the most common cause of bilateral facial nerve palsy?** | Lyme disease (*Borrelia burgdorferi*) |

## BELL'S PALSY

| | |
|---|---|
| **What is it?** | Sudden onset, unilateral facial weakness or paralysis in absence of CNS, ear, or cerebellopontine angle disease (i.e., no identifiable cause) |
| **What is the clinical course?** | Acute onset, with greatest muscle weakness reached within 3 weeks |
| **What is the incidence?** | Most common cause of **unilateral** facial weakness/paralysis |
| **What is the pathogenesis?** | Unknown; most widely accepted hypothesis is viral etiology (herpes virus); ischemic and immunologic factors are also implicated |
| **What is the common preceding event?** | URI |
| **What are the signs/symptoms?** | Pathology is related to swelling of the facial nerve; may present with total facial paralysis, altered lacrimation, increased tearing on affected side, change in taste if region above chorda tympani is affected, dry mouth, and hyperacusis. |
| **What is the treatment?** | Usually none is required, as most cases resolve spontaneously in 1 month; protect eye with drops and tape closed as needed; most otolaryngologists advocate steroids and acyclovir. Surgical decompression of CN VII is indicated if paralysis progresses or tests indicate deterioration. |
| **What is the prognosis?** | Overall, 90% of patients recover completely; if paralysis is incomplete, 95% to 100% will recover without sequelae. |

## SENSORINEURAL HEARING LOSS

| | |
|---|---|
| **What is it?** | Hearing loss from a lesion occurring in the cochlea or acoustic nerve rather than the external or middle ear |
| **What are the symptoms?** | Distortion of hearing, impaired speech discrimination, tinnitus |
| **What are the signs?** | Air conduction is better than bone conduction (positive Rinne test), Weber lateralizes to the side without the defect; audiogram most commonly shows greatest loss in high-frequency tones. |
| **What is the Weber vs. Rinne test?** | **Weber:** tuning fork on middle of head (lateral louder = either ipsilateral conductive loss or contralateral sensorineural) <br> **Rinnes:** tuning fork on mastoid and then next to ear (conductive loss louder on mastoid) |
| **What are the causes?** | Aging (presbycusis)—leading cause <br> Acoustic injury from sudden or prolonged exposure to loud noises <br> Perilymph fistula <br> Congenital (TORCH: maternal toxoplasmosis, rubella, CMV, herpes, and syphilis) <br> Ménière's disease <br> Drug/toxin-induced <br> Acoustic neuroma <br> Pseudotumor cerebri <br> CNS disease <br> Endocrine disorders <br> Sarcoidosis |
| **What is the most common cause in children?** | Meningitis (bacterial) |
| **What is the treatment?** | Treatment of underlying cause, hearing aids, lip reading, cochlear implant |

VERTIGO

| | |
|---|---|
| **What is it?** | The sensation of head/body movement, or movement of surroundings (usually rotational) |
| **What is the cause?** | Asymmetric neuronal activity between right and left vestibular systems |
| **What is the history of peripheral vertigo?** | Severe vertigo, nausea, vomiting, always accompanied by horizontal or rotatory nystagmus (fast component almost always to side opposite disease), other evidence of inner ear disease (tinnitus, hearing loss) |
| **What are the risk factors for peripheral vertigo?** | Frequently associated with a previously operated ear, a chronic draining ear, barotrauma, or head trauma |
| **What is the history of central vertigo?** | Found in brainstem or cerebellum: insidious onset, less intense and more subtle sensation of vertigo; occasionally, vertical nystagmus |
| **What are the steps in diagnostic evaluation?** | Depends on probability of central versus peripheral; careful neurologic and otologic examinations are required<br>May need FTA/VDRL (syphilis), temporal bone scans/CT/MRI, ENG, position testing, audiometric testing |
| **What is the most common etiology?** | Benign paroxysmal positional vertigo (BPPV); history of brief spells of severe vertigo with specific head positions |
| **What is the differential diagnosis?** | Central: vertebral basilar insufficiency (often in older patients with DJD of spine), Wallenberg syndrome, MS, epilepsy, migraine<br>Peripheral: BPPV, motion sickness, syphilis, Ménière's disease, vestibular neuronitis, labyrinthitis, acoustic neuroma, syphilis, perilymph fistula |
| **What is Tullio's phenomenon?** | Induction of vertigo by loud noises<br>Classically result of otosyphilis |

## MÉNIÈRE'S DISEASE

| | |
|---|---|
| **What is it?** | Disorder of the membranous labyrinth, causing fluctuating sensorineural hearing loss, episodic vertigo, nystagmus, tinnitus, and aural fullness, N/V |
| **What is the classic triad?** | Hearing loss, tinnitus, vertigo (H, T, V) |
| **What is the pathophysiology?** | Obscure, but most experts believe excessive production/defective resorption of endolymph. |
| **What is the medical treatment?** | Primarily medical: salt restriction, diuretics (thiazides), antinausea agents; occasionally diazepam is added; 80% of patients respond to medical management, antihistamines |
| **What are the indications for surgery?** | Surgery is offered to those who fail medical treatment or who have incapacitating vertigo (60% to 80% effective). |
| **What are the surgical options?** | 1. Shunt from membranous labyrinth to subarachnoid space<br>2. Vestibular neurectomy<br>3. Severe cases with hearing loss: labyrinthectomy |

## GLOMUS TUMORS

| | |
|---|---|
| **What are they?** | Benign, slow-growing tumors arising in glomus bodies found in the adventitial layer of blood vessels; often associated with cranial nerves IX and X in the middle ear |
| **What is the usual location?** | Middle ear, jugular bulb, course of CN IX to XII |
| **How common are they?** | Most common benign tumor of the temporal bone |
| **What is the treatment?** | Surgical resection, radiation therapy for poor operative candidates or for recurrences |

## NOSE AND PARANASAL SINUSES

EPISTAXIS

| | |
|---|---|
| **What is it?** | Bleeding from the nose |
| **What are the predisposing factors?** | Trauma, "nose picking," sinus infection, allergic or atrophic rhinitis, blood dyscrasias, tumor, environmental extremes (hot, dry climates, winters) |
| **What is the usual cause?** | Rupture of superficial mucosal blood vessels (Kiesselbach's plexus if anterior, sphenopalatine artery if posterior) |
| **What is the most common type?** | Anterior (90% of all epistaxis); usually the result of trauma |
| **Which type is more serious?** | Posterior; usually occurs in the elderly or is associated with a systemic disorder (hypertension, tumor, arteriosclerosis) |
| **What is the treatment?** | Direct pressure; if this fails, proceed to anterior nasal packing with gauze strips, followed if necessary by posterior packing with Foley catheter or lamb's wool; packs must be removed in less than 5 days to prevent infectious complications |
| **What is the treatment of last resort?** | Ligation or embolization of the spheno-palatine artery (posterior) or ethmoidal artery (anterior) |
| **What infectious disease syndrome is seen with nasal packing?** | Toxic shock syndrome: fever, shock, **rash** caused by exotoxin from *Staphylococcus aureus* |
| **What is the treatment of this syndrome?** | Supportive with removal of nasal packing, IV hydration, oxygen, and anti-staphylococcal antibiotics |

## ACUTE RHINITIS

| | |
|---|---|
| **What is it?** | Inflammation of nasal mucous membrane |
| **What is the most common cause?** | URI infection; rhinovirus is the most common agent in adults (other nonallergic causes: nasal deformities and tumors, polyps, atrophy, immune diseases, vasomotor problems) |

## ALLERGIC RHINITIS

| | |
|---|---|
| **What are the symptoms?** | Nasal stuffiness; watery rhinorrhea; paroxysms of morning sneezing; and itching of nose, conjunctiva, or palate |
| **How is the condition characterized?** | Early onset (before 20 years of age), familial tendency, other allergic disorders (eczema, asthma), elevated serum IgE, eosinophilia on nasal smear |
| **What are the findings on physical examination?** | Pale, boggy, bluish nasal turbinates coated with thin, clear secretions; in children, a transverse nasal crease sometimes results from repeated "allergic salute" |
| **What is the treatment?** | Allergen avoidance, antihistamines, decongestants; steroids or sodium cromylate in severe cases; desensitization via allergen immunotherapy is the only "cure" |

## ACUTE SINUSITIS

| | |
|---|---|
| **What is the typical history?** | Previously healthy patient with unrelenting progression of a viral URI or allergic rhinitis beyond the normal 5- to 7-day course |
| **What are the symptoms?** | Periorbital pressure/pain, nasal obstruction, nasal/postnasal mucopurulent discharge, fatigue, fever, headache |

**What are the signs?**

Tenderness over affected sinuses, pus in the nasal cavity; may also see reason for obstruction (septal deviation, spur, tight osteomeatal complex); transillumination is unreliable

**What is the pathophysiology?**

Thought to be secondary to decreased ciliary action of the sinus mucosa and edema causing obstruction of the sinus ostia, lowering intrasinus oxygen tension and predisposing patients to bacterial infection

**What are the causative organisms?**

Up to 50% of patients have negative cultures and cause is presumably (initially) viral; pneumococcus, *S. aureus,* group A streptococci, and *H. influenzae* are the most common bacteria cultured.

**What is the treatment?**

14-day course of antibiotics (penicillin G, amoxicillin, Ceclor®, and Augmentin® are commonly used), topical and systemic decongestants, and saline nasal irrigation

**What is the treatment for fungal sinusitis?**

Fungal sinusitis is commonly caused by *Mucor* and seen in immunosuppressed patients. Treatment is IV antifungals (e.g., amphotericin or caspofungin) and surgical debridement of all necrotic tissue.

## CHRONIC SINUSITIS

**What is it?**

Infection of nasal sinuses lasting longer than 4 weeks, or pattern of recurrent acute sinusitis punctuated by brief asymptomatic periods

**What is the pathology?**

Permanent mucosal changes secondary to inadequately treated acute sinusitis, consisting of mucosal fibrosis, polypoid growth, and inadequate ciliary action, hyperostosis (increased bone density on CT scan)

| | |
|---|---|
| **What are the symptoms?** | Chronic nasal obstruction, postnasal drip, mucopurulent rhinorrhea, low-grade facial and periorbital pressure/pain |
| **What are the causative organisms?** | Usually anaerobes (such as *Bacteroides, Veillonella, Rhinobacterium*); also *H. influenzae, Streptococcus viridans, Staphylococcus aureus, Staphylococcus epidermidis* |
| **What is the treatment?** | Medical management with decongestants, mucolytics, topical steroids, and antibiotics; if this approach fails, proceed to endoscopic or external surgical intervention |
| **What is FESS?** | **F**unctional **E**ndoscopic **S**inus **S**urgery |
| **What are the complications of sinusitis?** | Orbital cellulitis (if ethmoid sinusitis), meningitis, epidural or brain abscess (frontal sinus), cavernous sinus thrombosis (ethmoid or sphenoid), osteomyelitis (A.K.A. Pott's puffy tumor if frontal) |

## CANCER OF THE NASAL CAVITY AND PARANASAL SINUSES

| | |
|---|---|
| **What are the usual locations?** | Maxillary sinus (two-thirds)<br>Nasal cavity<br>Ethmoid sinus<br>Rarely in frontal or sphenoid sinuses |
| **What are the associated cell types?** | Squamous cell (80%)<br>Adenocellular (15%)<br>Uncommon: sarcoma, melanoma |
| **What rare tumor arises from olfactory epithelium?** | Esthesioneuroblastoma; usually arises high in the nose (cribriform plate) and is locally invasive |
| **What are the signs/ symptoms?** | Early—nasal obstruction, blood-tinged mucus, epistaxis<br>Late—localized pain, cranial nerve deficits, facial/palate asymmetry, loose teeth |

| | |
|---|---|
| **How is the diagnosis made?** | CT can adequately identify extent of the disease and local invasion. MRI is often also used to evaluate soft-tissue disease. |
| **What is the treatment?** | Surgery with or without x-ray therapy |
| **What is the prognosis?** | 5-year survival for T1 or T2 lesions approaches 70%. |

## JUVENILE NASOPHARYNGEAL ANGIOFIBROMA

| | |
|---|---|
| **What is it?** | The most commonly encountered vascular mass in the nasal cavity; locally aggressive but nonmetastasizing |
| **What is the usual history?** | Adolescent boys who present with nasal obstruction, recurrent massive epistaxis, possibly anosmia |
| **What is the usual location?** | Site of origin is the roof of the nasal cavity at the superior margin of sphenopalatine foramen |
| **Into what can the mass transform?** | Fibrosarcoma (rare cases reported) |
| **How is the diagnosis made?** | Carotid arteriography, CT; biopsy is contraindicated secondary to risk of uncontrollable hemorrhage |
| **What are indications for biopsy?** | **None!** |
| **What is the treatment?** | Surgery via lateral rhinotomy or sublabial maxillotomy with bleeding controlled by internal maxillary artery ligation or pre-operative embolization, in the setting of hypotensive anesthesia; preoperative irradiation has also been used to shrink the tumor |

## ORAL CAVITY AND PHARYNX

PHARYNGOTONSILLITIS

| | |
|---|---|
| **What is the common site of referred throat pain?** | EAR |
| **What is it?** | Acute or chronic infection of the naso-pharynx or oropharynx and/or Waldeyer's ring of lymphoid tissue (consisting of palatine, lingual, and pharyngeal tonsils and the adenoids) |
| **What is the etiology?** | Acute attacks can be viral (adenovirus, enterovirus, coxsackievirus, Epstein-Barr virus in infectious mononucleosis) or bacterial (group A β-hemolytic streptococci are the leading bacterial agent); chronic tonsillitis often with mixed population, including streptococci, staphylococci, and *M. catarrhalis* |
| **What are the symptoms?** | Acute—Sore throat, fever, local lymph-adenopathy, chills, headache, malaise<br>Chronic—Noisy mouth breathing, speech and swallowing difficulties, apnea, halitosis |
| **What are the signs?** | Viral—Injected tonsils and pharyngeal mucosa; exudate may occur, but less often than with bacterial tonsillitis<br>Bacterial—Swollen, inflamed tonsils with white-yellow exudate in crypts and on surface; cervical adenopathy |
| **How is the diagnosis made?** | CBC, throat culture, Monospot test |
| **What are the possible complications?** | Peritonsillar abscess (quinsy), retropharyngeal abscess (causing airway compromise), rheumatic fever, poststreptococcal glomerulonephritis (with β-hemolytic streptococci) |

| | |
|---|---|
| **What is the treatment?** | Viral—Symptomatic → acetaminophen, warm saline gargles, anesthetic throat spray<br>Bacterial—10 days PCN (erythromycin if PCN-allergic) |
| **What are the indications for tonsillectomy?** | Sleep apnea/cor pulmonale secondary to airway obstruction, suspicion of malignancy, hypertrophy causing malocclusion, peritonsillar abscess, recurrent acute or chronic tonsillitis |
| **What are the possible complications?** | Acute or delayed hemorrhage |

## PERITONSILLAR ABSCESS

| | |
|---|---|
| **What is the clinical setting?** | Inadequately treated recurrent acute or chronic tonsillitis |
| **What is the associated microbiology?** | Mixed aerobes and anaerobes (which may be PCN-resistant) |
| **What is the site of formation?** | Begins at the superior pole of the tonsil |
| **What are the symptoms?** | Severe throat pain, drooling dysphagia, odynophagia, trismus, cervical adenopathy, fever, chills, malaise |
| **What is the classic description of voice?** | "Hot-potato voice" |
| **What are the signs?** | Bulging, erythematous, edematous tonsillar pillar; swelling of uvula and displacement to contralateral side |
| **What is the treatment?** | IV antibiotics and surgical evacuation by incision and drainage; most experts recommend tonsillectomy after resolution of inflammatory changes |

## CANCER OF THE ORAL CAVITY

| | |
|---|---|
| **What is the usual cell type?** | Squamous cell (>90% of cases) |
| **What are the most common sites?** | **Lip,** tongue, floor of mouth, gingiva, cheek, and palate |
| **What is the etiology?** | Linked to smoking, alcohol, and smokeless tobacco products (alcohol and tobacco together greatly increase the risk) |
| **What is the frequency of the following conditions:** | |
| **Regional metastasis?** | About 30% |
| **Second primary?** | About 25% |
| **Nodal metastasis?** | Depends on size of tumor and ranges from 10% to 60%, usually to jugular and **jugulodigastric nodes, submandibular nodes** |
| **Distant metastasis?** | Infrequent |
| **How is the diagnosis made?** | Full history and physical examination, dental assessment, Panorex or bone scan if mandible is thought to be involved, CT/MRI for extent of tumor and nodal disease, FNA (often U/S guided) |
| **What is the treatment?** | Radiation, surgery, or both for small lesions; localized lesions can usually be treated surgically; larger lesions require combination therapy, possible mandibulectomy and neck dissection |
| **What is the prognosis?** | Depends on stage and site: Tongue: 20% to 70% survival Floor of mouth: 30% to 80% survival Most common cause of death in successfully treated head and neck cancer is development of a second primary (occurs in 20% to 40% of cases). |

## SALIVARY GLAND TUMORS

| | |
|---|---|
| **What is the frequency of gland involvement?** | Parotid gland (80%)<br>Submandibular gland (15%)<br>Minor salivary glands (5%) |
| **What is the potential for malignancy?** | Greatest in **minor salivary gland** tumors (80% are malignant) and least in parotid gland tumors (80% are benign); the smaller the gland, the greater the likelihood of malignancy |
| **How do benign and malignant tumors differ in terms of history and physical examination?** | Benign—mobile, nontender, no node involvement or facial weakness<br>Malignant—painful, fixed mass with evidence of local metastasis and facial paresis/paralysis |
| **What is the diagnostic procedure?** | FNA; never perform excisional biopsy of a parotid mass. Superficial parotidectomy is the procedure of choice for benign lesions of the lateral lobe. |
| **What is the treatment?** | Involves adequate surgical resection, sparing facial nerve if possible, neck dissection for node-positive necks |
| **What are the indications for postop XRT?** | Postoperative radiation therapy if high-grade cancer, recurrent cancer, residual disease, invasion of adjacent structures, any T3 or T4 parotid tumors |
| **What is the most common benign salivary tumor?** | **Pleomorphic adenoma** (benign mixed tumor) accounts for two-thirds of total (think: **P**leomorphic = **P**opular) |
| **What is the usual location?** | Parotid gland |
| **What is the clinical course?** | They are well-delineated and slow growing. |
| **What is the second most common benign salivary gland tumor?** | Warthin's tumor (1% of all salivary gland tumors) |

**What is the usual location?** 95% are found in parotid; 3% are bilateral.

**Describe the lesion.** Slow-growing, cystic mass is usually located in the tail of the superficial portion of the parotid; it rarely becomes malignant.

**What is the most common malignant salivary tumor?**

**Mucoepidermoid carcinoma** (10% of all salivary gland neoplasms) Think: **M**ucoepidermoid = **M**alignant
Most common parotid malignancy
Second most common submandibular gland malignancy

**What is the second most common malignant salivary tumor in adults?**

Adenoid cystic carcinoma
Less than 10% of all salivary gland neoplasms
Most common malignancy in submandibular and minor salivary glands
Second most common malignancy in parotid
Tends to have perineural invasion

## LARYNX ANATOMY

**Define the three parts.**
1. Glottis: begins halfway between the true and false cords (in the ventricle) and extends inferiorly 1.0 cm below the edge of the vocal folds
2. Supraglottis: extends from superior glottis to superior border of hyoid and tip of epiglottis
3. Subglottis: extends from lower border of glottis to inferior edge of cricoid cartilage

**Innervation?** Vagus nerve: superior laryngeal and recurrent laryngeal nerves; superior laryngeal supplies sensory to supraglottis and motor to inferior constrictor and cricothyroid muscle; recurrent laryngeal supplies sensory to glottis and subglottis and motor to all remaining intrinsic laryngeal muscles

## CROUP (LARYNGOTRACHEOBRONCHITIS)

| | |
|---|---|
| **What is it?** | A viral infection of the larynx and trachea, generally affecting children (boys > girls) |
| **What is the usual cause?** | Parainfluenza virus (think: crou**P** = **P**arainfluenza) |
| **What age group is affected most?** | 6 months to 3 years of age |
| **Is the condition considered seasonal?** | Yes; outbreaks most often occur in autumn. |
| **What are the precipitating events?** | Usually preceded by URI |
| **What is the classic symptom?** | Barking (seal-like), nonproductive cough |
| **What are the other symptoms?** | Respiratory distress, low-grade fever |
| **What are the signs?** | Tachypnea, inspiratory retractions, prolonged inspiration, inspiratory stridor, expiratory rhonchi/wheezes |
| **What is the differential diagnosis?** | Epiglottitis, bacterial tracheitis, foreign body, diphtheria, retropharyngeal abscess, peritonsillar abscess, asthma |
| **How is the diagnosis made?** | A-P neck x-ray shows classic "steeple sign," indicating subglottic narrowing; ABG may show hypoxemia plus hypercapnia. |
| **What is the treatment?** | **Keep child calm** (agitation only worsens obstruction); cool mist; steroids; aerosolized racemic EPI may be administered to reduce edema/airway obstruction |
| **What are the indications for intubation?** | If airway obstruction is severe or child becomes exhausted |

| | |
|---|---|
| **What is the usual course?** | Resolves in 3 to 4 days |
| **What type of secondary infection occurs?** | Secondary bacterial infection (streptococcal, staphylococcal) |

## EPIGLOTTITIS

| | |
|---|---|
| **What is it?** | Severe, rapidly progressive infection of the epiglottis |
| **What is the usual causative agent?** | *Haemophilus influenzae* type B |
| **What age group is affected?** | Children 2 to 5 years of age |
| **What are the signs/ symptoms?** | Sudden onset, high fever (40°C); "hot potato" voice; dysphagia ($\rightarrow$ drooling); no cough; patient prefers to sit upright, lean forward; patient appears toxic and stridulous |
| **How is the diagnosis made?** | Can usually be made clinically and does not involve direct observation of the epiglottis (which may worsen obstruction by causing laryngospasm) |
| **What is the treatment?** | Involves immediate airway support in the OR: intubation or possibly tracheostomy, medical treatment is comprised of steroids and IV antibiotics *against H. influenzae* |

## MALIGNANT LESIONS OF THE LARYNX

| | |
|---|---|
| **What is the incidence?** | Accounts for approximately 2% of all malignancies, more often in males |
| **What is the most common site?** | Glottis (two-thirds) |
| **What is the second most common type?** | Supraglottis (one-third) |
| **Which type has the worst prognosis?** | Subglottic tumors (infrequent) |

| | |
|---|---|
| **What are the risk factors?** | Tobacco, alcohol |
| **What is the pathology?** | 90% are squamous cell carcinoma. |
| **What are the symptoms?** | Hoarseness, throat pain, dysphagia, odynophagia, neck mass, (referred) ear pain |

## SUPRAGLOTTIC LESIONS

| | |
|---|---|
| **What is the usual location?** | Laryngeal surface of epiglottis |
| **What area is often involved?** | Pre-epiglottic space |
| **Extension?** | Tend to remain confined to supraglottic region, though may extend to vallecula or base of tongue |
| **What is the associated type of metastasis?** | High propensity for nodal metastasis |

## GLOTTIC LESIONS

| | |
|---|---|
| **What is the usual location?** | Anterior part of true cords |
| **Extension?** | May invade thyroid cartilage, cross midline to invade contralateral cord, or invade paraglottic space |
| **What is the associated type of metastasis?** | Rare nodal metastasis |
| **What is the treatment?** | Total or supraglottic laryngectomy, depending on location and extent of lesion; neck dissection if nodal involvement |
| | Radiation therapy or surgery is given for early (T1 or T2) lesions. Combination therapy (surgery + radiation) is given for advanced (T3 and T4) disease. |
| **What is the 5-year survival for:** | |
| **T1 lesions?** | 90% |
| **T2 lesions?** | 80% |

| | |
|---|---|
| **T3 lesions?** | 75% |
| **T4 lesions?** | 30% |

## NECK MASS

| | |
|---|---|
| **What is the usual etiology in infants?** | Congenital (branchial cleft cysts, thyroglossal duct cysts) |
| **What is the usual etiology in adolescents?** | Inflammatory (cervical adenitis is number one), with congenital also possible |
| **What is the usual etiology in adults?** | Malignancy (squamous is number one), especially if painless and immobile |
| **What is the "80% rule"?** | In general, 80% of neck masses are **benign** in children; 80% are **malignant** in adults older than 40 years of age. |
| **What are the seven cardinal symptoms of neck masses?** | Dysphagia, odynophagia, hoarseness, stridor (signifies upper airway obstruction), globus, speech disorder, referred ear pain (via CN V, IX, or X) |
| **What comprises the workup?** | Full head and neck examination, indirect laryngoscopy, CT and MRI, FNA for tissue diagnosis; biopsy contraindicated because it may adversely affect survival if malignant |
| **What is the differential diagnosis?** | Inflammatory: cervical lymphadenitis, cat-scratch disease, infectious mono-nucleosis, infection in neck spaces<br>Congenital: thyroglossal duct cyst (mid-line, elevates with tongue protrusion), branchial cleft cysts (lateral), dermoid cysts (midline submental), heman-gioma, cystic hygroma<br>Neoplastic: primary or metastatic |
| **What is the workup of node-positive squamous cell carcinoma and no primary site?** | Triple endoscopy (laryngoscopy, esophagoscopy, bronchoscopy) and blind biopsies |

| | |
|---|---|
| **What is the treatment?** | Surgical excision for congenital or neoplastic; two most important procedures for cancer treatment are radical and modified neck dissection |
| **What is the role of adjuvant treatment in head and neck cancer?** | Postoperative chemotherapy/XRT |

## RADICAL NECK DISSECTION

| | |
|---|---|
| **What is involved?** | Classically, removal of **nodes** from clavicle to mandible, sternocleidomastoid muscle, **submandibular gland,** tail of **parotid,** internal **jugular vein, digastric muscles, stylohyoid** and **omohyoid muscles, fascia** within the anterior and posterior triangles, CN XI, and cervical plexus sensory nerves |
| **What are the indications?** | 1. Clinically positive nodes that likely contain metastatic cancer<br>2. Clinically negative nodes in neck, but high probability of metastasis from a primary tumor elsewhere<br>3. A fixed cervical mass that is resectable |
| **What are the contraindications?** | 1. Distant metastasis<br>2. Fixation to structure that cannot be removed (e.g., carotid artery)<br>3. Low neck masses |

## MODIFIED NECK DISSECTION

| | |
|---|---|
| **What are the types:**<br>**Type I?** | Spinal accessory nerve preserved |
| **Type II?** | Spinal accessory and internal jugular vein preserved |
| **Type III?** | Spinal accessory, IJ, and sternocleidomastoid nerves preserved |
| **What are the advantages?** | Increased postoperative function and decreased morbidity (especially if bilateral), most often used in N0 |

lesions; these modifications are usually intraoperative decisions based on the location and extent of tumor growth

**What are the disadvantages?** May result in increased mortality from local recurrence

## FACIAL FRACTURES

### MANDIBLE FRACTURES

**What are the symptoms?** Gross disfigurement, pain, **malocclusion,** drooling

**What are the signs?** Trismus, fragment mobility and lacerations of gingiva, hematoma in floor of mouth

**What are the possible complications?** Malunion, nonunion, osteomyelitis, TMJ ankylosis

**What is the treatment?** Open or closed reduction
**MMF** = **M**axillo**M**andibular **F**ixation (wiring jaw shut)

### MIDFACE FRACTURES

**How are they evaluated?** Careful physical examination and CT

#### *Classification*

**Le Fort I?** Transverse maxillary fracture above the dental apices, which also traverses the pterygoid plate; palate is mobile, but nasal complex is stable

Le Fort I

**Le Fort II?**

Fracture through the frontal process of the maxilla, through the orbital floor and pterygoid plate; midface is mobile

Le Fort II

**Le Fort III?**

**Complete craniofacial separation;** differs from II in that it extends through the nasofrontal suture and frontozygomatic sutures

Le Fort III

**What is a "tripod" fracture?**

Fracture of the zygomatic complex; involves four fractures:
1. Frontozygomatic suture
2. Inferior orbital rim
3. Zygomaticomaxillary suture
4. Zygomaticotemporal suture

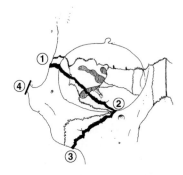

**What is a "blowout" fracture?**

Orbital fracture with "blowout" of supporting bony structural support of orbital floor; patient has enophthalmos (sunken-in eyeball)

**What is "entrapment"?**

Orbital fracture with "entrapment" of periorbital tissues within the fracture opening, including entrapment of extraocular muscles; loss of extraocular muscle mobility (e.g., lateral tracking) and diplopia (double vision)

**What is a "step off"?**

Fracture of the orbit with palpable "step off" of bony orbital rim (inferior or lateral)

**Are mandibular fractures usually a single fracture?**

No; because the mandible forms an anatomic ring, more than 95% of mandible fractures have more than one fracture site.

**What is the best x-ray study for mandibular fractures?**

Panorex

**What must be ruled out and treated with a broken nose (nasal fracture)?**

Septal hematoma; must drain to remove chance of a pressure-induced septal necrosis

## ENT WARD QUESTIONS

**How can otitis externa be distinguished from otitis media on examination?**

Otitis externa is characterized by severe pain upon manipulation of the auricle.

| | |
|---|---|
| **What causes otitis media?** | Most cases are caused by pneumococci and *H. influenzae*. |
| **What causes otitis externa?** | *Pseudomonas aeruginosa* |
| **What must be considered in unilateral serous otitis?** | Nasopharyngeal carcinoma |
| **What is the most common cause of facial paralysis?** | **Bell's palsy,** which has an unidentified etiology |
| **What is the single most important prognostic factor in Bell's palsy?** | Whether the affected muscles are completely paralyzed (if not, prognosis is > 95% complete recovery) |
| **What is the most common cause of parotid swelling?** | Mumps |
| **What is Heerfordt's syndrome?** | Sarcoidosis with parotid enlargement, facial nerve paralysis, and uveitis |
| **Which systemic disease causes salivary gland stones?** | Gout |
| **What is the most common salivary gland site of stone formation?** | Submandibular gland |
| **What is Mikulicz's syndrome?** | Any cause of bilateral enlargement of the parotid, lacrimal, and submandibular glands |
| **What are the three major functions of the larynx?** | 1. Airway protection 2. Airway/respiration 3. Phonation |
| **What is a cricothyroidotomy?** | Emergent surgical airway by incising the cricothyroid membrane |
| **Name the four major indications for a tracheostomy.** | 1. Prolonged mechanical ventilation (usually > 2 weeks) 2. Upper airway obstruction 3. Poor life-threatening pulmonary toilet 4. Severe obstructive sleep apnea |

**What is a ranula?**  Sublingual retention cyst arising from sublingual salivary glands

**What is Frey's syndrome?**  Flushing, pain, and diaphoresis in the auriculotemporal nerve distribution initiated by chewing

**What causes Frey's syndrome?**  Caused by abnormal regeneration of the sympathetic/parasympathetic nerves upon cutting the auriculotemporal nerve. These parasympathetic fibers, once destined for the parotid gland, find new targets in skin sweat glands. Thus, people sweat when eating.

**What is the classic triad of Ménière's disease?**  Hearing loss, tinnitus, vertigo (HTV)

**What is the most common posterior fossa tumor and where is it located?**  Acoustic neuromas, usually occurring at the cerebellopontine angle

**What is the most common site of sinus cancer?**  Maxillary sinus

**What tumor arises from olfactory epithelium?**  Esthesioneuroblastoma

**What cell type is most common in head and neck cancer?**  Squamous cell

**What are the most important predisposing factors to head and neck cancer?**  Excessive alcohol use and **tobacco** abuse of any form

**What is the most frequent site of salivary gland tumor?**  Parotid gland

**What is the most common salivary gland neoplasm:**
  **Benign?**  Pleomorphic adenoma

  **Malignant?**  Mucoepidermoid carcinoma

| | |
|---|---|
| **What is the classic feature of croup?** | Barking, seal-like cough |
| **What are the classic features of epiglottitis?** | "Hot potato" voice, sitting up, **drooling**, toxic appearance, high fever, **leaning forward** |
| **What comprises the workup of neck mass?** | Do **not** biopsy; obtain tissue **via FNA** and complete head and neck examination. |
| **What is Ramsay Hunt's syndrome?** | Painful facial nerve paralysis from herpes zoster of the ear |
| **What is the most common malignant neck mass in children, adolescents, and young adults?** | Lymphoma |
| **What is the most common primary malignant solid tumor of the head and neck in children?** | Rhabdomyosarcoma |
| **Throat pain is often referred to what body area?** | Ear |
| **What ENT condition is described as "crocodile tears"?** | Frey's syndrome! |
| **What is Brown's sign?** | Tympanic membrane pulsations that cease with positive pressure (from a "pneumatic" otoscope); seen with middle ear tumor mass |

# Chapter 71

# **Thoracic Surgery**

| | |
|---|---|
| **What does VATS stand for?** | **V**ideo **A**ssisted **T**horacic **S**urgery |

## THORACIC OUTLET SYNDROME (TOS)

| | |
|---|---|
| **What is it?** | Compression of the:<br>Subclavian artery<br>Subclavian vein or<br>Brachial plexus at the superior outlet of the thorax |
| **What are the causes (3)?** | 1. Various congenital anomalies, including cervical rib or abnormal fascial bands to the first rib, or abnormal anterior scalene muscle<br>2. Trauma:<br>Fracture of clavicle or first rib<br>Dislocation of humeral head<br>Crush injuries<br>3. Repetitive motor injuries (baseball pitchers) |
| **What are the symptoms?** | Paresthesias (neck, shoulder, arm, hand); 90% in ulnar nerve distribution<br>Weakness (neural/arterial)<br>Coolness of involved extremity (arterial)<br>Edema, venous distension, discoloration (venous) |
| **What is the most common problem seen with TOS?** | Neurologic symptoms |
| **Which nerve is most often involved?** | Ulnar nerve |
| **What are the signs?** | Paget-von Schroetter syndrome—venous thrombosis leading to edema, arm discoloration, and distension of the superficial veins<br>Weak brachial and radial pulses in the involved arm |

Hypesthesia/anesthesia

Occasionally, atrophy in the distribution of the ulnar nerve

Positive Adson maneuver/Tinel's sign

Edema

**What is the Adson maneuver?**

**Evaluates for arterial compromise**

Patient:

1. Extends neck (lifts head)
2. Takes a deep breath
3. Turns head toward examined side

Physician:

Monitors radial pulse on examined side

Test finding is positive if the radial pulse decreases or disappears during maneuver.

**What is Tinel's test?**

Tapping of the supraclavicular fossa producing paresthesias

**What is the treatment?**

Physical therapy (vast majority of cases)

Decompression of the thoracic outlet by resecting the first rib and cervical rib (if present) if physical therapy fails and as a last resort

## CHEST WALL TUMORS

### BENIGN TUMORS

**What are the most common types?**

1. Fibrous rib dysplasia (posterolateral rib)
2. Chondroma (at costochondral junction)
3. Osteochondroma (any portion of rib)

**What is the treatment?**

Wide excision and reconstruction with autologous or prosthetic grafts

### MALIGNANT TUMORS

**What are the most common types?**

1. Fibrosarcoma
2. Chondrosarcoma
3. Osteogenic sarcoma
4. Rhabdomyosarcoma
5. Myeloma
6. Ewing's sarcoma

| | |
|---|---|
| **What is the treatment?** | Excision with or without radiation |
| **What is Tietze's syndrome?** | Noninfectious costochondral cartilage inflammation |

## DISEASES OF THE PLEURA

### PLEURAL EFFUSION

| | |
|---|---|
| **What is it?** | Fluid in the pleural space |
| **What are the causes?** | 1. Pulmonary infections (pneumonia)<br>2. Congestive heart failure (CHF)<br>3. SLE or rheumatoid arthritis<br>4. Pancreatitis (sympathetic effusion)<br>5. Trauma<br>6. Pulmonary embolism<br>7. Renal disease<br>8. Cirrhosis<br>9. Malignancy (mesothelioma, lymphoma, metastasis)<br>10. Postpericardiotomy syndrome |
| **What are the symptoms?** | Dyspnea, pleuritic chest pain |
| **What are the signs?** | Decreased breath sounds, dullness to percussion, egophony at the upper limit |
| **What are the properties of a transudate?** | Specific gravity <1.016<br>Protein <3 g/dL<br>Few cells |
| **What are the properties of an exudate?** | Specific gravity >1.016<br>Protein >3 g/dL<br>Many cells |
| **What is the key diagnostic test?** | Thoracentesis (needle drainage) with studies including cytology |
| **What is the treatment?** | 1. Pigtail catheter or thoracostomy (chest tube)<br>2. Treat underlying condition<br>3. Consider sclerosis |

| | |
|---|---|
| **What is an empyema?** | Infected pleural effusion; must be drained, usually with chest tube(s)<br>Decortication may be necessary if the empyema is solid. |
| **What is a decortication?** | Thoracotomy and removal of an infected fibrous rind from around the lung (think of it as taking off a fibrous "cortex" from the lung) |

## LUNG ABSCESS

| | |
|---|---|
| **What are the signs/ symptoms?** | Fever, sputum, sepsis, fatigue |
| **What are the associated diagnostic studies?** | CXR: air-fluid level<br>CT scan to define position and to differentiate from an empyema<br>Bronchoscopy (looking for cancer/culture) |
| **What is the treatment?** | Antibiotics and bronchoscopy for culture and toilet, with or without surgery |
| **What are the indications for surgery?** | Underlying cancer/tumor<br>Refractory to antibiotics |
| **What are the surgical options?** | Lobectomy of lobe with abscess<br>Tube drainage |
| **What is middle lobe syndrome?** | Recurrent right middle lobe pneumonia caused most commonly by intermittent extrinsic bronchial obstruction |

## HEMOPTYSIS

| | |
|---|---|
| **What is it?** | Bleeding into the bronchial tree |
| **What are the causes?** | 1. Bronchitis (50%)<br>2. Tumor mass (20%)<br>3. TB (8%)<br>Other causes: bronchiectasis, pulmonary catheters, trauma |

| | |
|---|---|
| **Define MASSIVE hemoptysis.** | More than 600 cc/24 hours |
| **What comprises the workup?** | CXR<br>Bronchoscopy<br>Bronchial A-gram |
| **What is the treatment if massive?** | Bronchoscopy, intubation of unaffected side, Fogarty catheter occlusion of bleeding bronchus, bronchial A-gram with or without embolization, surgical resection of involved lung |
| **What is the treatment of moderate to mild bleeding?** | Laser coagulation, +/− epinephrine injection |

## SPONTANEOUS PNEUMOTHORAX

| | |
|---|---|
| **What is it?** | Atraumatic spontaneous development of a pneumothorax |
| **What are the causes?** | Idiopathic (primary), bleb disease-emphysema, etc. (secondary) |
| **What body habitus is associated with spontaneous pneumothorax?** | Thin and tall |
| **How is the diagnosis made?** | CXR |
| **What is the treatment?** | Chest tube |
| **What are the options if refractory, recurrent, or bilateral?** | Pleurodesis: scar the lung to the parietal pleura with a sclerosant (talc) via chest tube/thoracoscopy or by thoracotomy and mechanical abrasion |
| **Who might also need a pleurodesis after the first episode?** | Those whose lifestyles place them at increased risk for pneumothorax (e.g., pilots, scuba divers) |

# MESOTHELIOMA

## *Malignant Mesothelioma*

| | |
|---|---|
| **What is it?** | A primary pleural neoplasm |
| **What are the two types?** | 1. Localized<br>2. Diffuse (highly malignant) |
| **What are the risk factors?** | Exposure to asbestos<br>Smoking |
| **What are the symptoms?** | Localized: pleuritic pain, joint pain and swelling, dyspnea<br>Diffuse: chest pain, malaise, weight loss, cough |
| **What are the signs?** | Pleural effusion (present in only 10% to 15% of patients with local disease, almost always in diffuse disease [>75%]) |
| **What are the associated radiographic tests?** | X-ray may reveal a peripheral mass, often forming an obtuse angle with the chest wall; **CT is also performed.** |
| **How is the diagnosis made?** | Pleural biopsy, pleural fluid cytology |
| **What is the treatment if localized?** | Surgical excision |
| **What is the treatment if diffuse?** | Early stages may be resected, followed by radiation; for more advanced stages, radiation, chemotherapy, or both are done. |
| **What is the prognosis?** | Localized: poor<br>Diffuse: **dismal** (average life span after diagnosis is about 1 year) |

## *Benign Mesothelioma*

| | |
|---|---|
| **What is it?** | Benign pleural mesothelioma |
| **What pleura is usually involved?** | Visceral pleura |

| | |
|---|---|
| **What is the gross appearance?** | Pedunculated "broccoli or cauliflower" tumor on a stalk coming off of the lung |
| **What is the treatment?** | Surgical resection with at least 1 cm clear margin |
| **What is the prognosis?** | In contrast to malignant mesothelioma, the benign mesothelioma has an excellent prognosis with cure in the vast majority of cases (possibility of transformation into a malignant mesothelioma if inadequate resection). |

## DISEASES OF THE LUNGS

### BRONCHOGENIC CARCINOMA

| | |
|---|---|
| **What is the annual incidence of lung cancer in the United States?** | 170,000 new cases/year |
| **What is the number of annual deaths from lung cancer?** | 150,000; most common cancer death in the United States in men **and** women |
| **What is the number one risk factor?** | Smoking (85%!) |
| **Does asbestos exposure increase the risk in patients who smoke?** | Yes |
| **What type of lung cancer arises in nonsmoking?** | Adenocarcinoma |
| **Cancer arises more often in which lung?** | Right > left, upper lobes > lower lobes |
| **What are the signs/ symptoms?** | Change in a chronic cough<br>Hemoptysis, chest pain, dyspnea<br>Pleural effusion (suggests chest wall involvement)<br>Hoarseness (recurrent laryngeal nerve involvement)<br>Superior vena cava syndrome |

Diaphragmatic paralysis (phrenic nerve involvement)

Symptoms of metastasis/paraneoplastic syndrome

Finger clubbing

**What is Pancoast's tumor?**

Tumor at the apex of the lung or superior sulcus that may involve the brachial plexus, sympathetic ganglia, and vertebral bodies, leading to pain, upper extremity weakness, and Horner's syndrome

**What is Horner's syndrome?**

Injury to the cervical sympathetic chain: **M.A.P.:**

1. **M**iosis (small pupil)
2. **A**nhydrosis of ipsilateral face
3. **P**tosis

**What are the four most common sites of extrathoracic metastases?**

1. Bone
2. Liver
3. Adrenals
4. Kidney

**What are paraneoplastic syndromes?**

Syndromes that are associated with tumors but may affect distant parts of the body; they may be caused by hormones released from endocrinologically active tumors or may be of uncertain etiology

**Name five general types of paraneoplastic syndromes.**

1. Metabolic: Cushing's, SIADH, hypercalcemia
2. Neuromuscular: Eaton-Lambert, cerebellar ataxia
3. Skeletal: hypertrophic osteoarthropathy
4. Dermatologic: acanthosis nigricans
5. Vascular: thrombophlebitis

**What are the associated radiographic tests?**

CXR and CT scan

| **How is the tumor diagnosed?** | 1. Sputum cytology<br>2. Needle biopsy (CT or fluoro guidance)<br>3. Bronchoscopy with brushings, biopsies, or both<br>4. With or without mediastinoscopy, mediastinotomy, scalene node biopsy, or open lung biopsy for definitive diagnosis |
|---|---|

**For each tumor listed, recall its usual site in the lung and its natural course:**

| **Squamous cell?** | Two-thirds occur centrally in lung hilus; may also be a Pancoast's tumor; slow growth, late metastasis; associated with smoking (think: **S**quamous = **S**entral) |
|---|---|
| **Adenocarcinoma?** | Peripheral, rapid growth with hematogenous/nodal metastasis, associated with lung scarring |
| **Small (oat) cell?** | Central, highly malignant, usually not operable |
| **Large cell?** | Usually peripheral, very malignant |

**What are the stages of NON-small cell carcinoma of the lungs:**

| **Stage Ia?** | Tumor <3 cm, no nodes, no metastases (T1NoMo) |
|---|---|
| **Stage Ib?** | Tumor >3 cm, but no nodes and no metastases (T2NoMo) |
| **Stage IIa?** | Tumor <3 cm **and** positive nodes to lung or ipsilateral hilum; **no** metastases (T1N1Mo) |
| **Stage IIb?** | 1. Tumor >3 cm and positive nodes in lung or ipsilateral hilum (T2N1Mo)<br>2. Tumor that invades chest wall, diaphragm, mediastinal pleura, or pericardial sac (**no** mediastinal structures) and no nodes and **no** metastases (T3NoMo) |

**Stage IIIa?**

1. Tumor invades chest wall, diaphragm, or mediastinal pleura or pericardial sac **and** positive nodes in lung or ipsilateral hilum with **no** metastases (T3N1Mo).
2. Lymph node metastases to ipsilateral, mediastinal, or subcarinal nodes with **no** metastases and **no** mediastinal tumor invasion (T1N2Mo, T2N2Mo, T3N2Mo)

**Stage IIIb?**

**No** distant metastases but mediastinal invasion or lymph node metastases to contralateral hilum or mediastinum Supraclavicular/scalene nodes

**Stage IV?**

Distant metastasis

**What are the surgical contraindications by stage for NON-small cell carcinoma?**

Stage IV, Stage IIIb

**What is the role of chemotherapy?**

Induction chemotherapy prior to resection increases survival in NON-small cell cancer.

**What is the treatment by stage for NON-small cell lung carcinoma:**

    **Stage I?**

Surgical resection

    **Stage II?**

Surgical resection

    **Stage IIIa?**

Surgical resection if early IIIa, chemotherapy with or without XRT

    **Stage IIIb?**

Chemotherapy and XRT

    **Stage IV?**

Chemotherapy +/− XRT

**What is the treatment for isolated brain metastasis**

Surgical resection

**What is the approximate prognosis (5-year survival) after treatment of NON-small cell lung carcinoma by stage:**

**Stage Ia?**   80%

**Stage Ib?**   60%

**Stage IIa?**   35%

**Stage IIb?**   30%

**Stage IIIa?**   Approximately 20%

**Stage IIIb?**   <10%

**Stage IV?**   Basically 0%

**How is small cell carcinoma treated?**

Chemotherapy with or without x-ray therapy

**What are the six contraindications to surgery for lung cancer?**

Use the acronym "STOP IT:"
1. **S**uperior vena cava syndrome, **S**upraclavicular node metastasis, **S**calene node metastasis
2. **T**racheal carina involvement
3. **O**at cell carcinoma (treat with chemotherapy with or without radiation)
4. **P**ulmonary function tests shows FEV1 <1
5. Myocardial **I**nfarction (or cardiac cripple)
6. **T**umor elsewhere (metastatic disease)

**What postoperative FEV1 must you have?**

FEV1 >800 cc; thus, a preoperative FEV1 >2 is usually needed for a pneumonectomy
If FEV1 is <2, a ventilation perfusion scan should be performed.

**What is hypertrophic pulmonary osteoarthropathy?**

Periosteal proliferation and new bone formation at the end of long bones and in the bones of the hand (seen in 10% of patients with lung cancer)

## SOLITARY PULMONARY NODULES (COIN LESIONS)

| | |
|---|---|
| **What are they?** | Peripheral circumscribed pulmonary lesions |
| **What is the differential diagnosis?** | Granulomatous disease, benign neoplasms, malignancy |
| **What percentage are malignant?** | Overall, 5% to 10% (but >50% are malignant in smokers older than 50 years) |
| **Is there a gender risk?** | Yes; the incidence of coin lesions is 3 to 9 times higher and malignancy is nearly twice as common in men as in women. |
| **What are the symptoms?** | Usually asymptomatic with solitary nodules, but may include coughing, weight loss, chest pain, and hemoptysis |
| **What are the signs?** | Physical findings are uncommon; clubbing is rare; hypertrophic osteoarthropathy implies more than an 80% chance of malignancy. |
| **How is the diagnosis made?** | CXR, chest CT |
| **What is the significance of "popcorn" calcification?** | Most likely benign (i.e., hamartoma) |
| **What are the risk factors for malignancy?** | 1. Size: lesions >1 cm have a significant chance of malignancy, and those >4 cm are very likely to be malignant. 2. Indistinct margins (corona radiata) 3. Documented growth on follow-up x-ray (if no change in 2 years, most likely benign) 4. Increasing age |
| **What are the associated lab tests?** | 1. TB skin tests, etc. 2. Sputum cultures 3. Sputum cytology is diagnostic in 5% to 20% of cases. |
| **Which method of tissue diagnosis is used?** | Chest CT with needle biopsy, bronchoscopy (+/− transtracheal biopsy), excisional biopsy (open or thoracoscopic) |

| | |
|---|---|
| **What is the treatment?** | Surgical excision is the mainstay of treatment. |
| | Excisional biopsy is therapeutic for benign lesions, solitary metastasis, and for primary cancer in patients who are poor risks for more extensive surgery. |
| | Lobectomy for centrally placed lesions |
| | Lobectomy with node dissection for primary cancer (if resectable by preop evaluations) |
| **Which solitary nodule can be followed without a tissue diagnosis?** | Popcorn calcifications |
| | Mass unchanged for 2 years on previous CXR |
| **What is the prognosis?** | For malignant coin lesions <2 cm, 5-year survival is approximately 70%. |
| **What if the patient has an SPN and pulmonary hypertrophic osteoarthropathy?** | The patient has more than a 75% chance of having a carcinoma. |
| **What is hypertrophic pulmonary osteoarthropathy?** | Periosteal proliferation and new bone formation at the end of long bones and in bones of the hand |
| **What is its incidence?** | About 7% of patients with lung cancer (2% to 12%) |
| **What are the signs?** | Associated with clubbing of the fingers; diagnosed by x-ray of long bones, revealing periosteal bone hypertrophy |

## CARCINOID TUMOR

| | |
|---|---|
| **What is it?** | An APUD (amine-precursor uptake and decarboxylation) cell tumor of the bronchus |
| **What is its natural course in the lung?** | Slow growing (but may be malignant) |
| **What are the primary local findings?** | Wheezing and atelectasis caused by bronchial obstruction/stenosis |

| | |
|---|---|
| **What condition may it be confused with?** | Asthma |
| **How is the diagnosis made?** | Bronchoscopy reveals round red-yellow-purple mass covered by epithelium that protrudes into bronchial lumen. |
| **What is the treatment?** | Surgical resection (lobectomy with lymph node dissection)<br>Sleeve resection is also an option for proximal bronchial lesions. |
| **What is a sleeve resection?** | Resection of a ring segment of bronchus (with tumor inside) and then end to end anastomosis of the remaining ends, allowing salvage of lower lobe |
| **What is the prognosis (5-year survival) after complete surgical resection of carcinoid:** | |
| **Negative nodes?** | More than 90% are alive at 5 years. |
| **Positive nodes?** | Two-thirds are alive at 5 years. |
| **What is the most common benign lung tumor?** | Hamartoma (normal cells in a weird configuration) |

## PULMONARY SEQUESTRATION

| | |
|---|---|
| **What is it?** | Abnormal benign lung tissue with separate blood supply that **DOES NOT** communicate with the normal tracheobronchial airway |
| **Define the following terms:** | |
| **Interlobar** | Sequestration in normal lung tissue covered by normal visceral pleura |
| **Extralobar** | Sequestration not in normal lung covered by its own pleura |
| **What are the signs/symptoms?** | Asymptomatic, recurrent pneumonia |

**How is the diagnosis made?**   CXR, chest CT, A-gram, U/S with Doppler flow to ascertain blood supply

**What is the treatment in the following cases:**

    **Extralobar?**   Surgical resection

    **Intralobar?**   Lobectomy

**What is the major danger during surgery for sequestration?**   Anomalous blood supply from below the diaphragm (these can be cut and retract into the abdomen and result in exsanguination!)

Always document blood supply by A-gram or U/S with Doppler flow.

## DISEASES OF THE MEDIASTINUM

### MEDIASTINAL ANATOMY

**What structures lie in the following locations:**

    **Superior mediastinum?**   Aortic arch, great vessels, upper trachea, esophagus

    **Anterior mediastinum?**   Thymus, ascending aorta, lymph nodes

    **Middle mediastinum?**   Heart, lower trachea and bifurcation, lung hila, phrenic nerves, lymph nodes

    **Posterior mediastinum?**   Esophagus, descending aorta, thoracic duct, vagus and intercostal nerves, sympathetic trunks, azygous and hemizygous veins, lymph nodes

**What is the major differential diagnosis for tumors of the mediastinum:**

    **Anterior mediastinum?**   The classic **"four Ts": T**hyroid tumor, **T**hymoma, **T**errible lymphoma, **T**eratoma; also parathyroid tumor, lipoma, vascular aneurysms

| | |
|---|---|
| **Middle mediastinum?** | Lymphadenopathy (e.g., lymphoma, sarcoid), teratoma, fat pad, cysts, hernias, extension of esophageal mass, bronchogenic cancer |
| **Posterior mediastinum?** | Neurogenic tumors, lymphoma, aortic aneurysm, vertebral lesions, hernias |
| **What is the differential diagnosis for a neurogenic tumor?** | Schwannoma (A.K.A. neurolemmoma), neurofibroma, neuroblastoma, ganglioneuroma, ganglioneuroblastoma, pheochromocytoma |

## PRIMARY MEDIASTINAL TUMORS

### *Thymoma*

| | |
|---|---|
| **Where are they found in the mediastinum?** | Anterior |
| **How is the diagnosis made?** | CT |
| **What is the treatment?** | All thymomas should be surgically resected via midline sternotomy. |
| **What are the indications for *post*op radiation therapy?** | Invasive malignant tumor |
| **What are the indications for *pre*op chemotherapy?** | Tumor >6 cm and CT with invasion |
| **What percentage of thymomas are malignant?** | Approximately 25% |
| **How is a malignant thymoma diagnosed?** | At surgery with invasion into surrounding structures (not by histology!) |
| **What is myasthenia gravis?** | Autoimmune disease with antibodies against the muscle acetylcholine receptors |
| **What percentage of patients with myasthenia gravis have a thymoma?** | Approximately 15% |

| | |
|---|---|
| **What percentage of patients with thymoma have or will have myasthenia gravis?** | Approximately 75%! |

### Teratomas

| | |
|---|---|
| **What are they?** | Tumors of branchial cleft cells; the tumors contain ectoderm, endoderm, and mesoderm |
| **What is a dermoid cyst?** | A teratoma made up of ectodermal derivatives (e.g., teeth, skin, hair) |
| **Which age group is affected?** | Usually adolescents, but can occur at any age |
| **Where in the mediastinum do they occur?** | Anterior |
| **What are the characteristic x-ray findings?** | Calcifications or teeth; tumors may be cystic |
| **What percentage are malignant?** | Approximately 15% |
| **What is the treatment of benign dermoid cysts?** | Surgical excision |
| **What is the treatment of malignant teratoma?** | Preoperative chemotherapy until tumor markers are normal, then surgical resection |
| **Which tumor markers are associated with malignant teratomas?** | AFP, CEA |

### Neurogenic Tumors

| | |
|---|---|
| **What is the incidence?** | Most common mediastinal tumors in all age groups |
| **Where in the mediastinum do they occur?** | Posterior, in the paravertebral gutters |
| **What percentage are malignant?** | 50% in children<br>10% in adults |

| | |
|---|---|
| **What are the histologic types (5)? (Note cells of origin and whether benign or malignant)** | 1. Neurilemmoma or schwannoma (benign)—arise from Schwann cell sheaths of intercostal nerves<br>2. Neurofibroma (benign)—arise from intercostal nerves; can degenerate into:<br>3. Neurosarcoma (malignant)<br>4. Ganglioneuroma (benign)—from sympathetic chain<br>5. Neuroblastoma (malignant)—also from sympathetic chain |

## LYMPHOMA

| | |
|---|---|
| **Where in the mediastinum do they occur?** | Anywhere, but most often in the anterosuperior mediastinum or hilum in the middle mediastinum |
| **What percentage of lymphomas involve mediastinal nodes?** | Approximately 50% |
| **What are the symptoms?** | Cough, fever, chest pain, weight loss, SVC syndrome, chylothorax |
| **How is the diagnosis made?** | 1. CXR, CT<br>2. Mediastinoscopy or mediastinotomy with node biopsy |
| **What is the treatment?** | Nonsurgical (chemotherapy, radiation, or both) |

## MEDIASTINITIS

### *Acute Mediastinitis*

| | |
|---|---|
| **What is it?** | Acute suppurative mediastinal infection |
| **Name the six etiologies.** | 1. Esophageal perforation (Boerhaave's syndrome)<br>2. Postoperative wound infection<br>3. Head and neck infections<br>4. Lung or pleural infections<br>5. Rib or vertebral osteomyelitis<br>6. Distant infections |

| | |
|---|---|
| **What are the clinical features?** | Fever, chest pain, dysphagia (especially with esophageal perforation), respiratory distress, leukocytosis |
| **What is the treatment?** | 1. Wide drainage<br>2. Treatment of primary cause<br>3. Antibiotics |

### *Chronic Mediastinitis*

| | |
|---|---|
| **What is it?** | Mediastinal fibrosis secondary to *chronic* granulomatous infection |
| **What is the most common etiology?** | Histoplasma capsulatum |
| **What are the clinical features?** | 50% are asymptomatic; symptoms are related to compression of adjacent structures: SVC syndrome, bronchial and esophageal strictures, constrictive pericarditis. |
| **How is the diagnosis made?** | CXR or CT may be helpful, but surgery/biopsy often makes the diagnosis. |
| **What is the treatment?** | Antibiotics; surgical removal of the granulomas is rarely helpful |

## SUPERIOR VENA CAVA SYNDROME

| | |
|---|---|
| **What is it?** | Obstruction of the superior vena cava, usually by extrinsic compression |
| **What is the number one cause?** | Malignant tumors cause approximately 90% of cases; lung cancer is by far the most common; other tumors include thymoma, lymphoma, and Hodgkin's disease. |
| **What are the clinical manifestations?** | 1. Blue discoloration and puffiness of the face, arms, and shoulders<br>2. CNS manifestations may include headache, nausea, vomiting, visual distortion, stupor, and convulsions.<br>3. Cough, hoarseness, and dyspnea |

| | |
|---|---|
| **What is the treatment?** | 1. Diuretics and fluid restriction<br>2. Prompt radiation therapy with or without chemotherapy for any causative cancer |
| **What is the prognosis?** | SVC obstruction itself is fatal in less than 5% of cases; mean survival time in patients with malignant obstruction is about 7 months. |

## DISEASES OF THE ESOPHAGUS

### ANATOMIC CONSIDERATIONS

| | |
|---|---|
| **What is the primary function of the UES?** | Swallowing |
| **What is the primary function of the LES?** | Prevention of reflux |
| **The esophageal venous plexus drains inferiorly into the gastric veins. Why is this important?** | The gastric veins are part of the portal venous system; portal hypertension can thus be referred to the esophageal veins, leading to varices. |
| **Identify the esophageal muscle type:** | |
| **Proximal 1/3** | Skeletal muscle |
| **Middle 1/3** | Smooth muscle > skeletal muscle |
| **Distal 1/3** | Smooth muscle |
| **Identify the blood supply to the esophagus:** | |
| **Proximal 1/3** | Inferior thyroid, anterior intercostals |
| **Middle 1/3** | Esophageal arteries, bronchial arteries |
| **Distal 1/3** | Left gastric artery, left inferior phrenic artery |
| **What is the length of the esophagus?** | Approximately 25 cm in the adult (40 cm from teeth to LES) |

| | |
|---|---|
| **Why is the esophagus notorious for anastomotic leaks?** | The esophagus has no serosa (same as the distal rectum). |
| **What nerve runs with the esophagus?** | The vagus nerve |

## ZENKER'S DIVERTICULUM

| | |
|---|---|
| **What is it?** | A pharyngoesophageal diverticulum; a false diverticulum containing mucosa and submucosa at the UES at the pharyngoesophageal junction through Killian's triangle |

**Zenker's diverticulum**

| | |
|---|---|
| **What is the disease's "claim to fame"?** | It is the most common esophageal diverticulum. |
| **What are the signs/ symptoms?** | Dysphagia, neck mass, halitosis, food regurgitation, heartburn |
| **How is the diagnosis made?** | Barium swallow |
| **What is the treatment?** | 1. Diverticulectomy<br>2. Cricopharyngeus myotomy, if >2 cm |

## ACHALASIA

| | |
|---|---|
| **What is it?** | 1. Failure of the LES to relax during swallowing<br>2. Loss of esophageal **peristalsis** |

| | |
|---|---|
| **What are the proposed etiologies?** | 1. Neurologic (ganglionic degeneration of Auerbach's plexus, vagus nerve, or both); possibly infectious in nature<br>2. Chagas' disease in South America |
| **What are the associated long-term conditions?** | Esophageal carcinoma secondary to Barrett's esophagus from food stasis |
| **What are the symptoms?** | Dysphagia for both solids and liquids, followed by regurgitation; dysphagia for liquids is worse |

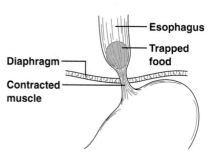

| | |
|---|---|
| **What are the diagnostic findings?** | Radiographic contrast studies reveal dilated esophageal body with narrowing inferiorly.<br>**Manometry:** motility studies reveal increased pressure in the LES and failure of the LES to relax during swallowing |
| **What is the treatment?** | 1. Balloon dilation of the LES<br>2. Medical treatment of reflux versus Belsey Mark IV 270° fundoplication (do not perform 360° Nissen)<br>3. Myotomy of the lower esophagus and LES |

## DIFFUSE ESOPHAGEAL SPASM

| | |
|---|---|
| **What is it?** | Strong, nonperistaltic contractions of the esophageal body; sphincter function is usually normal |
| **What is the associated condition?** | Gastroesophageal reflux |

| | |
|---|---|
| **What are the symptoms?** | Spontaneous chest pain that radiates to the back, ears, neck, jaw, or arms |
| **What is the differential diagnosis?** | Angina pectoris<br>Psychoneurosis<br>Nutcracker esophagus |
| **What are the associated diagnostic tests?** | **Esophageal manometry:** Motility studies reveal repetitive, high-amplitude contractions with normal sphincter response.<br>Upper GI may be normal, but 50% show segmented spasms or corkscrew esophagus.<br>Endoscopy |
| **What is the classic finding on esophageal contrast study (UGI)?** | "Corkscrew esophagus" |
| **What is the treatment?** | Medical (antireflux measures, Ca channel blockers, nitrates)<br>Long esophagomyotomy in refractory cases |

## NUTCRACKER ESOPHAGUS

| | |
|---|---|
| **What is it also known as?** | Hypertensive peristalsis |
| **What is it?** | Very strong peristaltic waves |
| **What are the symptoms?** | Spontaneous chest pain that radiates to the back, ears, neck, jaw, or arms |
| **What is the differential diagnosis?** | Angina pectoris<br>Psychoneurosis<br>Diffuse esophageal spasm |
| **What are the associated diagnostic tests?** | 1. Esophageal manometry: motility studies reveal repetitive, high-amplitude contractions with normal sphincter response<br>2. Results of UGI may be normal (rule out mass).<br>3. Endoscopy |

| | |
|---|---|
| **What is the treatment?** | Medical (antireflux measures, Ca channel blockers, nitrates)<br>Long esophagomyotomy in refractory cases |

## ESOPHAGEAL REFLUX

| | |
|---|---|
| **What is it?** | Reflux of gastric contents into the lower esophagus resulting from the decreased function of the LES |
| **What are the causes?** | 1. Decreased LES tone<br>2. Decreased esophageal motility<br>3. Hiatal hernia<br>4. Gastric outlet obstruction<br>5. NGT |
| **Name four associated conditions/factors.** | 1. Sliding hiatal hernia<br>2. Tobacco and alcohol<br>3. Scleroderma<br>4. Decreased endogenous gastrin production |
| **What are the symptoms?** | Substernal pain, heartburn, regurgitation; symptoms are worse when patient is supine and after meals |
| **How is the diagnosis made?** | 1. pH probe in the lower esophagus reveals acid reflux.<br>2. EGD shows esophagitis.<br>3. Manometry reveals decreased LES pressure.<br>4. Barium swallow |
| **What is the treatment?** | Initially medical: $H_2$-blockers, antacids, metoclopramide, omeprazole<br>Elevation of the head of the bed; small, multiple meals |
| **Which four complications require surgery?** | 1. Failure of medical therapy<br>2. Esophageal strictures<br>3. Progressive pulmonary insufficiency secondary to documented nocturnal aspiration<br>4. Barrett's esophagus |

**Describe each of the following types of surgery:**

**Nissen**

360° fundoplication: wrap fundus of stomach all the way around the esophagus

**Belsey Mark IV**

270° fundoplication: wrap fundus of stomach, but not all the way around

**Hill**

Tighten arcuate ligament around esophagus and tack stomach to diaphragm

**Lap Nissen**

Nissen via laparoscope

**Lap Toupet**

Lap fundoplication posteriorly with less than 220 to 250° wrap used with decreased esophageal motility; disadvantage is more postoperative reflux

**What is Barrett's esophagus?**

Replacement of the lower esophageal squamous epithelium with columnar epithelium secondary to reflux

**Why is it significant?**

This lesion is premalignant.

**What is the treatment?**

People with significant reflux should be followed with regular EGDs with biopsies, $H_2$-blockers, and antireflux precautions; many experts believe that patients with severe dysplasia should undergo esophagectomy.

## CAUSTIC ESOPHAGEAL STRICTURES

**Which agents may cause strictures if ingested?**

Lye, oven cleaners, drain cleaners, batteries, sodium hydroxide tablets (Clinitest)

**How is the diagnosis made?**

History; EGD is clearly indicated early on to assess the extent of damage (<24 hrs); scope to level of severe injury (deep ulcer) only, water soluble contrast study for deep ulcers to rule out perforation

| | |
|---|---|
| **What is the initial treatment?** | 1. NPO/IVF/$H_2$-blocker<br>2. Do **not** induce emesis.<br>3. Corticosteroids (controversial—probably best for shallow/moderate ulcers), antibiotics (penicillin/gentamicin) for moderate ulcers<br>4. Antibiotic for deep ulcers<br>5. Upper GI at 10 to 14 days |
| **What is the treatment if stricture develops?** | Dilation with Maloney dilator/balloon catheter<br>In severe refractory cases, esophagectomy with colon interposition or gastric pull up |
| **What is the long-term follow-up?** | Because of increased risk of esophageal squamous cancer (especially with ulceration), patients need endoscopies every other year. |
| **What is a Maloney dilator?** | Mercury-filled rubber dilator |

## ESOPHAGEAL CARCINOMA

| | |
|---|---|
| **What are the two main types?** | 1. Adenocarcinoma at the GE junction<br>2. Squamous cell carcinoma in most of the esophagus |
| **What is the most common histology?** | **Worldwide:** squamous cell carcinoma (95%!)<br>**USA:** adenocarcinoma |
| **What is the age and gender distribution?** | Most common in the sixth decade of life; men predominate, especially black men |
| **What are the etiologic factors (5)?** | 1. Tobacco<br>2. Alcohol<br>3. GE reflux<br>4. Barrett's esophagus<br>5. Radiation |
| **What are the symptoms?** | Dysphagia, weight loss<br>Others symptoms include chest pain, back pain, hoarseness, symptoms of metastasis |

| | |
|---|---|
| **What comprises the workup?** | 1. UGI<br>2. EGD<br>3. Transesophageal ultrasound (TEU)<br>4. CT scan of chest/abdomen |
| **What is the differential diagnosis?** | Leiomyoma, metastatic tumor, lymphomas, benign stricture, achalasia, diffuse esophageal spasm, GERD |
| **How is the diagnosis made?** | 1. Upper GI localizes tumor.<br>2. EGD obtains biopsy and assesses resectability.<br>3. Full metastatic workup (CXR, bone scan, CT, LFTs) |

**Describe the stages of esophageal cancer:**

| | |
|---|---|
| **Stage I** | Tumor: invades **lamina propria** or **submucosa**<br>Nodes: negative |
| **Stage IIa** | Tumor: invades muscularis propria or adventitia<br>Nodes: negative |
| **Stage IIb** | Tumor: **any tumor** that invades up to the muscularis propria<br>Nodes: positive regional nodes |
| **Stage III** | Tumor: invades adventitia<br>Nodes: positive regional nodes OR<br>Tumor: invades adjacent structures<br>Nodes: positive or negative nodes |
| **Stage IV** | Distant metastasis |
| **What is the treatment?** | Esophagectomy with gastric pull-up or colon interposition |
| **What is an Ivor-Lewis procedure?** | Laparotomy and right thoracotomy with gastroesophageal anastomosis in the chest after esophagectomy |

| | |
|---|---|
| **What is a "blunt esophagectomy"?** | Esophagectomy with "blunt" transhiatal dissection of esophagus from abdomen and gastroesophageal anastomosis in the neck |
| **What is the operative mortality rate?** | About 5% |
| **Has radiation therapy and/or chemotherapy been shown to decrease mortality?** | No |
| **What is the postop complication rate?** | ≈ 33%! |

**What is the prognosis (5-year survival) by stage:**

| | |
|---|---|
| I? | 80% |
| II? | 33% |
| III? | 15% |
| IV? | Basically 0% |

---

# Chapter 72

# Cardiovascular Surgery

**What do the following abbreviations stand for:**

| | |
|---|---|
| AI? | **A**ortic **I**nsufficiency/regurgitation |
| AS? | **A**ortic **S**tenosis |
| ASD? | **A**trial **S**eptal **D**efect |
| CABG? | **C**oronary **A**rtery **B**ypass **G**rafting |
| CAD? | **C**oronary **A**rtery **D**isease |
| CPB? | **C**ardio**P**ulmonary **B**ypass |
| IABP? | **I**ntra-**A**ortic **B**alloon **P**ump |

| | |
|---|---|
| **LAD?** | **L**eft **A**nterior **D**escending coronary artery |
| **IMA?** | **I**nternal **M**ammary **A**rtery |
| **MR?** | **M**itral **R**egurgitation |
| **PTCA?** | **P**ercutaneous **T**ransluminal **C**oronary **A**ngioplasty (balloon angioplasty) |
| **VAD?** | **V**entricular **A**ssist **D**evice |
| **VSD?** | **V**entricular **S**eptal **D**efect |

**Define the following terms:**

| | |
|---|---|
| **Stroke volume (SV)** | mL of blood pumped per heartbeat (SV = CO/HR) |
| **Cardiac output (CO)** | Amount of blood pumped by the heart each minute: heart rate × SV |
| **Cardiac Index (CI)** | CO/BSA (body surface area) |
| **Ejection fraction** | Percentage of blood pumped out of the left ventricle: SV ÷ end diastolic volume (nl 55% to 70%) |
| **Compliance** | Change in volume/change in pressure |
| **SVR** | **S**ystemic **V**ascular **R**esistance = $\dfrac{MAP - CVP}{CO \times 80}$ |
| **Preload** | Left ventricular end diastolic pressure or volume |
| **Afterload** | Arterial resistance the heart pumps against |
| **PVR** | **P**ulmonary **V**ascular **R**esistance = $PA_{(mean)} - PCWP/CO \times 80$ |
| **MAP** | **M**ean **A**rterial **P**ressure = Diastolic BP + 1/3 (Systolic BP − Diastolic BP) |
| **What is a normal CO?** | 4 to 8 L/minute |
| **What is a normal CI?** | 2.5 to 4 L/minute |

| | |
|---|---|
| **What are the ways to increase CO?** | "Remember **M.R. PAIR**":<br>1. **M**echanical assistance (IABP, VAD)<br>2. **R**ate—Increase heart rate<br>3. **P**reload—Increase preload<br>4. **A**fterload—Decrease afterload<br>5. **I**notropes—Increase contractility<br>6. **R**hythm—Normal sinus |
| **When does most of the coronary blood flow take place?** | During diastole (66%) |
| **Name the three major coronary arteries.** | 1. Left anterior descending (LAD)<br>2. Circumflex<br>3. Right coronary |
| **What are the three main "cardiac electrolytes"?** | 1. Calcium (inotropic)<br>2. Potassium (dysrhythmias)<br>3. Magnesium (dysrhythmias) |

## ACQUIRED HEART DISEASE

### CORONARY ARTERY DISEASE (CAD)

| | |
|---|---|
| **What is it?** | Atherosclerotic occlusive lesions of the coronary arteries; segmental nature makes CABG possible |
| **What is the incidence?** | CAD is the #1 killer in the Western world; more than 50% of cases are triple vessel diseases involving the LAD, circumflex, and right coronary arteries. |
| **What are the symptoms?** | If ischemia occurs (low flow, vasospasm, thrombus formation, plaque rupture, or a combination), patient may experience chest pain; crushing, substernal shortness of breath; nausea/upper abdominal pain; sudden death; or may be asymptomatic with fatigue. |
| **Who classically gets "silent" MIs?** | Patients with diabetes (autonomic dysfunction) |

**What are the risk factors?**

HTN
Smoking
High (> 240) cholesterol/lipids
Obesity
Diabetes mellitus
Family history

**Which diagnostic tests should be performed?**

Exercise stress testing (± thallium)
Echocardiography
Localize dyskinetic wall segments
Valvular dysfunction
Estimate ejection fraction
Cardiac catheterization with coronary angiography and left ventriculography (definitive test)

**What is the treatment?**

Medical therapy (β-blockers, aspirin, nitrates, HTN medications), angioplasty (PTCA), surgical therapy: CABG

## CABG

**What is it?**

**C**oronary **A**rtery **B**ypass **G**rafting

Vein grafts

**What are the indications?**

Left main disease
Three-vessel disease (main arteries—not branches)
Unstable or disabling angina unresponsive to medical therapy
Postinfarct angina
Coronary artery rupture, dissection, thrombosis after PTCA

| | |
|---|---|
| **What procedures are most often used in the treatment?** | Coronary arteries grafted (usually 3 to 6): internal mammary pedicle graft and saphenous vein free graft are most often used (IMA 95% 10-year patency vs. 50% with saphenous) |
| **What other vessels are occasionally used for grafting?** | Radial artery, inferior epigastric vein |
| **What are the possible complications?** | Hemorrhage<br>Tamponade<br>MI, dysrhythmias<br>Infection<br>Graft thrombosis<br>Sternal dehiscence<br>Postpericardiotomy syndrome, stroke |
| **What is the operative mortality?** | Between 1% and 3% for elective CABG (vs. 5% to 10% for acute MI) |
| **What medications should almost every patient be given after CABG?** | Aspirin, beta-blocker |
| **Can a CABG be performed off cardiopulmonary bypass?** | Yes, today they are performed with or without bypass. |

## POSTPERICARDIOTOMY SYNDROME

| | |
|---|---|
| **What is it?** | Pericarditis after pericardiotomy (unknown etiology), occurs weeks to 3 months postoperatively |
| **What are the signs/ symptoms?** | Fever<br>Chest pain, atrial fibrillation<br>Malaise<br>Pericardial friction rub<br>Pericardial effusion/pleural effusion |
| **What is the treatment?** | NSAIDs, with or without steroids |
| **What is pericarditis after an MI called?** | Dressler's syndrome |

## CARDIOPULMONARY BYPASS (CPB)

**What is it?**

Pump and oxygenation apparatus remove blood from SVC and IVC and return it to the aorta, bypassing the heart and lungs and allowing cardiac arrest for open heart procedures, heart transplant, lung transplant, or heart-lung transplant, as well as procedures on the proximal great vessels.

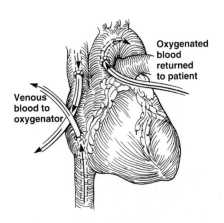

**Oxygenated blood returned to patient**

**Venous blood to oxygenator**

**Is anticoagulation necessary?**

Yes, just before and during the procedure, with heparin

**How is anticoagulation reversed?**

Protamine

**What are the six ways to manipulate cardiac output after CPB?**

Rate, rhythm, afterload, preload, inotropes, mechanical (IABP and VAD)

**What mechanical problems can decrease CO after a CPB procedure?**

Cardiac tamponade, pneumothorax

**What is "tamponade physiology"?**

↓ Cardiac output, ↑ heart rate, hypotension, **CVP = wedge pressure**

**What are the possible complications?**

Trauma to formed blood elements (especially thrombocytopenia and platelet dysfunction)
Pancreatitis (low flow)
Heparin rebound
CVA
Failure to wean from bypass
Technical complications (operative technique)
MI

**What are the options for treating postop CABG mediastinal bleeding?**

Protamine, ↑ PEEP, FFP, platelets, aminocaproic acid

**What is heparin rebound?**

Increased anticoagulation after CPB from increased heparin levels, as increase in peripheral blood flow after CPB returns heparin residual that was in the peripheral tissues

**What is the method of lowering SVR after CPB?**

Warm the patient, administer sodium nitroprusside (SNP) and dobutamine

**What are the options if a patient cannot be weaned from CPB?**

Inotropes (e.g., epinephrine)
VAD, IABP

**What percentage of patients go into AFib after CPB?**

Up to 33%

**What is the workup of a postoperative patient with AFib?**

Rule out PTX (CXR), acidosis (ABG), electrolyte abnormality (LABS), and ischemia (EKG).

**What is a MIDCAB?**

**M**inimally **I**nvasive **D**irect **C**oronary **A**rtery **B**ypass—LIMA to LAD bypass without CPB and through a small thoracotomy

**What is TMR?**

**T**rans**M**yocardial laser **R**evascularization-laser through groin catheter makes small holes (intramyocardial sinusoids) in cardiac muscle to allow blood to nourish the muscle

| | |
|---|---|
| **What is OPCAB?** | **O**ff **P**ump **C**oronary **A**rtery **B**ypass— median sternotomy but no bypass pump |
| **TMR is modeled after what type of heart?** | Reptile and human fetus! |

## AORTIC STENOSIS (AS)

| | |
|---|---|
| **What is it?** | Destruction and calcification of valve leaflets, resulting in obstruction of left ventricular outflow |
| **What are the causes?** | Calcification of bicuspid aortic valve Rheumatic fever Acquired calcific AS (7th to 8th decades) |
| **What are the symptoms?** | Angina (5 years life expectancy if untreated) Syncope (3 years life expectancy if untreated) CHF (2 years life expectancy if untreated) Often asymptomatic until late |
| **What is the memory aid for the aortic stenosis complications?** | **A**ortic **S**tenosis **C**omplications = **A**ngina **S**yncope **C**HF—5,3,2 |
| **What are the signs?** | Murmur: crescendo-decrescendo systolic second right intercostal space with radiation to the carotids Left ventricular heave or lift from left ventricular hypertrophy |
| **What tests should be performed?** | CXR, ECG, echocardiography Cardiac catheterization—needed to plan operation |
| **What is the surgical treatment?** | Valve replacement with tissue or mechanical prosthesis |
| **What are the indications for surgical repair?** | If patient is symptomatic or valve cross-sectional area is <0.75 cm² (normal 2.5 to 3.5 cm²) and/or gradient >50 mm Hg |

**What are the pros/cons of mechanical valve?**

Mechanical valve is more durable, but requires lifetime anticoagulation.

**What is the treatment option in poor surgical candidates?**

Balloon aortic "valvuloplasty" (percutaneous)

**Why is a loud murmur often a good sign?**

Implies a high gradient, which indicates preserved LV function

**Why might an AS murmur diminish over time?**

It may imply a decreasing gradient from a decline in LV function.

## AORTIC INSUFFICIENCY (AI)

**What is it?**

Incompetency of the aortic valve

**What are the causes?**

Bacterial endocarditis (*Staphylococcus aureus, Streptococcus viridans*)
Rheumatic fever
Annular ectasia from collagen vascular disease (especially Marfan's syndrome)

**What are the predisposing conditions?**

Bicuspid aortic valve, connective tissue disease

**What are the symptoms?**

Palpitations from dysrhythmias and dilated left ventricle
Dyspnea/orthopnea from left ventricular failure
Angina from decreased diastolic BP and coronary flow (*Note:* most coronary blood flow occurs during diastole and aorta rebound.)

**What are the signs?**

Murmur: blowing, decrescendo diastolic at left sternal border
Austin-Flint murmur: reverberation of regurgitant flow
Increased pulse pressure: "pistol shots," "water-hammer" pulse palpated over peripheral arteries, Corrigan's pulse

**What is Corrigan's pulse?**

1. Low diastolic blood pressure
2. Wide pulse pressure
(A.K.A. water-hammer pulse)

| | |
|---|---|
| **Which diagnostic tests should be performed?** | 1. CXR: increasing heart size can be used to follow progression<br>2. Echocardiogram<br>3. Catheterization (definitive) |
| **What is the treatment?** | Aortic valve replacement |
| **What are the indications for surgical treatment?** | Symptomatic patients (CHF, PND, etc.), left ventricle dilatation, decreasing LV function, decreasing EF, acute AI onset |
| **What is the prognosis?** | Low operative risk; surgery gives symptomatic improvement and may improve longevity |

## MITRAL STENOSIS (MS)

| | |
|---|---|
| **What is it?** | Calcific degeneration and narrowing of the mitral valve resulting from rheumatic fever in most cases |
| **What are the symptoms?** | 1. Dyspnea from increased left atrial pressure, causing pulmonary edema (i.e., CHF)<br>2. Hemoptysis (rarely life-threatening)<br>3. Hoarseness from dilated left atrium impinging on the recurrent laryngeal nerve<br>4. Palpations (AFib) |
| **What are the signs?** | Murmur: crescendo diastolic rumble at apex<br>Irregular pulse from AFib caused by dilated left atrium<br>Stroke caused by systemic emboli from left atrium (AFib and obstructed valve allow blood to pool in the left atrium and can lead to thrombus formation) |
| **Which diagnostic tests should be performed?** | Echocardiogram<br>Catheterization |
| **What are the indications for intervention?** | 1. Symptoms (severe)<br>2. Pulmonary HTN and mitral valve area $<1$ cm$^2$/m$^2$<br>3. Recurrent thromboembolism |

| | |
|---|---|
| **What are the treatment options?** | 1. Open commissurotomy (open heart operation)<br>2. Balloon valvuloplasty: percutaneous<br>3. Valve replacement |
| **What is the medical treatment for mild symptomatic patients?** | Diuretics |
| **What is the prognosis?** | More than 80% of patients are well at 10 years with successful operation. |

## MITRAL REGURGITATION (MR)

| | |
|---|---|
| **What is it?** | Incompetence of the mitral valve |
| **What are the causes?** | Severe mitral valve prolapse (some prolapse is found in 5% of the population, with women ≥ men)<br>Rheumatic fever<br>Post-MI from papillary muscle dysfunction/rupture<br>Ruptured chordae |
| **What are the most common causes?** | Rheumatic fever (#1 worldwide), ruptured chordae/papillary muscle dysfunction |
| **What are the symptoms?** | Often insidious and late: dyspnea, palpitations, fatigue |
| **What are the signs?** | Murmur: holosystolic, apical radiating to the axilla |
| **What are the indications for treatment?** | 1. Symptoms<br>2. LV >45 mm end-systolic dimension (left ventricular dilation) |
| **What is the treatment?** | 1. Valve replacement<br>2. Annuloplasty: suture a prosthetic ring to the dilated valve annulus |
| **What is a normal EF?** | From 55% to 70% |

## ARTIFICIAL VALVE PLACEMENT

| | |
|---|---|
| **What is it?** | Replacement of damaged valves with tissue or mechanical prosthesis |
| **What are the types of artificial valves?** | Tissue and mechanical |
| **What are the pros and cons:** | |
| **Tissue?** | NO anticoagulation but shorter duration (20–40% need replacement in 10 years); good for elderly |
| **Mechanical?** | Last longer (>15 years) but require ANTICOAGULATION) |
| **Contraindications for tissue valve?** | Dialysis (calcify), youth |
| **Contraindications for mechanical valve?** | Pregnancy (or going to be pregnant due to anticoagulation), bleeding risk (alcoholic, PUD) |
| **What is the operative mortality?** | From 1% to 5% in most series |
| **What must patients with an artificial valve receive before dental procedures?** | Antibiotics |
| **Define the Ross procedure.** | Aortic valve replacement with a pulmonary **auto**graft (i.e., patient's own valve!) |

## INFECTIOUS ENDOCARDITIS

| | |
|---|---|
| **What is it?** | Microbial infection of heart valves |
| **What are the predisposing conditions?** | Pre-existing valvular lesion, procedures that lead to bacteremia/IV drug use |
| **What are the common causative agents?** | *S. viridans:* associated with abnormal valves<br>*S. aureus:* associated with IV drug use<br>*S. epidermidis:* associated with prosthetic valves |

| | |
|---|---|
| **What are the signs/ symptoms?** | Murmur (new or changing) <br> Petechiae <br> Splinter hemorrhage (fingernails) <br> Roth spots (on retina) <br> Osler nodes (raised, **painful** on soles and palms; **O**sler = **O**uch!) <br> Janeway lesions (similar to Osler nodes, but flat and **painless**) (Janeway = pain **away**) |
| **Which diagnostic tests should be performed?** | Echocardiogram, TEE <br> Serial blood cultures (definitive) |
| **What is the treatment?** | Prolonged IV therapy with bactericidal antibiotics, to which infecting organisms are sensitive |
| **What is the prognosis?** | Infection can progress, requiring valve replacement |

## CONGENITAL HEART DISEASE

### VENTRICULAR SEPTAL DEFECT (VSD)

| | |
|---|---|
| **What is its claim to fame?** | Most common congenital heart defect |
| **What is it?** | Failure of ventricular septum to completely close; **80% of cases involve the membranous portion of the septum,** resulting in left-to-right shunt, increased pulmonary blood flow, and CHF if pulmonary to systemic flow is >2:1 |
| **What is pulmonary vascular obstructive disease?** | Pulmonary artery hyperplasia from increased pulmonary pressure caused by a left to right shunt (e.g., VSD) |
| **What is Eisenmenger's syndrome?** | Irreversible pulmonary HTN from chronic changes in pulmonary arterioles and increased right heart pressures; cyanosis develops when the shunt reverses (becomes right to left across the VSD) |
| **What is the treatment of Eisenmenger's syndrome?** | The only option is heart-lung transplant; otherwise, the disease is untreatable. |

| | |
|---|---|
| **What is the incidence of VSD?** | 30% of heart defects (most common defect) |

## PATENT DUCTUS ARTERIOSUS (PDA)

| | |
|---|---|
| **What is it?** | Physiologic right-to-left shunt in fetal circulation connecting the pulmonary artery to the aorta bypassing fetal lungs; often, this shunt persists in the neonate |
| **What are the factors preventing closure?** | Hypoxia, increased prostaglandins, prematurity |
| **What are the symptoms?** | Often asymptomatic <br> Poor feeding <br> Respiratory distress <br> CHF with respiratory infections |
| **What are the signs?** | Acyanotic, unless other cardiac lesions are present; continuous "machinery" murmur |
| **Which diagnostic tests should be performed?** | Physical examination <br> Echocardiogram (to rule out associated defects) <br> Catheter (seldom required) |
| **What is the medical treatment?** | Indomethacin is an NSAID: prostaglandin (PG) inhibitor (PG keeps PDA open). |
| **What is the treatment?** | Surgical ligation or cardiac catheterization closure at 6 months to 2 years of age |

## TETRALOGY OF FALLOT (TOF)

| | |
|---|---|
| **What is it?** | Misalignment of the infundibular septum in early development, leading to the characteristic tetrad: <br> 1. Pulmonary stenosis/obstruction of right ventricular outflow <br> 2. Overriding aorta <br> 3. Right ventricular hypertrophy <br> 4. VSD |

| | |
|---|---|
| **What are the symptoms?** | Hypoxic spells (squatting behavior increases SVR and increases pulmonary blood flow) |
| **What are the signs?** | Cyanosis<br>Clubbing<br>Murmur: SEM at left third intercostal space |
| **Which diagnostic tests should be performed?** | CXR: small, "boot-shaped" heart and decreased pulmonary blood flow<br>Echocardiography |
| **What is the prognosis?** | 95% survival at specialized centers |

## IHSS

| | |
|---|---|
| **What is IHSS?** | **I**diopathic **H**ypertrophic **S**ubaortic **S**tenosis |
| **What is it?** | Aortic outflow obstruction from septal tissue |
| **What is the usual presentation?** | Similar to aortic stenosis |

## COARCTATION OF THE AORTA

| | |
|---|---|
| **What is it?** | Narrowing of the thoracic aorta, with or without intraluminal "shelf" (infolding of the media); usually found near ductus/ligamentum arteriosum |
| **What are the three types?** | 1. Preductal (fatal in infancy if untreated)<br>2. Juxtaductal<br>3. Postductal |
| **What percentage are associated with other cardiac defects?** | 60% (bicuspid aortic valve is most common) |
| **What is the major route of collateral circulation?** | Subclavian artery to the IMA to the intercostals to the descending aorta |

**What are the risk factors?**
Turner's syndrome, male > female

**What are the symptoms?**
Headache
Epistaxis
Lower extremity fatigue → claudication

**What are the signs?**
Pulses: decreased lower extremity pulses
Murmurs:
1. Systolic—from turbulence across coarctation, often radiating to infrascapular region
2. Continuous—from dilated collaterals

**Which diagnostic tests should be performed?**
CXR
    "3" sign is aortic knob, coarctation, and dilated poststenotic aorta
    Rib notching is bony erosion from dilated intercostal collaterals
Echocardiogram
Cardiac catheterization if cardiac defects

**What is the treatment?**
Surgery:
Resection with end-to-end anastomosis
Subclavian artery flap
Patch graft (rare)
Interposition graft
Endovascular repair an option in adults

**What are the indications for surgery?**
Symptomatic patient
Asymptomatic patient older than 3 to 4 years

**What are the possible postoperative complications?**
Paraplegia
"Paradoxic" HTN
Mesenteric necrotizing panarteritis (GI bleeding), Horner's syndrome, injury to recurrent laryngeal nerve

**What are the long-term concerns?**
Aortic dissection, HTN

## TRANSPOSITION OF THE GREAT VESSELS

| | |
|---|---|
| **What is it?** | Aorta originates from the right ventricle and the pulmonary artery from the left ventricle; fatal without PDA, ASD, or VSD to allow communication between the left and right circulations |
| **What is the incidence?** | From 5% to 8% of defects |
| **What are the signs/ symptoms?** | Most common lesion that presents with cyanosis and CHF in neonatal period (> 90% by day 1) |
| **Which diagnostic tests should be performed?** | CXR: "egg-shaped" heart contour Catheterization (definitive) |
| **What is the treatment?** | Arterial switch operation—aorta and pulmonary artery are moved to the correct ventricle and the coronaries are reimplanted |

## EBSTEIN'S ANOMALY

| | |
|---|---|
| **What is it?** | Tricuspid valve is placed abnormally low in the right ventricle, forming a large right atrium and a small right ventricle, leading to tricuspid regurgitation and decreased right ventricular output |
| **What are the risk factors?** | 400 times the risk if the mother has taken lithium |

## VASCULAR RINGS

| | |
|---|---|
| **What are they?** | Many types; represent an anomalous development of the aorta/pulmonary artery from the embryonic aortic arch that surrounds and obstructs the trachea/ esophagus |
| **How are they diagnosed?** | Barium swallow, MRI |
| **What are the signs/ symptoms?** | Most prominent is stridor from tracheal compression |

## CYANOTIC HEART DISEASE

| | |
|---|---|
| **What are the causes?** | The five "Ts" of cyanotic heart disease:<br>**T**etralogy of Fallot<br>**T**runcus arteriosus<br>**T**otally anomalous pulmonary venous return (TAPVR)<br>**T**ricuspid atresia<br>**T**ransposition of the great vessels |

## CARDIAC TUMORS

| | |
|---|---|
| **What is the most common benign lesion?** | Myxoma in adults |
| **What is the most common location?** | Left atrium with pedunculated morphology |
| **What is the most common malignant tumor in children?** | Rhabdomyosarcoma |

## DISEASES OF THE GREAT VESSELS

## THORACIC AORTIC ANEURYSM

| | |
|---|---|
| **What is it?** | Aneurysm of the thoracic aorta |
| **What is the cause?** | Vast majority result from atherosclerosis, connective tissue disease. |
| **What is the major differential diagnosis?** | Aortic dissection |
| **What percentage of patients have aneurysms of the aorta at a different site?** | About 33%! (rule out AAA) |
| **What are the signs/ symptoms?** | Most are asymptomatic.<br>Chest pain, stridor, hemoptysis (rare), recurrent laryngeal nerve compression |
| **What is the most common way to diagnose?** | Routine CXR |
| **Which diagnostic tests should be performed?** | CXR, CT, MRI, aortography |

| | |
|---|---|
| **What are the indications for treatment?** | >6 cm in diameter<br>Symptoms<br>Rapid increase in diameter<br>Rupture |
| **What is the treatment?** | Replace with graft, open or endovascular stent |
| **What are the dreaded complications after treatment of a thoracic aortic aneurysm?** | Paraplegia (up to 20%)<br>Anterior spinal syndrome |
| **What is anterior spinal syndrome?** | Syndrome characterized by:<br>Paraplegia<br>Incontinence (bowel/bladder)<br>Pain and temperature sensation loss |
| **What is the cause?** | Occlusion of the great radicular artery of **Adamkiewicz,** which is one of the intercostal/lumbar arteries from T8 to L4 |

## AORTIC DISSECTION

| | |
|---|---|
| **What is it?** | Separation of the walls of the aorta from an intimal tear and disease of the tunica media; a false lumen is formed and a "reentry" tear may occur, resulting in "double-barrel" aorta |
| **What are the aortic dissection classifications?** | DeBakey classification<br>Stanford classification |
| **Define the DeBakey classifications:** | |
| **DeBakey type I** | Involves ascending **and** descending aorta |

**DeBakey type II**

Involves ascending aorta only

**DeBakey type III**

Involves descending aorta only

**Define the Stanford classifications:**
    **Type A**

Ascending aorta (requires surgery)
± Descending aorta (includes DeBakey types I and II)

| | |
|---|---|
| **Type B** | Descending aorta only (nonoperative, except for complications) (same as DeBakey type III) |

| | |
|---|---|
| **What is the etiology?** | HTN (most important)<br>Marfan's syndrome<br>Bicuspid aortic valve<br>Coarctation of the aorta<br>Cystic medial necrosis<br>Proximal aortic aneurysm |
| **What are the signs/ symptoms?** | **Abrupt onset of severe chest pain, most often radiating/tearing to the back;** onset is typically more abrupt than that of MI; the pain can migrate as the dissection progresses; patient describes a **"tearing pain"** |
| **Note three other sequelae.** | 1. Cardiac tamponade; Beck's triad—distant heart sounds, increased CVP with JVD, decreased blood pressure<br>2. Aortic insufficiency—diastolic murmur<br>3. Aortic arterial branch occlusion/shearing, leading to ischemia in the involved circulation (i.e., unequal pulses, CVA, paraplegia, renal insufficiency, bowel ischemia, claudication) |
| **Which diagnostic tests are indicated?** | CXR:<br>  1. Widened mediastinum<br>  2. Pleural effusion<br>TEE<br>CTA (CT angiography)<br>Aortography (definitive gold standard but time-consuming!) |

| | |
|---|---|
| **What is a dissecting aortic aneurysm?** | A misnomer! Not an aneurysm! |

**What is the treatment of the various types:**

| | |
|---|---|
| **Types I and II (Stanford type A)?** | Surgical because of risk of:<br>1. Aortic insufficiency<br>2. Compromise of cerebral and coronary circulation<br>3. Tamponade<br>4. Rupture |
| **Type III (Stanford type B)?** | Medical (control BP), unless complicated by rupture or significant occlusions |
| **Describe the surgery for an aortic dissection. (Type I, II Stanford A)** | Open the aorta at the proximal extent of dissection, and then sew—graft to— intimal flap and adventitia circumferentially (endovascular an option). |
| **What is the preoperative treatment?** | Control BP with sodium nitroprusside and β-blockers (e.g., esmolol; β-blockers decrease shear stress). |
| **What is the postoperative treatment?** | Lifetime control of BP and monitoring of aortic size |
| **What is the possible cause of MI in a patient with aortic dissection?** | Dissection involves the coronary arteries or underlying LAD. |

**What are the ECG signs of the following disorders:**

| | |
|---|---|
| **Atrial fibrillation?** | Irregularly irregular |

**PVC?**

Premature ventricular complex: Wide QRS

**Ventricular aneurysm?**

ST elevation

**Ischemia?**

ST elevation/ST depression/flipped T waves

**Infarction?**

Q waves

**Pericarditis?**

ST elevation throughout leads

**RBBB?**

**R**ight **B**undle **B**ranch **B**lock: wide QRS and "rabbit ears" or R-R in V1 or V2

**LBBB?**

**L**eft **B**undle **B**ranch **B**lock: wide QRS and "rabbit ears" or R-R in V5 or V6

**Wolff-Parkinson-White?**

Delta wave = slurred upswing on QRS

**First degree A-V block?**

Prolonged P-R interval (0.2 second)

**Second degree A-V block?**

Dropped QRS; not all P waves transmit to produce ventricular contraction

| | |
|---|---|
| **Wenckebach phenomenon?** | Second-degree block with progressive delay in P-R interval prior to dropped beat |
| **Third-degree A-V block?** | Complete A-V dissociation; random P wave and QRS |

## MISCELLANEOUS

| | |
|---|---|
| **What is Mondor's disease?** | Thrombophlebitis of the thoracoepigastric veins |
| **What is a VAD?** | **V**entricular **A**ssist **D**evice |
| **How does an IABP work?** | The **I**ntra-**A**ortic **B**alloon **P**ump has a balloon tip resting in the aorta. The balloon inflates in diastole, increasing diastolic BP and coronary blood flow. In systole the balloon deflates, creating a negative pressure, lowering afterload, and increasing systolic BP. |
| **What electrolyte must be monitored during diuresis after CPB?** | $K^+$ |
| **How is extent/progress of postbypass diuresis followed?** | I's and O's, CXR, JVD, edema, daily weight |
| **What is an Austin Flint murmur?** | Diastolic murmur of AI secondary to regurgitant turbulent flow |
| **Where is the least oxygenated blood in the body?** | Coronary sinus |
| **What is the most common cause of a cardiac tumor?** | Metastasis |

# Chapter 73    **Transplant Surgery**

**Define the following terms:**

**Autograft**

Same individual is both donor and recipient.

**Isograft**

Donor and recipient are genetically identical (identical twins).

**Allograft**

Donor and recipient are genetically dissimilar, but of the same species.

**Xenograft**

Donor and recipient belong to different species.

**Orthotopic**

Donor organ is placed in normal anatomic position (liver, heart).

**Heterotopic**

Donor organ is placed in a different site than the normal anatomic position (kidney, pancreas).

**Paratopic**

Donor organ is placed close to original organ.

**Chimerism**

Sharing cells between the graft and donor.

## BASIC IMMUNOLOGY

**What are histocompatibility antigens?**

Distinct (genetically inherited) cell surface proteins of the human leukocyte antigen system (HLA)

**Why are they important?**

They are targets (class I antigens) and initiators (class II antigens) of immune response to donor tissue (i.e., distinguishing self from nonself).

**Which cells have class I antigens?**

All nucleated cells (think: class 1 = all cells and thus "one for all")

| | |
|---|---|
| **Which cells have class II antigens?** | Macrophages, monocytes, B cells, activated T cells, endothelial cells |
| **What are the gene products of MHC called in humans?** | HLA (human leukocyte antigen) |
| **What is the location of the MHC complex?** | Short arm of chromosome 6 |
| **What is a haplotype?** | The combination of HLA genes on a chromosome inherited from one parent. Therefore, two siblings have a 25% chance of being "haploidentical." |
| **Does HLA matching matter in organ transplantation?** | With recent improvements in immunosuppression (i.e., cyclosporine), the effect is largely obscured, but it still does matter. The most important ones to match in order to improve renal allograft survival are HAL-B and HLA-DR. |

## CELLS

### T CELLS

| | |
|---|---|
| **What is the source?** | Thymus |
| **What is the function?** | Cell-mediated immunity/rejection |
| **What are the types?** | Th (CD4): helper T—help B cells become plasma cells <br> Ts (CD8): suppressor T—regulate immune response <br> Tc (CD8): cytotoxic T—kill cell by direct contact |

### B CELLS

| | |
|---|---|
| **What is the function?** | Humoral immunity |
| **What is the cell type that produces antibodies?** | B cells differentiate into plasma cells. |

## MACROPHAGE

| | |
|---|---|
| **What is it?** | A monocyte in parenchymal tissue |
| **What is its function?** | Processes foreign protein and presents it to lymphocytes |
| **What is it also known as?** | Antigen-presenting cell (APC) |
| **Briefly describe the events leading to antibody production.** | 1. Macrophage engulfs antigen and presents it to Th cells; the macrophage produces IL-1.<br>2. The Th cells then produce IL-2, and the Th cells proliferate.<br>3. The Th cells then activate (via IL-4) B cells that differentiate into plasma cells, which produce antibodies against the antigen presented. |

## IMMUNOSUPPRESSION

| | |
|---|---|
| **Who needs to be immunosuppressed?** | All recipients (except autograft or isograft) |
| **What are the major drugs used for immunosuppression?** | Corticosteroids, azathioprine, cyclosporine/tacrolimus |
| **What are the other drugs?** | OKT3, ATGAM, mycophenolate |
| **What is the advantage of "triple therapy"?** | Employs three immunosuppressive drugs; therefore, a lower dose of each can be used, decreasing the toxic side effects of each |
| **What is "induction therapy"?** | High doses of immunosuppression to "induce" immunosuppression |

## CORTICOSTEROIDS

| | |
|---|---|
| **Which is most commonly used in transplants?** | Prednisone |
| **How does it function?** | Primarily blocks production of IL-1 by macrophage and stabilizes lysosomal membrane of macrophage |

| | |
|---|---|
| **What is the associated toxicity?** | "Cushingoid," alopecia, striae, HTN, diabetes, pancreatitis, ulcer disease, osteomalacia, aseptic necrosis (especially of the femoral head) |

**What is the relative potency of the following corticosteroids:**

| | |
|---|---|
| **Cortisol?** | 1 |
| **Prednisone?** | 4 |
| **Methylprednisolone?** | 5 |
| **Dexamethasone?** | 25 |

## AZATHIOPRINE (AZA [IMURAN®])

| | |
|---|---|
| **How does it function?** | Prodrug that is cleaved into mercaptopurine; inhibits synthesis of DNA and RNA, leading to decreased cellular (T/B cells) production |
| **What is the associated toxicity?** | Toxic to bone marrow (leukopenia + thrombocytopenia), hepatotoxic, associated with pancreatitis |
| **When should a lower dose of AZA be administered?** | When WBC is <4 |
| **What is the associated drug interaction?** | Decrease dose if patient is also on allopurinol, because allopurinol inhibits the enzyme xanthine oxidase, which is necessary for the breakdown of azathioprine. |

## CYCLOSPORINE (CSA)

| | |
|---|---|
| **What is its function?** | "Calcineurin inhibitor" inhibits production of IL-2 by Th cells |
| **What is the associated toxicity?** | Toxicity for cyclosporine includes the 11 "**H**'s" and three "**N**'s": **H**epatitis, **H**ypertrichosis, gingival **H**yperplasia, **H**yperlipidemia (worse than FK), **H**yperglycemia, **H**ypertension (worse |

than FK), **H**emolytic uremic syndrome,
**H**yperkalemia, **H**ypercalcemia,
**H**ypomagnesemia, **H**yperuricemia,
**N**ephrotoxicity, **N**eurotoxicity (headache,
tremor), **N**eoplasia (lymphoma, KS,
squamous cell skin cancers)

| | |
|---|---|
| **What drugs increase CSA levels?** | Diltiazem<br>Ketoconazole<br>Erythromycin, fluconazole, **ranitidine** |
| **What drugs decrease CSA levels?** | By inducing the p450 system: dilantin, Tegretol®, rifampin, isoniazid, barbiturates |
| **What are the drugs of choice for HTN from CSA?** | Clonidine, calcium channel blockers |

## ATGAM/ANTITHYMOCYTE GLOBULIN

| | |
|---|---|
| **How does it function?** | Antibody against thymocytes, lymphocytes (polyclonal) |
| **When is it typically used?** | For induction |
| **What is the associated toxicity?** | Thrombocytopenia, leukopenia, serum sickness, rigors, fever, anaphylaxis, increased risk of viral infection, arthralgia |

## OKT3

| | |
|---|---|
| **How does it work?** | MONOclonal antibody that binds CD3 receptor (on T cells) |
| **What is a major problem with multiple doses?** | Blocking antibodies develop, and OKT3 is less effective each time it is used. |
| **What are basiliximab and daclizumab?** | Anti-CD25 monoclonal antibodies |

## TACROLIMUS

| | |
|---|---|
| **What is tacrolimus also known as?** | Prograf®(FK506) |

| | |
|---|---|
| **How does it work?** | Similar to CSA—"calcineurin inhibitor" blocks IL-2 receptor expression, inhibits T cells |
| **What is its potency compared to CSA?** | 100 times more potent than CSA |
| **What are its side effects?** | Nephrotoxicity and CNS toxicity (tremor, seizure, parasthesia, coma), hyperkalemia, alopecia, diabetes |

## SIROLIMUS

| | |
|---|---|
| **What is sirolimus also known as?** | Rapamycin, Rapamune® |
| **How does it work?** | Like CSA and tacrolimus, it does not bind to and inhibit calcineurin, rather it blocks T-cell signaling. |
| **Toxicity?** | Hypertriglyceridemia, thrombocytopenia, wound/healing problems, anemia, oral ulcers |

## MYCOPHENOLATE MOFETIL (MMF)

| | |
|---|---|
| **What is MMF also known as?** | CellCept® |
| **How does it work?** | Inhibitor of inosine monophosphate dehydrogenase required for de novo purine synthesis which expanding T and B cells depend on; also inhibits adhesion molecule and antibody production |

## OVERVIEW OF IMMUNOSUPPRESSION MECHANISMS

What drug acts at the
following sites:

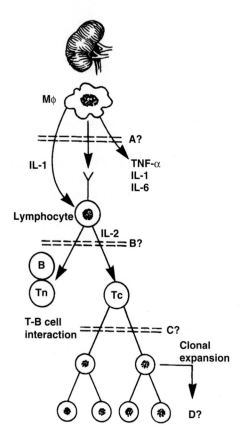

| A? | Corticosteroids |
| B? | CSA/tacrolimus |
| C? | AZA |
| D? | OKT3/ATGAM |

## MATCHING OF DONOR AND RECIPIENT

| | |
|---|---|
| **How is ABO crossmatching performed?** | Same procedure as in blood typing |
| **What is the purpose of lymphocytotoxic cross-matching?** | Tests for HLA antibodies in serum; most important in kidney and pancreas transplants |
| **How is the test performed?** | Mix recipient serum with donor lymphocyte and rabbit complement. |
| **Is HLA crossmatching important?** | Yes, for kidney and pancreas transplants |

## REJECTION

| | |
|---|---|
| **How many methods of rejection are there?** | Two: humoral and cell-mediated |
| **Name the types of rejection.** | Hyperacute, accelerated acute, acute, chronic |
| **What are the associated time courses by type?** | Hyperacute—immediate in OR<br>Accelerated acute—7 to 10 days post-transplant<br>Acute—weeks to months post-transplant<br>Chronic—months to years post-transplant |
| **What happens in hyperacute rejection?** | Antigraft antibodies in recipient recognize foreign antigen immediately after blood perfuses transplanted organ. |
| **What happens in acute rejection?** | T-cell mediated rejection |
| **What type of rejection is responsible for chronic rejection?** | Cellular, antibody (humoral), or both |
| **What is the treatment of hyperacute rejection?** | Remove transplanted organ |

| | |
|---|---|
| **What is the treatment of acute rejection?** | High-dose steroids/OKT3 |
| **What is the treatment of chronic rejection?** | Not much (irreversible) or retransplant |

## ORGAN PRESERVATION

| | |
|---|---|
| **What is the storage temperature of an organ?** | 4°C—keep on ice in a cooler |
| **Why should it be kept cold?** | Cold decreases the rate of chemical reactions; decreased energy use minimizes effects of hypoxia and ischemia. |
| **What is U-W solution?** | University of Wisconsin solution; used to perfuse an organ prior to removal from the donor |
| **What is in it?** | Potassium phosphate, buffers, starch, steroids, insulin, electrolytes, adenosine |
| **Why should it be used?** | Lengthens organ preservation time |

## MAXIMUM TIME BETWEEN HARVEST AND TRANSPLANT OF ORGAN

| | |
|---|---|
| **Heart?** | 6 hours |
| **Lungs?** | 6 hours |
| **Pancreas?** | 24 hours |
| **Liver?** | 24 hours |
| **Kidney?** | Up to 72 hours |

## KIDNEY TRANSPLANT

| | |
|---|---|
| **In what year was the first transplant performed in man?** | 1954 |
| **By whom?** | Joseph E. Murray—1990 Nobel Prize winner in Medicine |

| | |
|---|---|
| **What are the indications for kidney transplant?** | Irreversible renal failure from: |
| | 1. Glomerulonephritis (leading cause) |
| | 2. Pyelonephritis |
| | 3. Polycystic kidney disease |
| | 4. Malignant HTN |
| | 5. Reflux pyelonephritis |
| | 6. Goodpasture's syndrome (antibasement membrane) |
| | 7. Congenital renal hyperplasia |
| | 8. Fabry's disease |
| | 9. Alport's syndrome |
| | 10. Renal cortical necrosis |
| | 11. Damage caused by type 1 diabetes mellitus |
| **Define renal failure.** | GFR <20% to 25% of normal; as GFR drops to 5% to 10% of normal, uremic symptoms begin (e.g., lethargy, seizures, neuropathy, electrolyte disorders) |
| **What is the most common cause for kidney transplant?** | **Diabetes** (25%) |

## STATISTICS

| | |
|---|---|
| **What are the sources of donor kidneys?** | Cadaveric (70%)<br>Living related donor (LRD; 30%) |
| **What survival rate is associated with cadaveric source?** | 90% at 1 year if HLA matched; 80% at 1 year if not HLA matched; 75% graft survival at 3 years |
| **What survival rate is associated with LRD?** | Between 90% and 95% patient survival at 3 years; 75% to 85% graft survival at 3 years |
| **What are the tests for compatibility?** | ABO, HLA typing |
| **If a choice of left or right donor kidney is available, which is preferred?** | Left—longer renal vein allows for easier anastomosis |
| **Should the placement of the kidney be hetero- or orthotopic?** | Heterotopic—retroperitoneal in the right lower quadrant or left lower quadrant above the inguinal ligament |

**Why?**

Preserves native kidneys, allows easy access to iliac vessels, places ureter close to the bladder, easy to biopsy kidney

**Define anastomoses of a heterotopic kidney transplant.**

1. Renal artery to iliac artery
2. Renal vein to iliac vein
3. Ureter to bladder

**What is the correct placement of the ureter?**

Submucosally through the bladder wall—decreases reflux

**What is the differential diagnosis of post–renal transplant fluid collection?**

**HAUL:**
**H**ematoma
**A**bscess
**U**rinoma
**L**ymphocele

**Why keep native kidneys?**

Increased morbidity if they are removed

**What is the indication for removal of native kidneys?**

Uncontrollable HTN, ongoing renal sepsis

## REJECTION

**What is the red flag that indicates rejection?**

Increasing creatinine

| | |
|---|---|
| **What is the differential diagnosis of increased creatinine?** | (Remember: "**-tion**") obstruc**tion,** dehydra**tion,** infec**tion,** intoxica**tion** (CSA); plus lymphocele, ATN |
| **What are the signs/ symptoms?** | Fever, malaise, HTN, ipsilateral leg edema, pain at transplant site, oliguria |
| **What is the workup for the following tests:** | |
| **U/S with Doppler?** | Look for fluid collection around the kidney, hydronephrosis, flow in vessels. |
| **Radionuclide scan?** | Look at flow and function. |
| **Biopsy?** | Distinguish between rejection and cyclosporine toxicity. |
| **What is the time course for return of normal renal function after transplant?** | LRD—3 to 5 days<br>Cadaveric—7 to 15 days |

## LIVER TRANSPLANT

| | |
|---|---|
| **Who performed the first liver transplant?** | Thomas Starzl (1963) |
| **What are the indications?** | Liver failure from:<br>1. Cirrhosis (leading indication in adults)<br>2. Budd-Chiari<br>3. Biliary atresia (leading indication in children)<br>4. Neonatal hepatitis<br>5. Chronic active hepatitis<br>6. Fulminant hepatitis with drug toxicity—acetaminophen<br>7. Sclerosing cholangitis<br>8. Caroli's disease<br>9. Subacute hepatic necrosis<br>10. Congenital hepatic fibrosis<br>11. Inborn errors of metabolism<br>12. Fibrolamellar hepatocellular carcinoma |

**What is the MELD score?**

The "**M**odel for **E**nd Stage **L**iver **D**isease" is the formula currently used to assign points for prioritizing position on the waiting list for cadaveric liver transplant. The MELD score is based on INR, bilirubin, and creatinine with extra points given for the presence of liver cancer.

**What is the test for compatibility?**

ABO typing

**What is the placement?**

Orthotopic

**What are the options for biliary drainage?**

1. Donor common bile to recipient common bile duct end to end
2. Roux-en-Y choledochojejunostomy

**What is the "piggyback technique"?**

The recipient vena cava is left in place. The donor infrahepatic IVC is oversewn. The donor superior IVC is anastomosed onto a cuff made from the recipient hepatic veins. Allows for greater hemodynamic stability of the recipient during OLT.

**How does Living Donor Liver Transplantation (LDLT) work?**

An adult donates a left lateral segment to a child or an adult donates a right lobe to another adult.

**What is a split liver transplant?**

A cadaveric liver is harvested and divided into two "halves" for two recipients. Usually a left lateral segment for a child and a right lobe for an adult.

**What is chronic liver rejection called?**

"Vanishing bile duct syndrome"

## REJECTION

**What are the red flags indicating rejection?**

Decreased bile drainage, increased serum bilirubin, increased LFTs

**What is the site of rejection?**

Rejection involves the biliary epithelium first and later the vascular endothelium.

**What is the workup with the following tests:**

**U/S with Doppler?** — Look at flow in portal vein, hepatic artery; rule out thrombosis, leaky anastomosis, infection (abscess).

**Cholangiogram?** — Look at bile ducts (easy to do; patients usually have a T-tube if they have primary biliary anastomosis).

**Biopsy?** — Especially important 3 to 6 weeks postoperatively, when CMV is of greatest concern

**Does hepatorenal syndrome renal function improve after liver transplant?** — Yes

## SURVIVAL STATISTICS

**What is the 1-year survival rate?** — Approximately 80% to 85%

**What percentage of patients require retransplant?** — Approximately 20%

**Why?** — Usually primary graft dysfunction, rejection, infection, vascular thrombosis, or recurrence of primary disease

## PANCREAS TRANSPLANT

**Who performed the first pancreas transplant?** — Richard C. Lillehei and William D. Kelly (1966)

**What are the indications?** — Type I (juvenile) diabetes mellitus associated with severe complications (renal failure, blindness, neuropathy) or very poor glucose control

**What are the tests for compatibility?** — ABO, DR matching (class II)

**What is the placement?** — Heterotopic, in iliac fossa or paratopic

**Where is anastomosis of the exocrine duct in heterotopic placement?**

To the bladder

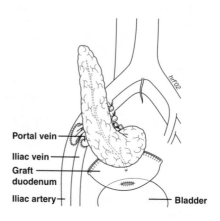

Portal vein
Iliac vein
Graft duodenum
Iliac artery
Bladder

**Why?**

Measures the amount of amylase in urine, gives an indication of pancreatic function (i.e., high urine amylase indicates good pancreatic function)

**What is the associated electrolyte complication?**

Loss of bicarbonate

**Where is anastomosis of the exocrine duct in paratopic placement?**

To the jejunum

**Why?**

It is close by and physiologic.

**What is the advantage of paratopic placement?**

Endocrine function drains to the portal vein directly to the liver, and pancreatic contents stay within the GI tract (no need to replace bicarbonate).

**What are the red flags indicating rejection?**

Hyperamylasemia, hyperglycemia, hypoamylasuria, graft tenderness

**Why should the kidney and pancreas be transplanted together?**

Kidney function is a better indicator of rejection; also better survival of graft is associated with kidney-pancreas transplant than pancreas alone.

**Why is hyperglycemia not a good indicator for rejection surveillance?**

Hyperglycemia appears relatively late with pancreatic rejection

## HEART TRANSPLANT

**Who performed the first heart transplant?**

Christiaan Barnard (1967)

**What are the indications?**

Age birth to 65 years with terminal acquired heart disease—class IV of New York Heart Association classification (inability to do any physical activity without discomfort = 10% chance of surviving 6 months)

**What are the contraindications?**

Active infection
Poor pulmonary function
Increased pulmonary artery resistance

**What are the tests for compatibility?**

ABO, size

**What is the placement?**

Orthotopic anastomosis of atria, aorta, pulmonary artery

**What is sewn together in a heart transplant?**

The donor heart atriums, pulmonary artery, and aorta are sewn to the recipient heart atriums, pulmonary artery, and aorta.

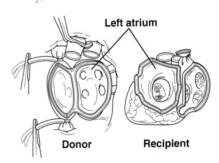

Left atrium

Donor        Recipient

**What are the red flags of rejection?**

Fever, hypotension or hypertension, increased T4/T8 ratio

| | |
|---|---|
| **What are the tests for rejection?** | Endomyocardial biopsy—much more important than clinical signs/symptoms; patient undergoes routine biopsy |
| **What are survival statistics for:** | |
|     **1 year?** | 85% |
|     **5 years?** | 65% |

## INTESTINAL TRANSPLANTATION

| | |
|---|---|
| **What is it?** | Transplantation of the small bowel |
| **What are transplant anastomoses?** | Donor SMA to recipient aorta<br>Donor SMV to recipient portal vein |
| **What are indications?** | Short gut syndrome and inability to sustain TPN (liver failure, lack of venous access, etc.) |
| **What percentage of intestinal transplant recipients have an episode of rejection in the first 6 months?** | > 90% |
| **What is a common postoperative problem other than rejection?** | GVHD (graft versus host disease) from large lymphoid tissue in transplanted intestines |
| **What is the most common cause of death postoperatively?** | **Sepsis** |
| **How is rejection surveillance conducted?** | Endoscopic biopsies |
| **What is graft survival for:** | |
|     **1 year?** | 65% |
|     **3 years?** | 50% |
|     **5 years?** | 15% |

## LUNG TRANSPLANT

| | |
|---|---|
| **Who performed the first lung transplant?** | James Hardy (1963) |
| **What are the indications?** | Generally, a disease that substantially limits activities of daily living and is likely to result in death within 12 to 18 months:<br>Pulmonary fibrosis<br>COPD<br>Eosinophilic granuloma<br>Primary pulmonary HTN<br>Eisenmenger's syndrome<br>Cystic fibrosis |
| **What are the contraindications?** | Current smoking<br>Active infection |
| **What tests comprise the pretransplant assessment of the recipient?** | 1. Pulmonary—PFTs, V/Q scan<br>2. Cardiac—Echo, cath, angiogram<br>3. Exercise tolerance test |
| **What are the donor requirements?** | 1. 55 years of age or younger<br>2. Clear chest film<br>3. PA oxygen tension of 300 on 100% oxygen and 5 cm PEEP<br>4. No purulent secretions on bronchoscopy |
| **What are necessary anastomoses?** | Bronchi, PA, pulmonary veins (Bronchial artery is not necessary.) |
| **What are the postop complications?** | Bronchial necrosis/stricture, reperfusion, pulmonary edema, rejection |
| **What are the red flags of rejection (4)?** | 1. Decreased arterial $O_2$ tension<br>2. Fever<br>3. Increased fatigability<br>4. Infiltrate on x-ray |
| **What is chronic lung rejection called?** | Obliterative bronchiolitis (OB) |

**What are the survival rates:**

   **1 year?**                      71%

   **5 yrs?**                        45%

## TRANSPLANT COMPLICATIONS

| | |
|---|---|
| **What are four major complications?** | 1. Infection<br>2. Rejection<br>3. Post-transplant lymphoproliferative disease<br>4. Complications of steroids |

### INFECTION

| | |
|---|---|
| **What are the usual agents?** | DNA viruses, especially CMV, HSV, VZV |
| **When should CMV infection be suspected?** | More than 21 days post-transplant |
| **What is the time of peak incidence of CMV infections?** | 4 to 6 weeks post-transplant |
| **What are the signs/symptoms of CMV?** | Fever, neutropenia, signs of rejection of transplant; also can present as viral pneumonitis, hepatitis, colitis |
| **How is CMV diagnosed?** | Biopsy of transplant to differentiate rejection, cultures of blood, urine |
| **What is the treatment of CMV?** | Ganciclovir, with or without immunoglobin; foscarnet |
| **What are the complications of ganciclovir?** | Bone marrow suppression |
| **What are the signs/symptoms of HSV?** | Herpetic lesions, shingles, fever, neutropenia, rejection of transplant |
| **What is the treatment of HSV?** | Acyclovir until patient is asymptomatic |

MALIGNANCY

| | |
|---|---|
| **What are the most common types?** | Skin/lip cancer (40%), B-cell cancer, cervical cancer in women, T-cell lymphoma, Kaposi's sarcoma |
| **Which epithelial cancers are important after transplant?** | Skin/lip cancer, especially basal cell and squamous cell |
| **What is post-transplant lymphoma associated with?** | Multiple doses of OKT3<br>EBV<br>Young > elderly |
| **What is the treatment for post-transplant lympho-proliferative disease (PTLD)?** | 1. Drastically reduce immunosuppression<br>2. ± Radiation<br>3. ± Chemotherapy |

# Chapter 74

# Orthopaedic Surgery

## ORTHOPAEDIC TERMS

**What do the following abbreviations stand for:**

| | |
|---|---|
| ORIF? | **O**pen **R**eduction **I**nternal **F**ixation |
| ROM? | **R**ange **O**f **M**otion |
| FROM? | **F**ull **R**ange **O**f **M**otion |
| ACL? | **A**nterior **C**ruciate **L**igament |
| PCL? | **P**osterior **C**ruciate **L**igament |
| MCL? | **M**edial **C**ollateral **L**igament |
| PWB? | **P**artial **W**eight **B**earing |
| FWB? | **F**ull **W**eight **B**earing |
| WBAT? | **W**eight **B**earing **A**s **T**olerated |
| THA? | **T**otal **H**ip **A**rthroplasty |
| TKA? | **T**otal **K**nee **A**rthroplasty |
| THR? | **T**otal **H**ip **R**eplacement |
| TKR? | **T**otal **K**nee **R**eplacement |

| | |
|---|---|
| **PROM?** | **P**assive **R**ange **O**f **M**otion |
| **AROM?** | **A**ctive **R**ange **O**f **M**otion |
| **AFO?** | **A**nkle **F**oot **O**rthotic |
| **AVN?** | **AV**ascular **N**ecrosis |

**Define the following terms:**

| | |
|---|---|
| **Supination** | Palm up |
| **Pronation** | Palm down |
| **Plantarflexion** | Foot down at ankle joint (plant foot in ground) |
| **Foot dorsiflexion** | Foot up at ankle joint |
| **Adduction** | Movement toward the body (**ADD**uction = **ADD** to the body) |
| **Abduction** | Movement away from the body |
| **Inversion** | Foot sole faces midline |
| **Eversion** | Foot sole faces laterally |
| **Volarflexion** | Hand flexes at wrist joint toward flexor tendons |
| **Wrist dorsiflexion** | Hand flexes at wrist joint toward extensor tendons |
| **Allograft bone** | Bone from human donor other than patient |
| **Reduction** | Maneuver to restore proper alignment to fracture or joint |
| **Closed reduction** | Reduction done without surgery (e.g., casts, splints) |
| **Open reduction** | Surgical reduction |
| **Fixation** | Stabilization of a fracture after reduction by means of surgical placement of hardware that can be external or internal (e.g., pins, plates, screws) |

**Tibial pin**

Pin placed in the tibia for treating femur or pelvic fractures by applying skeletal traction.

**Unstable fracture or dislocation**

Fracture or dislocation in which further deformation will occur if reduction is **not** performed

**Varus**

Extremity abnormality with apex of defect pointed away from midline (e.g., genu varum = bowlegged; with valgus, this term can also be used to describe fracture displacement)

Think: knees are very **varied** apart

**Valgus**

Extremity abnormality with apex of defect pointed toward the midline (e.g., genu valgus = knock-kneed)

**Dislocation**

Total loss of congruity and contact between articular surfaces of a joint

**Subluxation**

Loss of congruity between articular surfaces of a joint; articular contact still remains

**Arthroplasty**

Total joint replacement (most last 10 to 15 years)

**Arthrodesis**

Joint fusion with removal of articular surfaces

**Osteotomy**

Cutting bone (usually wedge resection) to help realigning of joint surfaces

**Non-union**

Failure of fractured bone ends to fuse

**Define each of the following:**

**Diaphysis**

Main shaft of long bone

**Metaphysis**

Flared end of long bone

**Physis**

Growth plate, found only in immature bone

## TRAUMA GENERAL PRINCIPLES

**Define extremity examination in fractured extremities.**

1. Observe entire extremity (e.g., open, angulation, joint disruption).
2. Neurologic (sensation, movement)
3. Vascular (e.g., pulses, cap refill)

**Which x-rays should be obtained?**

Two views (also joint above and below fracture)

**How are fractures described?**

1. Skin status (open or closed)
2. Bone (by thirds: proximal/middle/distal)
3. Pattern of fracture (e.g., comminuted)
4. Alignment (displacement, angulation, rotation)

**How do you define the degree of angulation, displacement, or both?**

Define lateral/medial/anterior/posterior displacement and angulation of the distal fragment(s) in relation to the proximal bone.

**Identify each numbered structure:**

1. Diaphysis
2. Metaphysis
3. Physis
4. Epiphysis

## FRACTURES

**Define the following patterns of fracture:**

**Closed fracture**

Intact skin over fracture/hematoma

**Open fracture**

Wound overlying fracture, through which fracture fragments are in continuity with outside environment; high risk of infection
*Note*: Called compound fracture in the past

**Simple fracture**

One fracture line, two bone fragments

**Comminuted fracture**

Results in more than two bone fragments; also known as fragmentation

Comminuted fracture

**Transverse fracture**

Fracture line perpendicular to long axis of bone

Transverse fracture

**Oblique fracture**

Fracture line creates an oblique angle with long axis of bone

Oblique fracture

**Spiral fracture**

Severe oblique fracture in which fracture plane rotates along the long axis of bone; caused by a twisting injury

Spiral fracture

**Longitudinal fracture**

Fracture line parallel to long axis of bone

**Impacted fracture**

Fracture resulting from compressive force; end of bone is driven into contiguous metaphyseal region without displacement

**Pathologic fracture**

Fracture through abnormal bone (e.g., tumor-laden or osteoporotic bone)

**Stress fracture**

Fracture in normal bone from cyclic loading on bone

**Greenstick fracture**          Incomplete fracture in which cortex on
                                 only one side is disrupted; seen in children

Greenstick fracture

**Torus fracture**               Impaction injury in children in which
                                 cortex is buckled but not disrupted
                                 (A.K.A. buckle fracture)

**Avulsion fracture**            Fracture in which tendon is pulled from
                                 bone, carrying with it a bone chip

Avulsion fracture

**Periarticular fracture**       Fracture close to but not involving the
                                 joint

**Intra-articular fracture**     Fracture through the articular surface of
                                 a bone (usually requires ORIF)

**Define the following specific
fractures:**
  **Colles' fracture**           **Distal radius** fracture with dorsal
                                 displacement and angulation, usually
                                 from falling on an outstretched hand;
                                 (a common fracture!)

**Smith's fracture**

"Reverse Colles' fracture"—distal radial fracture with volar displacement and angulation, usually from falling on the **dorsum** of the hand (uncommon)

**Jones' fracture**

Fracture at the base of the fifth metatarsal diaphysis

**Bennett's fracture**

Fracture-dislocation of the base of the first metacarpal with disruption of the carpometacarpal joint

**Boxer's fracture**

Fracture of the metacarpal neck, "classically" of the small finger

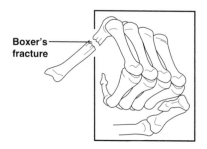

Boxer's fracture

| | |
|---|---|
| **Night stick fracture** | Ulnar fracture |
| **Clay shoveler's avulsion fracture** | Fracture of spinous process of C6-C7 |
| **Hangman's fracture** | Fracture of the pedicles of C2 |
| **Transcervical fracture** | Fracture through the neck of the femur |
| **Tibial plateau fracture** | Intra-articular fracture of the proximal tibia (the plateau is the flared proximal end) |
| **Monteggia fracture** | Fracture of the proximal third of the ulna with dislocation of the radial head |
| **Galeazzi fracture** | Fracture of the radius at the junction of the middle and distal thirds accompanied by disruption of the distal radioulnar joint |
| **Tibial "plateau" fracture** | Proximal tibial fracture |

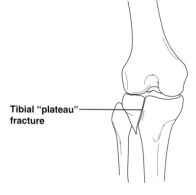

Tibial "plateau" fracture

**"Pilon" fracture**                    Distal tibial fracture

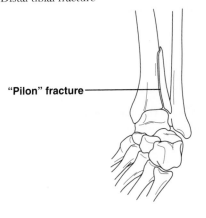

"Pilon" fracture———

**Pott's fracture**                     Fracture of distal fibula

**Pott's disease**                      Tuberculosis of the spine

## ORTHOPAEDIC TRAUMA

**What are the major
orthopaedic emergencies?**

1. Open fractures/dislocations
2. Vascular injuries (e.g., knee dislocation)
3. Compartment syndromes
4. Neural compromise, especially spinal injury
5. Osteomyelitis/septic arthritis; acute, i.e., when aspiration is indicated
6. Hip dislocations—require immediate reduction or patient will develop avascular necrosis; "reduce on the x-ray table"
7. Exsanguinating pelvic fracture (binder, external fixator)

**What is the main risk
when dealing with an open
fracture?**

Infection

**Which fracture has the
highest mortality?**

Pelvic fracture (up to 50% with open pelvic fractures)

**What factors determine the extent of injury?**

1. Age: suggests susceptible point in musculoskeletal system:
   Child—growth plate
   Adolescent—ligaments
   Elderly—metaphyseal bone
2. Direction of forces
3. Magnitude of forces

**What is the acronym for indications for OPEN reduction?**

**"NO CAST":**
**N**onunion
**O**pen fracture

**C**ompromise of blood supply
**A**rticular surface malalignment
**S**alter-Harris grade III, IV fracture
**T**rauma patients who need early ambulation

**How are open fractures classified:**
**Grade I?**

<1-cm laceration

**Grade II?**

>1-cm and <10-cm laceration

**Grade IIIA?**

Open fracture with massive tissue devitalization/loss

**Grade IIIB?**

Open fracture with massive tissue devitalization/loss and extensive periosteal stripping or extensive gross contamination

**Grade IIIC?**

Open fracture with massive tissue devitalization/loss and major vascular injury requiring repair

**What is the initial treatment of an open fracture?**

1. Prophylactic antibiotics to include IV gram-positive ± anaerobic coverage
   Grade I—cefazolin (Ancef®)
   Grade II or III—cefoxitin/gentamicin
2. Surgical débridement
3. Inoculation against tetanus
4. Lavage wound <6 hours postincident with high-pressure sterile irrigation
5. Open reduction of fracture and stabilization (e.g., use of external fixation)

**What structures are at risk with a humeral fracture?**

Radial nerve, brachial artery

**What must be done when both forearm bones are broken?**

Because precise movements are needed, open reduction and internal fixation are musts.

**How have femoral fractures been repaired traditionally?**

Traction for 4 to 6 weeks

**What is the newer technique?**

Intramedullary rod placement

**What are the advantages?**

Nearly immediate mobility with decreased morbidity/mortality

**What is the chief concern following tibial fractures?**

Recognition of associated compartment syndrome

**What is suggested by pain in the anatomic snuff-box?**

Fracture of scaphoid bone (A.K.A. navicular fracture)

**What is the most common cause of a "pathologic" fracture in adults?**

Osteoporosis

## COMPARTMENT SYNDROME

**What is acute compartment syndrome?**

Increased pressure within an osteofascial compartment that can lead to ischemic necrosis

**How is it diagnosed?**

Clinically, using intracompartmental pressures is also helpful (especially in unresponsive patients). Fasciotomy is clearly indicated if pressure in the compartment is >40 mm Hg (30 to 40 mm Hg is a gray area).

**What are the causes?**

Fractures, vascular compromise, reperfusion injury, compressive dressings; can occur after any musculoskeletal injury

| | |
|---|---|
| **What are common causes of forearm compartment syndrome?** | Supracondylar humerus fracture, brachial artery injury, radius/ulna fracture, crush injury |
| **What is Volkmann's contracture?** | The final sequela of forearm compartment syndrome; **contracture** of the forearm flexors from replacement of dead muscle with fibrous tissue |
| **What is the most common site of compartment syndrome?** | Calf (four compartments: anterior, lateral, deep posterior, superficial posterior compartments) |
| **What situations should immediately alert one to be on the lookout for a developing compartment syndrome?** | 1. Supracondylar elbow fractures in children<br>2. Proximal/midshaft tibial fractures<br>3. Electrical burns<br>4. Arterial/venous disruption |
| **What are the symptoms of compartment syndrome?** | Pain, paresthesias, paralysis |
| **What are the signs of compartment syndrome?** | Pain on passive movement (out of proportion to injury), cyanosis or pallor, hypoesthesia (decreased sensation, decreased two point discrimination), firm compartment |
| **Can a patient have a compartment syndrome with a palpable or Doppler-detectable distal pulse?** | YES! |
| **What are the possible complications of compartment syndrome?** | Muscle necrosis, nerve damage, contractures, myoglobinuria |
| **What is the initial treatment of the orthopaedic patient developing compartment syndrome?** | Bivalve and split casts, remove constricting clothes/dressings, place extremity at heart level |
| **What is the definitive treatment of compartment syndrome?** | Fasciotomy within 4 hours (6 to 8 hours maximum) if at all possible |

MISCELLANEOUS TRAUMA INJURIES AND COMPLICATIONS

| | |
|---|---|
| **Name the motor and sensation tests used to assess the following peripheral nerves:** | |
| **Radial** | Wrist extension; dorsal web space; sensation: between thumb and index finger |
| **Ulnar** | Little finger abduction; sensation: little finger-distal ulnar aspect |
| **Median** | Thumb opposition or thumb pinch sensation: index finger-distal radial aspect |
| **Axillary** | Arm abduction; sensation: deltoid patch on lateral aspect of upper arm |
| **Musculocutaneous** | Elbow (biceps) flexion; lateral forearm sensation |
| **How is a peripheral nerve injury treated?** | Controversial, although clean lacerations may be repaired primarily; most injuries are followed for 6 to 8 weeks (EMG) |
| **What fracture is associated with a calcaneus fracture?** | L-spine fracture (usually from a fall) |
| **Name the nerves of the brachial plexus.** | Think: "morning rum" or **"A.M. RUM"** = **A**xillary, **M**edian, then **R**adial, **U**lnar, and **M**usculocutaneous nerves |
| **What are the indications for operative exploration with a peripheral nerve injury?** | 1. Loss of nerve function *after* reduction of fracture<br>2. No EMG signs of nerve regeneration after 8 weeks (nerve graft) |

## DISLOCATIONS

### SHOULDER

| | |
|---|---|
| **What is the most common type?** | 95% are anterior (posterior are associated with seizures or electrical shock). |
| **Which structures are at risk?** | Axillary nerve and axillary artery |

| | |
|---|---|
| **How is it diagnosed?** | Indentation of soft tissue beneath acromion |
| **What is the treatment?** | 1. Reduction via gradual traction<br>2. Immobilization for 3 weeks in internal rotation<br>3. ROM exercises |

## ELBOW

| | |
|---|---|
| **What is the most common type?** | Posterior |
| **Which structures are at risk?** | Brachial artery, ulnar nerve, median nerve |
| **What is the treatment?** | Reduce and splint for 7 to 10 days. |

## HIP

| | |
|---|---|
| **When should hip dislocations be reduced?** | Immediately, to decrease risk of avascular necrosis; "reduce on the x-ray table!" |
| **What is the most common cause of a hip dislocation?** | High velocity trauma (e.g., MVA) |
| **What is the most common type?** | Posterior—"dashboard dislocation"—often involves fracture of posterior lip of acetabulum |
| **Which structures are at risk?** | Sciatic nerve; blood supply to femoral head—avascular necrosis (AVN) |
| **What is the treatment?** | Closed or open reduction |

## KNEE

| | |
|---|---|
| **What are the common types?** | Anterior or posterior |
| **Which structures are at risk?** | Popliteal artery and vein, peroneal nerve—especially with posterior dislocation, ACL, PCL (*Note:* need arteriogram) |

**What is the treatment?**　　Immediate attempt at relocation (do not wait to x-ray), arterial repair, and then ligamentous repair (delayed or primary)

## THE KNEE

**What are the ligaments of the knee?**　　Anterior cruciate ligament (ACL), posterior cruciate ligament (PCL), medial collateral ligament (MCL), lateral collateral ligament (LCL), patellar ligament

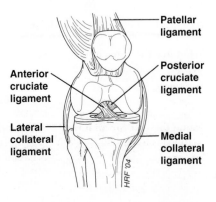

**What is the "anterior drawer test" of the knee?**　　Test to ascertain the anterior stability of the knee and integrity of the ACL
Knee is placed in 90° flexion and pulled forward (like opening a drawer). If tibia is pulled forward, test is positive and consistent with an ACL tear.

| | |
|---|---|
| **What is the meniscus of the knee?** | The cartilage surface of the tibia plateau (lateral and medial meniscus); tears are repaired usually by arthroscopy with removal of torn cartilage fragments |
| **What is Mcmurray's sign?** | Seen with a medial meniscus tear: medial tenderness of knee with flexion and internal rotation of the knee |
| **What is the "unhappy triad"?** | Lateral knee injury resulting in ACL tear, MCL tear, and a medial meniscus injury |

## ACHILLES TENDON RUPTURE

| | |
|---|---|
| **What are the signs of an Achilles tendon rupture?** | Severe calf pain, also bruised swollen calf, two ends of ruptured tendon may be felt, patient will have weak plantar flexion from great toe flexors that should be intact |
| **Name the test for an intact Achilles tendon.** | **Thompson's test:** a squeeze of the gastrocnemius muscle results in plantar flexion of the foot |

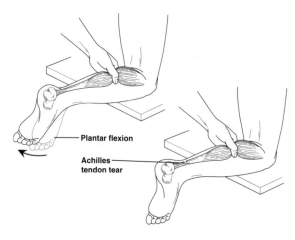

## ROTATOR CUFF

| | |
|---|---|
| **What muscles form the rotator cuff?** | 1. **S**upraspinatus (acronym = **"SITS"**) <br> 2. **I**nfraspinatus <br> 3. **T**eres minor <br> 4. **S**ubscapularis |

| | |
|---|---|
| **When do tears usually occur?** | Fifth decade |
| **What is the usual history?** | Intermittent shoulder pain especially with **overhead** activity, followed by an episode of acute pain corresponding to a tendon tear; weak abduction |
| **What is the treatment?** | Most tears: symptomatic pain relief Later: if poor muscular function persists, surgical repair is indicated |
| **What is Volkmann's contracture?** | Contracture of forearm flexors secondary to **forearm compartment syndrome** |
| **What is the usual cause of Volkmann's contracture?** | Brachial artery injury, **supracondylar humerus fracture,** radius/ulnar fracture, crush injury, etc. |

## MISCELLANEOUS

| | |
|---|---|
| **Define the following terms:** | |
| **Dupuytren's contracture** | Thickening and contracture of palmar fascia; incidence increases with age |
| **Charcot's joint** | Joint arthritis from peripheral neuropathy |
| **Tennis elbow** | Tendonitis of the lateral epicondyle of the humerus (classically seen in tennis players) |
| **Turf toe** | Hyperextension of the great toe (tear of the tendon of the flexor hallucis brevis); classically seen in football players |
| **Shin splints** | Exercise-induced anterior compartment hypertension (compartment syndrome); seen in runners |
| **Heel spur** | Plantar fasciitis with abnormal bone growth in the plantar fascia Classically seen in runners and walkers |
| **Nightstick fracture** | Ulnar fracture |
| **Kienbock's disease** | Avascular necrosis of the lunate |

**What is traumatic myositis?**　Abnormal bone deposit in a muscle after blunt trauma deep muscle contusion (benign)

**How does a "cast saw" cut the cast but not the underlying skin?**　It is an "oscillating" saw (designed by Dr. Homer Stryker in 1947) that goes back and forth cutting anything hard while moving the skin back and forth without injuring it.

## ORTHOPAEDIC INFECTIONS

### OSTEOMYELITIS

**What is osteomyelitis?**　Inflammation/infection of bone marrow and adjacent bone

**What are the most likely causative organisms?**　Neonates: *Staphylococcus aureus,* gram-negative *streptococcus*
Children: *S. aureus, Haemophilus influenzae,* streptococci
Adults: *S. aureus*
Immunocompromised/drug addicts: *S. aureus* gram-negative
Sickle cell: *Salmonella*

**What is the most common organism isolated in osteomyelitis in the general adult population?**　*S. aureus*

**What is the most common isolated organism in patients with sickle cell disease?**　*Salmonella*

**What is seen on physical examination?**　Tenderness, decreased movement, swelling

**What are the diagnostic steps?**　History and physical examination, needle aspirate, blood cultures, CBC, ESR, bone scan

**What are the treatment options?**　Antibiotics with or without surgical drainage

| | |
|---|---|
| **What is a Marjolin's ulcer?** | Squamous cell carcinoma that arises in a chronic sinus from osteomyelitis |

## SEPTIC ARTHRITIS

| | |
|---|---|
| **What is septic arthritis?** | Inflammation of a joint beginning as synovitis and ending with destruction of articular cartilage if left untreated |
| **What are the causative agents?** | Same as in osteomyelitis, except that gonococcus is a common agent in the adult population |
| **What are the findings on physical examination?** | Joint pain, decreased motion, joint swelling, joint warm to the touch |
| **What are the diagnostic steps?** | Needle aspirate (look for pus; culture plus Gram stain), x-ray, blood cultures, ESR |
| **What is the treatment?** | Decompression of the joint via needle aspiration and IV antibiotics; hip, shoulder, and spine must be surgically incised, débrided, and drained |

## ORTHOPAEDIC TUMORS

| | |
|---|---|
| **What is the most common type in adults?** | Metastatic! |
| **What are the common sources?** | Breast, lung, prostate, kidney, thyroid, and multiple myeloma |
| **What is the usual presentation?** | Bone pain or as a pathologic fracture |
| **What is the most common primary malignant bone tumor?** | Multiple myeloma (45%) |
| **What is the differential diagnosis of a possible bone tumor?** | 1. Metastatic disease<br>2. Primary bone tumors<br>3. Metabolic disorders (e.g., hyperparathyroidism)<br>4. Infection |

| | |
|---|---|
| **What are the benign bone tumors (8)?** | 1. Osteochondroma<br>2. Enchondroma<br>3. Unicameral/aneurysmal bone cysts<br>4. Osteoid osteoma<br>5. Chondroblastoma<br>6. Fibroxanthoma<br>7. Fibrous dysplasia<br>8. Nonossifying fibroma |
| **What are the malignant bone tumors (7)?** | 1. Multiple myeloma<br>2. Osteosarcoma<br>3. Chondrosarcoma<br>4. Ewing's sarcoma<br>5. Giant cell tumor (locally malignant)<br>6. Malignant melanoma<br>7. Metastatic |
| **Compare benign and malignant bone tumors in terms of:** | |
| **Size** | Benign—small; <1 cm<br>Malignant— >1 cm |
| **Bone reaction** | Benign—sclerotic bone reaction<br>Malignant—little reaction |
| **Margins** | Benign—sharp<br>Malignant—poorly defined |
| **Invasive** | Benign—confined to bone<br>Malignant—often extends to surrounding tissues |
| **Are most pediatric bone tumors benign or malignant?** | 80% are benign (most common is osteochondroma). |
| **Are most adult bone tumors benign or malignant?** | 66% are malignant (most commonly metastatic). |
| **What are the diagnostic steps?** | 1. PE/lab tests<br>2. Radiographs<br>3. CT scan, technetium scan, or both<br>4. Biopsy |

| | |
|---|---|
| **What are radiographic signs of malignant tumors?** | Large size<br>Aggressive bone destruction, poorly<br>    defined margins<br>Ineffective bone reaction to tumor<br>Extension to soft tissues |
| **What are the radiographic signs of benign tumor?** | Small<br>Well circumscribed, sharp margins<br>Effective bone reaction to the tumor<br>    (sclerotic periostitis)<br>No extension—confined to bone |
| **What are some specific radiographic findings of the following:**<br>    **Osteosarcoma?** | "Sunburst pattern" |
|     **Fibrous dysplasia** | Bubbly lytic lesion "ground glass" |
|     **Ewing's sarcoma** | "Onion skinning" |
| **What is the mainstay of treatment for bone tumors?** | Surgery (excision plus débridement)<br>for both malignant and benign lesions;<br>radiation therapy and chemotherapy as<br>adjuvant therapy for many malignant<br>tumors |

## OSTEOSARCOMA

| | |
|---|---|
| **What is the usual age at presentation?** | Between 10 and 20 years |
| **What is the gender distribution?** | Men > women |
| **What is the most common location?** | Approximately two-thirds in the distal femur, proximal tibia |
| **What is the radiographic sine qua non?** | Bone formation somewhere within tumor |
| **What is the treatment?** | Resection (limb sparing if possible) plus chemotherapy |
| **What is the 5-year survival rate?** | Approximately 70% |

| | |
|---|---|
| **What is the most common site of metastasis?** | Lungs |
| **What is the most common benign bone tumor?** | **Osteochondroma;** it is cartilaginous in origin and may undergo malignant degeneration |
| **What is a chondrosarcoma?** | Malignant tumor of cartilaginous origin; presents in middle-aged and older patients and is unresponsive to chemotherapy and radiotherapy |

## EWING'S SARCOMA

| | |
|---|---|
| **What is the usual presentation?** | Pain, swelling in involved area |
| **What is the most common location?** | Around the knee (distal femur, proximal tibia) |
| **What is the usual age at presentation?** | Evenly spread among those younger than 20 years of age |
| **What are the associated radiographic findings?** | Lytic lesion with periosteal reaction termed "onion skinning," which is calcified layering<br><br>Central areas of tumor can undergo liquefaction necrosis, which may be confused with purulent infection (particularly in a child with fever, leukocytosis, and bone pain). |
| **What is a memory aid for Ewing's sarcoma?** | "**TKO** Ewing":<br>**T**wenty years old or younger<br>**K**nee joint<br>"**O**nion skinning" |
| **What is the 5-year survival rate?** | 50% |
| **How can Ewing's sarcoma mimic the appearance of osteomyelitis?** | Bone cysts |

| | |
|---|---|
| **What is a unicameral bone cyst?** | Fluid-filled cyst most commonly found in the proximal humerus in children 5 to 15 years of age |
| **What is the usual presentation?** | Asymptomatic until pathologic fracture |
| **What is the treatment?** | Steroid injections |
| **What is an aneurysmal bone cyst?** | A hemorrhagic lesion that is locally destructive by expansile growth, but does not metastasize |
| **What is the usual presentation?** | Pain and swelling; pathologic fractures are rare |
| **What is the treatment?** | Curettage and bone grafting |

## ARTHRITIS

| | |
|---|---|
| **Which arthritides are classified as degenerative?** | Osteoarthritis<br>Post-traumatic arthritis |
| **What signs characterize osteoarthritis?** | Heberden's nodes/Bouchard's nodes<br>**Symmetric** destruction, usually of the hip, knee, or spine |
| **What are Bouchard's nodes?** | Enlarged PIP joints of the hand from cartilage/bone growth |
| **What are Heberden's nodes?** | Enlarged DIP joints of the hand from cartilage/bone growth |
| **What is post-traumatic arthritis?** | Usually involves one joint of past trauma |
| **What are the treatment options for degenerative arthritis?** | 1. NSAIDS for acute flare-ups, **not** for long-term management<br>2. Local corticosteroid injections<br>3. Surgery |

| | |
|---|---|
| **What are the characteristics of rheumatoid arthritis?** | Autoimmune reaction in which invasive pannus attacks hyaline articular cartilage, rheumatoid factor (anti-IgG/IgM) in 80% of patients, three times more common in women, skin nodules (e.g., rheumatoid nodule) |
| **What is pannus?** | Inflammatory exudate overlying synovial cells inside the joint |
| **What are the classic hand findings with rheumatoid arthritis?** | Wrist: radial deviation<br>Fingers: ulnar deviation |
| **What are the surgical management options for joint/bone diseases?** | 1. Arthroplasty<br>2. Arthrodesis (fusion)<br>3. Osteotomy |
| **What is the major difference between gout and pseudogout?** | Gout: caused by urate deposition, negative birefringent, needle crystal<br>Pseudogout: caused by calcium pyrophosphate positive birefringent square crystals (think: **P**ositive **S**quare crystals = **PS**eudogout) |
| **What is a Charcot's joint?** | Arthritic joint from peripheral neuropathy |

## PEDIATRIC ORTHOPAEDICS

| | |
|---|---|
| **What are the major differences between pediatric and adult bones?** | Children: increased bone flexibility and bone healing (thus, many fractures are treated closed, whereas an adult would require O.R.I.F.), physis (weak point) |
| **What types of fractures are unique to children?** | Greenstick fracture<br>Torus fracture<br>Fracture through physis |

### SALTER CLASSIFICATION

| | |
|---|---|
| **What does it describe?** | Fractures in children involving physis |
| **What does it indicate high risk of?** | Potential growth arrest |

**Define the following terms:**

**Salter I**                     Through physeal plate only

**Salter II**                    Involves physis and metaphysis

**Salter III**                   Involves physis and epiphysis

**Salter IV**                    Extends from metaphysis through physis,
                                 into epiphysis

**Salter V**                     Axial force crushes physeal plate

**Define the following
fractures by Salter-Harris
grade:**

                   Salter III

                   Salter IV

                   Salter I

Salter V

Salter II

**What acronym can help you remember the Salter classifications?**

**"SALTR":**
**S**eparated = type I
**A**bove = type II
**L**ower = type III
**T**hrough = type IV
**R**uined = type V

**What is the simple numerical method for remembering the Salter-Harris classification?**

| | |
|---|---|
| **Why is the growth plate of concern in childhood fractures?** | The growth plate represents the "weak link" in the child's musculoskeletal system. Fractures involving the growth plate of long bones may compromise normal growth, so special attention should be given to them. |
| **What is a chief concern when oblique/spiral fractures of long bones are seen in children?** | Child abuse is a possibility; other signs of abuse should be investigated. |
| **What is usually done during reduction of a femoral fracture?** | A small amount of overlap is allowed because increased vascularity from injury may make the affected limb longer if overlap is not present. Treatment after reduction is a spica cast. |
| **What is unique about ligamentous injury in children?** | Most "ligamentous" injuries are actually fractures involving the growth plate! |
| **What two fractures have a high incidence of associated compartment syndrome?** | 1. Tibial fractures<br>2. Supracondylar fractures of humerus (Volkmann's contracture) |

## CONGENITAL HIP DISLOCATION

| | |
|---|---|
| **What is the epidemiology?** | Female > male, firstborn children, breech<br>Presentation, 1–1000 births |
| **What percentage are bilateral?** | 10% |
| **How is the diagnosis made?** | Barlow's maneuver, Ortolani's sign<br>Radiographic confirmation is required. |
| **What is Barlow's maneuver?** | Detects unstable hip: patient is placed in the supine position and attempt is made to push femurs posteriorly with knees at 90°/hip flexed and hip will dislocate (think: push **B**ack = **B**arlow) |

| | |
|---|---|
| **What is Ortolani's sign?** | The "clunk" produced by relocation of a dislocated femoral head when the examiner abducts the flexed hip and lifts the greater trochanter anteriorly; detects a dislocated hip (think: **O**ut = **O**rtolani's) |
| **What is the treatment?** | Pavlik harness—maintains hip reduction with hips flexed at 100° to 110° |

## SCOLIOSIS

| | |
|---|---|
| **What is the definition?** | Lateral curvature of a portion of the spine<br>Nonstructural: corrects with positional change<br>Structural: does not correct |
| **What are the treatment options?** | 1. Observation<br>2. Braces (Milwaukee brace)<br>3. Surgery |
| **What are the indications for surgery for scoliosis?** | Respiratory compromise<br>Rapid progressive<br>Curves more than 40°<br>Failure of brace |

## MISCELLANEOUS

| | |
|---|---|
| **Define the following terms:**<br>    **Legg-Calvé-Perthes disease** | Idiopathic avascular necrosis of femoral head in children |
|     **Slipped capital femoral epiphysis** | Migration of proximal femoral epiphysis on the metaphysis in children. The proximal femoral epiphysis externally rotates and displaces anteriorly from the capital femoral epiphysis, which stays reduced in the acetabulum.<br>*Note*: Hip pain in children often presents as knee pain. |
|     **Blount's disease** | Idiopathic varus bowing of tibia |
|     **Nursemaid's elbow** | Dislocation of radial head (from pulling toddler's arm) |

| | |
|---|---|
| **Little League elbow** | Medial epicondylitis |
| **Osgood-Schlatter's disease** | Apophysitis of the tibial tubercle resulting from repeated powerful contractions of the quadriceps; seen in adolescents with an open physis<br>Treatment of mild cases: activity restriction<br>Treatment of severe cases: cast |
| **What is the most common pediatric bone tumor?** | Osteochondroma (remember, 80% of bone tumors are benign in children) |

# Chapter 75     Neurosurgery

## HEAD TRAUMA

| | |
|---|---|
| **What is the incidence?** | 70,000 fatal injuries/year in the United States, 500,000 head injuries per year |
| **What percentage of trauma deaths result from head trauma?** | 50% |

**Identify the dermatomes:**

| | |
|---|---|
| **What is the Glasgow Coma Scale (GCS)?** | The GCS is an objective assessment of the level of consciousness after trauma. |

## GCS SCORING SYSTEM

**Eyes?**

**Eye Opening (E)**
4—opens spontaneously
3—opens to voice (command)
2—opens to painful stimulus
1—does not open eyes
(Think: "4 eyes")

**Motor?**

**Motor Response (M)**
6—obeys commands
5—localizes painful stimulus
4—withdraws from pain
3—decorticate posture
2—decerebrate posture
1—no movement
(Think: 6-cylinder motor)

**Verbal?**

**Verbal Response (V)**
5—appropriate and oriented
4—confused
3—inappropriate words
2—incomprehensible sounds
1—no sounds
(Think: Jackson 5 = verbal 5)

**What indicates coma by GCS score?**

<8 (think: "less than eight—it may be too late")

**What does unilateral, dilated, nonreactive pupil suggest?**

Focal mass lesion with ipsilateral herniation with compression of CN III

**What do bilateral fixed and dilated pupils suggest?**

Diffusely increased ICP

**What are the four signs of basilar skull fracture?**

1. **Raccoon eyes**—periorbital ecchymoses
2. **Battle's sign**—postauricular ecchymoses
3. **Hemotympanum**
4. **CSF** rhinorrhea/otorrhea

**What is the initial radiographic imaging in trauma?**

1. Head CT (if LOC or GCS < 15)
2. C-spine CT
3. T/L spine AP and lateral

**Should the trauma head CT be with or without IV contrast?**

Without!

**What is normal ICP?**

Between 5 and 15 mm $H_2O$

**What is the worrisome ICP?**

More than 20 mm $H_2O$

**What determines ICP (Monroe-Kelly hypothesis)?**

1. Volume of brain
2. Volume of blood
3. Volume of CSF

**What is the CPP?**

**C**erebral **P**erfusion **P**ressure = mean arterial pressure—ICP (normal CPP is >70)

**What is Cushing's reflex?**

Physiologic response to increased ICP:
1. Hypertension
2. Bradycardia
3. Decreased RR

**What are the general indications to monitor ICP after trauma?**

1. GCS <9
2. Altered level of consciousness or unconsciousness with multiple system trauma
3. Decreased consciousness with focal neurologic examination abnormality

**What is Kocher's point?**

Landmark for placement of ICP monitor bolt:

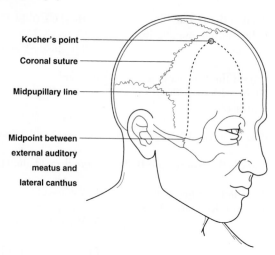

Kocher's point
Coronal suture
Midpupillary line
Midpoint between external auditory meatus and lateral canthus

| | |
|---|---|
| **What nonoperative techniques are used to decrease ICP?** | 1. **Elevate** head of bed (HOB) 30° (if spine cleared)<br>2. Diuresis-mannitol (osmotic diuretic), Lasix®, limit fluids<br>3. Intubation ($PCO_2$ control)<br>4. Sedation<br>5. Pharmacologic paralysis<br>6. Ventriculostomy (CSF drainage) |
| **What is the acronym for the treatment of elevated ICP?** | **ICP HEAD:**<br><br>**I**NTUBATE<br>**C**ALM (sedate)<br>**P**LACE DRAIN (ventriculostomy)/ PARALYSIS<br><br>**H**YPERVENTILATE TO $PCO_2 \approx 35$<br>**E**LEVATE head<br>**A**DEQUATE BLOOD PRESSURE (CPP >70)<br>**D**IURETIC (e.g., mannitol) |
| **Can a tight c-collar cause increased ICP?** | Yes (it blocks venous drainage from brain!) |
| **Why is prolonged hyperventilation dangerous?** | It may result in severe vasoconstriction and ischemic brain necrosis! Use only for very brief periods. |

| | |
|---|---|
| **What is a Kjellberg?** | Decompressive bifrontal craniectomy (pronounced "shellberg") with removal of frontal bone placed in freezer for possible later replacement |
| **How does cranial nerve examination localize the injury in a comatose patient?** | The CNs proceed caudally in the brain stem as numbered. Presence of corneal reflex (CN 5 + 7) indicates intact pons. Intact gag reflex (CN 9 + 10) shows functioning upper medulla. Be aware that CN 6 palsy is often a false localizing sign. |
| **What is acute treatment of seizures after head trauma?** | Benzodiazepines (Ativan®) |
| **What is seizure prophylaxis after severe head injury?** | Give phenytoin for 7 days. |
| **What is the significance of hyponatremia (low sodium level) after head injury?** | S.I.A.D.H. must be ruled out; remember, **S.I.A.D.H. S**odium **I**s **A**lways **D**own **H**ere |

## EPIDURAL HEMATOMA

| | |
|---|---|
| **What is an epidural hematoma?** | Collection of blood between the skull and dura |
| **What causes it?** | Usually occurs in association with a skull fracture as bone fragments lacerate meningeal arteries |
| **What artery is associated with epidural hematomas?** | **Middle meningeal artery** |
| **What is the most common sign of an epidural hematoma?** | More than 50% have ipsilateral blown pupil. |
| **What is the classic history with an epidural hematoma?** | LOC followed by a "lucid interval" followed by neurologic deterioration |
| **What are the classic CT findings with an epidural hematoma?** | Lenticular (lens)-shaped hematoma (think: **E**pidural = **LE**nticular) |

| | |
|---|---|
| **What is the surgical treatment for an epidural hematoma?** | Surgical evacuation |
| **What are the indications for surgery with an epidural hematoma?** | Any symptomatic epidural hematoma; any epidural hematoma >1 cm |

## SUBDURAL HEMATOMA

| | |
|---|---|
| **What is it?** | Blood collection under the dura |
| **What causes it?** | Tearing of "bridging" veins that pass through the space between the cortical surface and the dural venous sinuses or injury to the brain surface with resultant bleeding from cortical vessels |
| **What are the three types of subdurals?** | 1. Acute—symptoms within 48 hours of injury<br>2. Subacute—symptoms within 3 to 14 days<br>3. Chronic—symptoms after 2 weeks or longer |
| **What is the treatment of epidural and subdural hematomas?** | The mass effect (pressure) must be reduced. Craniotomy with clot evacuation is usually required. |

**What classic CT findings appear on head CT for a subdural hematoma?**

Curved, crescent-shaped hematoma (think: s**U**bdural = c**U**rved)

## TRAUMATIC SUBARACHNOID HEMORRHAGE

**What is it?**

Head trauma resulting in blood below the arachnoid membrane and above the pia

**What is the treatment?**

Anticonvulsants and observation

## CEREBRAL CONTUSION

**What is it?**

Hemorrhagic contusion of brain parenchyma

**What are coup and contrecoup injuries?**

Coup—injury at the site of impact
Contrecoup—injury at the site opposite the point of impact

**What is DAI?**

**D**iffuse **A**xonal **I**njury (shear injury to brain parenchyma) from rapid deceleration injury; 33% mortality; long-term coma

**What is the best diagnostic test for DAI?**

MRI

## SKULL FRACTURE

| | |
|---|---|
| **What is a depressed skull fracture?** | A fracture in which one or more fragments of the skull are forced below the inner table of the skull |
| **What are the indications for surgery?** | 1. Contaminated wound requiring cleaning and débridement<br>2. Severe deformity<br>3. Impingement on cortex<br>4. Open fracture<br>5. CSF leak |
| **What is the treatment for open skull fractures?** | 1. Antibiotics<br>2. Seizure prophylaxis (phenytoin)<br>3. Surgical therapy |

## SPINAL CORD TRAUMA

| | |
|---|---|
| **What are the two general types of injury?** | 1. Complete—no motor/sensory function below the level of injury<br>2. Incomplete—residual function below the level of injury |
| **Define "spinal shock."** | Loss of all reflexes and motor function, hypotension, bradycardia |
| **Define "sacral sparing."** | Sparing of sacral nerve level: anal sphincter intact, toe flexion, perianal sensation |
| **What initial studies/ intervention are important?** | 1. ABCs—obtain airway and ventilate if needed<br>2. Maintain BP (IVF, pressors if refractory to fluids)<br>3. NG tube—prevents aspiration<br>4. Foley<br>5. High-dose steroids—proven to improve outcome if given <8 hours post injury<br>6. Complete cervical x-rays and those of lower levels as indicated by examination |
| **What are the diagnostic studies?** | Plain films, CT, MRI |

**What are the indications for emergent surgery with spinal cord injury?**

Unstable vertebral fracture
Incomplete injury with extrinsic compression
Spinal epidural or subdural hematoma

**What is the indication for IV high-dose steroids with spinal cord injury?**

Controversial: Blunt spinal cord injury with neurologic deficit (methylprednisolone: high-dose bolus [30 mg/kg] followed by continuous infusion [5.4 mg/kg] for 23 hours)

**Have steroids been proven to help after PENETRATING spine injury?**

No

**Describe the following conditions:**

    **Anterior cord syndrome**

Affects corticospinal and lateral spinothalamic tracts, paraplegia, loss of pain/temperature sensation, preserved touch/vibration/proprioception

    **Central cord syndrome**

Preservation of some lower extremity motor and sensory ability with upper extremity weakness

| | |
|---|---|
| **Brown-Séquard syndrome** | Hemisection of cord resulting in ipsilateral motor weakness and touch/proprioception loss with contralateral pain/temperature loss |

| | |
|---|---|
| **Posterior cord syndrome** | Injury to posterior spinal cord with loss of proprioception distally |
| **How can the findings associated with Brown-Séquard syndrome be remembered?** | Think: CAPTAIN Brown-Séquard = "CPT": Contralateral Pain Temperature loss |
| **Define the following terms:** | |
| **Jefferson's fracture** | Fracture through **C1** arches from axial loading (unstable fracture) |
| **Hangman's fracture** | Fracture through the pedicles of **C2** from hyperextension; usually stable Think: hangman (C2) is below stature of President T. Jefferson (C1) |
| **Odontoid fracture** | Fracture of the odontoid process of C2 (view with open-mouth odontoid x-ray) |
| **Priapism** | Penile erection seen with spinal cord injury |
| **Chance fracture** | Transverse vertebral fracture |
| **Clay shoveler's fracture** | Fracture of spinous process of C7 |

**Odontoid fractures**

A: Type I—fracture through tip of dens
B: Type II—fracture through base of dens
C: Type III—fracture through body of C2

## TUMORS

### GENERAL

**What is the incidence of CNS tumors?**

Approximately 1% of all cancers; third leading cause of cancer deaths in people 15 to 34 years of age; second leading cause of cancer deaths in children

**What is the usual location of primary tumors in adults/ children?**

In adults, roughly two-thirds of tumors are supratentorial, one-third are infratentorial; the reverse is true in children (i.e., 2/3 infratentorial)

**What is the differential diagnosis of a ring-enhancing brain lesion?**

Metastatic carcinoma, abscess, GBM, lymphoma

**What are the adverse effects of tumors on the brain?**

1. Increased ICP
2. Mass effect on cranial nerves
3. Invasion of brain parenchyma, disrupting nuclei/tracts
4. Seizure foci
5. Hemorrhage into/around tumor mass

**What are the signs/ symptoms of brain tumors?**

1. Neurologic deficit (66%)
2. Headache (50%)
3. Seizures (25%)
4. Vomiting (classically in the morning)

**How is the diagnosis made?**

CT or MRI is the standard diagnostic study.

| | |
|---|---|
| **What are the surgical indications?** | 1. Establishing a tissue diagnosis<br>2. Relief of increased ICP<br>3. Relief of neurologic dysfunction caused by tissue compression<br>4. Attempt to cure in the setting of localized tumor |
| **What are the most common intracranial tumors in adults?** | Metastatic neoplasms are most common; among primaries, gliomas are number 1 (50%) and meningiomas are number 2 (25%). |
| **What are the most common in children?** | 1. Medulloblastomas (33%)<br>2. Astrocytomas (33%)<br>3. Ependymomas (10%) |

## GLIOMAS

| | |
|---|---|
| **What is a glioma?** | A general name for several tumors of neuroglial origin (e.g., astrocytes, ependymal, oligodendrocytes) |
| **What are the characteristics of a LOW-grade astrocytoma?** | Nuclear atypia, high mitotic rate, high signal on T2 weighted images, nonenhancing with contrast CT |
| **What is the most common primary brain tumor in adults?** | Glioblastoma multiforme (GBM) (Think: **GBM** = **G**reatest **B**rain **M**alignancy) |
| **What are its characteristics?** | Poorly defined, highly aggressive tumors occurring in the white matter of the cerebral hemispheres; spread extremely rapidly |
| **What is the average age of onset?** | Fifth decade |
| **What is the treatment?** | Surgical debulking followed by radiation therapy |
| **What is the prognosis?** | Without treatment, more than 90% of patients die within 3 months of diagnosis. With treatment, 90% die within 2 years. |

## MENINGIOMAS

| | |
|---|---|
| **What is the layer of origination?** | Arachnoid cap cells |
| **What are the risk factors?** | Radiation exposure<br>Neurofibromatosis 2<br>Female sex |
| **What are the associated histologic findings?** | Psammoma bodies (concentric calcifications), Whorl formations (onion skin pattern) |
| **What is the histologic malignancy determination?** | Brain parenchymal invasion |
| **What is the peak age of occurrence?** | Between 40 and 50 years |
| **What is the gender ratio?** | Females predominate almost 2:1. |
| **What is the clinical presentation?** | Variable depending on location; lateral cerebral convexity tumors can cause focal deficits or headache; sphenoid tumors can present with seizures; posterior fossa tumors with CN deficits; olfactory groove tumors with anosmia |
| **What is the treatment?** | Preoperative embolization and surgical resection |

## CEREBELLAR ASTROCYTOMAS

| | |
|---|---|
| **What is the peak age of occurrence?** | Between 5 and 9 years |
| **What is the usual location?** | Usually in the cerebellar hemispheres; less frequently in the vermis |
| **What are the signs/ symptoms?** | Usually lateral cerebellar signs occur: ipsilateral incoordination or dysmetria (patient tends to fall to side of tumor), as well as nystagmus and ataxia; CN deficits are also frequently present, especially in CNs VI and VII. |

| | |
|---|---|
| **What are the treatment and prognosis?** | Completely resectable in 75% of cases, which usually results in a cure; overall 5-year survival rate exceeds 90% |

## MEDULLOBLASTOMA

| | |
|---|---|
| **What is the peak age of occurrence?** | First decade (3 to 7 years) |
| **What is the cell of origin?** | External granular cells of cerebellum |
| **What is the most common location?** | Cerebellar vermis in children; cerebellar hemispheres of adolescents and adults |
| **What are the signs/ symptoms?** | Headache, vomiting, and other signs of increased ICP; also usually truncal ataxia |
| **What are the treatment and prognosis?** | Best current treatment includes surgery to debulk the tumor, cranial and spinal radiation, and chemotherapy; 5-year survival rate is more than 50%. |

## PITUITARY TUMORS

| | |
|---|---|
| **What is the most common pituitary tumor?** | Prolactinoma |
| **What is the most common presentation of a prolactinoma?** | Bitemporal hemianopsia (lateral visual fields blind) |
| **What are the blood prolactin levels with a prolactinoma?** | Greater than 300 mg/L is diagnostic for prolactinoma (>100 mg/L is abnormal) |
| **Medical treatment of a prolactinoma?** | Bromocriptine |
| **Surgical treatment for a prolactinoma?** | Transsphenoidal resection of the pituitary tumor (in cases refractory to bromocriptine) |
| **What is the treatment of a recurrent prolactinoma after surgical resection?** | Radiation therapy |

## VASCULAR NEUROSURGERY

### SUBARACHNOID HEMORRHAGE (SAH)

**What are the usual causes?**

Most cases are due to **trauma;** of nontraumatic SAH, the leading cause is ruptured **berry aneurysm,** followed by arteriovenous malformations

**What is a berry aneurysm?**

Saccular outpouching of vessels in the circle of Willis, usually at bifurcations

**What is the usual location of a berry aneurysm?**

Anterior communicating artery is number one (30%), followed by posterior communicating artery and middle cerebral artery.

**What medical disease increases the risk of berry aneurysms?**

Polycystic kidney disease and connective tissue disorders (e.g., Marfan's syndrome)

**What is an AVM?**

A congenital abnormality of the vasculature with connections between the **arterial** and **venous** circulations without interposed capillary network

**Where do they occur?**

More than 75% are supratentorial.

**What are the signs/ symptoms of SAH?**

Classic symptom is **"the worst headache of my life."** Meningismus is documented by neck pain and positive Kernig's and Brudzinski's signs. Occasionally LOC, vomiting, nausea, photophobia

**What comprises the workup of SAH?**

If SAH is suspected, head CT should be the first test ordered to look for subarachnoid blood. LP may show xanthochromic CSF, but is not necessary if CT is definitive. This test should be followed by arteriogram to look for aneurysms or AVMs.

**What are the possible complications of SAH?**

1. Brain edema leading to increased ICP
2. Rebleeding (most common in the first 24 to 48 hours posthemorrhage)
3. **Vasospasm** (most common cause of morbidity and mortality)

| | |
|---|---|
| **What is the treatment for vasospasm?** | Nimodipine (calcium channel blocker) |
| **What is the treatment of aneurysm?** | Surgical treatment by placing a metal clip on the aneurysm is the mainstay of therapy. Alternatives include balloon occlusion or coil embolization. |
| **What is the treatment of AVM?** | Many are on the brain surface and accessible operatively. Preoperative embolization can reduce the size of the AVM. For surgically inaccessible lesions, radiosurgery (gamma knife) has been effective in treating AVMs less than 3 cm in diameter. |

## INTRACEREBRAL HEMORRHAGE

| | |
|---|---|
| **What is it?** | Bleeding into the brain parenchyma |
| **What is the etiology?** | Number one is hypertensive/ atherosclerotic disease giving rise to Charcot-Bouchard aneurysms (small tubular aneurysms along smaller terminal arteries); other causes include coagulopathies, AVMs, amyloid angiopathy, bleeding into a tumor, and trauma. |
| **Where does it occur?** | Two-thirds occur in the basal ganglia; putamen is the structure most commonly affected. |
| **How often does blood spread to the ventricular system?** | Two-thirds of cases |
| **What is the usual presentation?** | Two-thirds present with coma; large putamen bleeding classically presents with contralateral hemiplegia and hemisensory deficits, lateral gaze preference, aphasia, and homonymous hemianopsia. |
| **What is the associated diagnostic study?** | CT |

| | |
|---|---|
| **What are the surgical indications?** | CN III palsy, progressive alteration of consciousness |
| **What is the prognosis?** | Poor, especially with ventricular or diencephalons involvement |

## SPINE

### LUMBAR DISC HERNIATION

| | |
|---|---|
| **What is it?** | Extrusion of the inner portion of the intervertebral disc (nucleus pulposus) through the outer annulus fibrosis, causing impingement on nerve roots exiting the spinal canal |
| **Which nerve is affected?** | The nerve exiting at the level below (e.g., an L4-L5 disc impinges on the L5 nerve exiting between L5-S1) |
| **Who is affected?** | Middle-aged and older individuals |
| **What is the usual cause?** | Loss of elasticity of the posterior longitudinal ligaments and annulus fibrosis as a result of aging |
| **What are the most common sites?** | L5-S1 (45%) <br> L4-L5 (40%) |
| **What is the usual presenting symptom?** | Low back pain |
| **What are the signs:** <br> **L5-S1?** | Decreased ankle jerk reflex <br> Weakness of plantar flexors in foot <br> Pain in back/midgluteal region to posterior calf to lateral foot <br> Ipsilateral radiculopathy on straight leg raise |
| **L4-L5?** | Decreased biceps femoris reflex <br> Weak extensors of foot |

**L3-L4?**

Decrease or absence of knee jerks, weakness of the quadriceps femoris, pain in lower back/buttock, pain in lateral thigh and anterior thigh

Pain in hip/groin region to posterolateral thigh, lateral leg, and medial toes

**What is cauda equina syndrome?**

Herniated disc compressing multiple S1, S2, S3, S4 nerve roots, resulting in bowel/bladder incontinence, "saddle anesthesia" over buttocks/perineum, low back pain, sciatica

**What is "sciatica"?**

Radicular or nerve root pain

**How is the diagnosis made?**

CT, CT myelogram, or MRI

**What is the treatment?**

Conservative—bed rest and analgesics

Surgical—partial hemilaminectomy and discectomy (removal of herniated disc)

**What are the indications for emergent surgery?**

1. Cauda equina syndrome
2. Progressive motor deficits

## CERVICAL DISC DISEASE

**What is it?**

Basically the same pathology as previously described, except in the cervical region; the disc impinges on the nerve exiting the canal at the same level of the disease (e.g., a C6-C7 disc impinges on the C7 nerve root exiting at the C6-C7 foramen)

**What are the most common sites?**

C6-C7 (70%)
C5-C6 (20%)
C7-T1 (10%)

**What are the signs/ symptoms:**
    **C7?**

Decreased triceps reflex/strength, weakness of forearm extension

Pain from neck, through triceps and into index and middle finger

| | |
|---|---|
| **C6?** | Decreased biceps and brachioradialis reflex<br>Weakness in forearm flexion<br>Pain in neck, radial forearm, and thumb |
| **C8?** | Weakness in intrinsic hand muscles, pain in fourth/fifth fingers |
| **What is Spurling's sign?** | Reproduction of radicular pain by having the patient turn his head to the affected side and applying axial pressure to the top of the head |
| **How is the diagnosis made?** | CT or MRI |
| **What is the treatment?** | Anterior or posterior discectomy with fusion PRN |
| **What are the symptoms of central cervical cord compression from disc fragments?** | Myelopathic syndrome with LMN signs at level of compression and UMN signs distally; e.g., C7 compression may cause bilateral loss of triceps reflex and bilateral hyperreflexia, clonus, and Babinski signs in lower extremities |

## SPINAL EPIDURAL ABSCESS

| | |
|---|---|
| **What is the etiology?** | Hematogenous spread from skin infections is most common; also, distant abscesses/infections, UTIs, postoperative infections, spine surgery, epidural anesthesia |
| **What is the commonly associated medical condition?** | Diabetes mellitus |
| **What are the most common sites?** | 1. Thoracic<br>2. Lumbar<br>3. Cervical |
| **What is the most common organism?** | *Staphylococcus aureus* |

| | |
|---|---|
| **What are the signs/ symptoms?** | Fever; severe pain over affected area and with flexion/extension of spine; weakness can develop, ultimately leading to paraplegia; 15% of patients have a back furuncle |
| **How is the diagnosis made?** | MRI is test of choice. |
| **Which test is contraindicated?** | LP, because of the risk of seeding CSF with bacteria, causing meningitis |
| **What is the treatment?** | Surgical drainage and appropriate antibiotic coverage |
| **What is the prognosis?** | Depends on preop condition; severe neurologic deficits (e.g., paraplegia) show little recovery; 15% to 20% of cases are fatal |

## PEDIATRIC NEUROSURGERY

### HYDROCEPHALUS

| | |
|---|---|
| **What is it?** | Abnormal condition consisting of an increased volume of CSF along with distension of CSF spaces |
| **What are the three general causes?** | 1. Increased production of CSF<br>2. Decreased absorption of CSF<br>3. Obstruction of normal flow of CSF (90% of cases) |
| **What is the normal daily CSF production?** | Approximately 500 mL |
| **What is the normal volume of CSF?** | Approximately 150 mL in the average adult |
| **Define "communicating" versus "noncommunicating" hydrocephalus.** | Communicating—unimpaired connection of CSF pathway from lateral ventricle to subarachnoid space<br>Noncommunicating—complete or incomplete obstruction of CSF flow within or at the exit of the ventricular system |

| | |
|---|---|
| **What are the specific causes of hydrocephalus?** | 1. Congenital malformation<br>Aqueductal stenosis<br>Myelomeningocele<br>2. Tumors obstructing CSF flow<br>3. Inflammation causing impaired absorption of fluid<br>Subarachnoid hemorrhage<br>Meningitis<br>4. Choroid plexus papilloma causing increased production of CSF |
| **What are the signs/ symptoms?** | Signs of increased ICP: HA, nausea, vomiting, ataxia, increasing head circumference exceeding norms for age |
| **How is the diagnosis made?** | CT, MRI, measurement of head circumference |
| **What is the treatment?** | 1. Remove obvious offenders.<br>2. Perform bypass obstruction with ventriculoperitoneal shunt or ventriculoatrial shunt. |
| **What is the prognosis if untreated?** | 50% mortality; survivors show decreased IQ (mean = 69); neurologic sequelae: ataxia, paraparesis, visual deficits |
| **What are the possible complications of treatment?** | 1. Blockage/shunt malfunction<br>2. Infection |
| **What is hydrocephalus ex vacuo?** | Increased volume of CSF spaces from brain atrophy, not from any pathology in the amount of CSF absorbed or produced |
| **What is a "shunt series"?** | A series of x-rays covering the entire shunt length—looking for shunt disruption/kinking to explain malfunction of shunt |

## SPINAL DYSRAPHISM/NEURAL TUBE DEFECTS

| | |
|---|---|
| **What is the incidence?** | Approximately 1/1000 live births in the United States |

| | |
|---|---|
| **What are the race/gender demographics?** | More common in white patients and female patients |
| **Define spina bifida occulta.** | Defect in the development of the posterior portion of the vertebrae |
| **What are the signs/ symptoms?** | Usually asymptomatic, though it may be associated with other spinal abnormalities; usually found incidentally on x-rays |
| **What is the most common clinically significant defect?** | Myelomeningocele: herniation of nerve roots and spinal cord through a defect in the posterior elements of the vertebra(e); the sac surrounding the neural tissue may be intact, but more commonly is ruptured and therefore exposes the CNS to the external environment. |
| **What are the most common anatomic sites?** | #1 lumbar region; #2 lower thoracic region; #3 upper sacral region |
| **What are the signs/ symptoms?** | Variable from mild skeletal deformities to a complete motor/sensory loss; bowel/ bladder function is difficult to evaluate, but often is affected and can adversely affect survival. |
| **What is the treatment?** | With open myelomeningoceles, patients are operated on immediately to prevent infection. |
| **What is the prognosis?** | Approximately 95% survival for the first 2 years, compared with 25% in patients not undergoing surgical procedures |
| **Which vitamin is thought to lower the rate of neural tube defects in utero?** | Folic acid |

## CRANIOSYNOSTOSIS

| | |
|---|---|
| **What is it?** | Premature closure of one or more of the sutures between the skull plates |
| **What is the incidence?** | 1/200 live births in the United States |

| | |
|---|---|
| **What are the types?** | Named for the suture that is fused (e.g., sagittal, coronal, lambdoid); sagittal craniosynostosis accounts for more than 50% of all cases; more than one suture can be fused, and all or part of a suture may be affected. |
| **How is the diagnosis made?** | Physical examination can reveal ridges along fused sutures and lessened suture mobility. Plain x-rays can show a lack of lucency along the fused suture, but are rarely required. |
| **What are the indications for surgery?** | Most often the reasons are cosmetic, as the cranial vault will continue to deform with growth. Occasionally, a child will present with increased ICP secondary to restricted brain growth. |
| **What is the timing of surgery?** | Usually 3 to 4 months of age; earlier surgery increases the risk of anesthesia; later surgeries are more difficult because of the worsening deformities and decreasing malleability of the skull. |
| **What is the operative mortality?** | Less than 1% |

## MISCELLANEOUS

| | |
|---|---|
| **What is the most common bacteria causing postneurosurgery meningitis?** | *Staphylococcus aureus* (skin flora) |
| **What classically presents as the "worst headache of my life"?** | Spontaneous subarachnoid hemorrhage |
| **What classically has a "lucid interval"?** | Epidural hemorrhage |
| **What is the most common location of a hypertensive intracerebral hemorrhage?** | Putamen |

| | |
|---|---|
| **What is Horner's syndrome?** | Cervical sympathetic chain lesion: "**M.A.P.**":<br>**M**iosis<br>**A**nhydrosis of ipsilateral face<br>**P**tosis |
| **What is a third-nerve palsy?** | Think: the third nerve does three things:<br>1. Diplopia<br>2. Ptosis<br>3. Mydriasis |
| **What is Millard-Gubler syndrome?** | Pons infarction:<br>1. VI nerve palsy<br>2. VII nerve palsy<br>3. Contralateral hemiplegia |
| **What is syringomyelia?** | Central pathologic cavitations of the spinal cord |

# Chapter 76 Urology

**Define the following terms:**

| | |
|---|---|
| **Cystogram** | Contrast study of the bladder |
| **Ureteral stents** | Plastic tubes placed via cystoscope into the ureters for stenting, identification, etc. |
| **Cystoscope** | Scope placed into the urethra and into the bladder to visualize the bladder |
| **Perc nephrostomy** | Catheter placed through the skin into the kidney pelvis to drain urine with distal obstruction, etc. |
| **Retrograde pyelogram** | Dye injected into the ureter up into the kidney and films taken |
| **RUG** | **R**etrograde **U**rethro**G**ram (dye injected into the urethra and films taken; rules out urethral injury, usually in trauma patients) |

**Gomco clamp** — Clamp used for circumcision; protects penis glans

**Bell clapper's deformity** — Condition of congenital absence of gubernaculum attachment to scrotum

**Fournier's gangrene** — Extensive tissue necrosis/infection of the perineum in patients with diabetes

**Foley catheter** — Straight bladder catheter placed through the urethra

**Coudé catheter** — Basically, a Foley catheter with hook on the end to get around a large prostate

**Suprapubic catheter** — Bladder catheter placed through the skin above the pubic symphysis into the bladder

**Posthitis** — Foreskin infection

**Hydrocele** — Clear fluid in the processus vaginalis membrane

**Communicating hydrocele** — Hydrocele that communicates with peritoneal cavity and, thus, gets smaller and larger as fluid drains and then reaccumulates

**Noncommunicating hydrocele**

Hydrocele that does not communicate with the peritoneal cavity; hydrocele remains the same size

**Varicocele**

Abnormal dilation of the pampiniform plexus to the spermatic vein in the spermatic cord; described as a "bag of worms"

**Spermatocele**

Dilatation of epididymis or vas deferens

**Epididymitis**

Infection of the epididymis

**Prehn's sign**

Elevation of the painful testicle that reduces the pain of epididymitis

**TRUS**

**T**rans **R**ectal **U**ltra**S**ound

**DRE**

**D**igital **R**ectal **E**xamination

**Orchitis**

Inflammation/infection of the testicle

**Pseudohermaphroditism**

Genetically **one** sex; partial or complete opposite-sex genitalia

**Urgency**

Overwhelming sensation to void immediately

**Dysuria**

Painful urination (usually burning sensation)

**Frequency**

Urination more times than usual

| | |
|---|---|
| **Polyuria** | Urination in larger amounts than usual |
| **Nocturia** | Awakening to urinate |
| **Hesitancy** | Delay in urination |
| **Pneumaturia** | Air passed with urine via the urethra |
| **Pyuria** | WBSs in urine; UTI >10 WBC/HPF |
| **Cryptorchidism** | Undescended testicle |
| **IVP** | **I**ntra**V**enous **P**yelogram (dye is injected into the vein, collects in the renal collecting system, and an x-ray is taken) |
| **Hematuria** | RBCs in urine |
| **Space of Retzius** | Anatomic extraperitoneal space in front of the bladder |
| **Enuresis** | Involuntary urination while asleep |
| **Incontinence** | Involuntary urination |
| **TURP** | **T**rans**U**rethral **R**esection of the **P**rostate |
| **PVR** | **P**ost**V**oid **R**esidual |
| **Priapism** | Prolonged, painful erection |
| **Paraphimosis** | Foreskin held (stuck) in the retracted position |
| **Phimosis** | Inability to retract the foreskin |
| **Balanitis** | Inflammation/infection of the glans penis |
| **Balanoposthitis** | Inflammation/infection of the glans and prepuce of the penis |
| **UTI** | **U**rinary **T**ract **I**nfection |
| **Peyronie's disease** | Abnormal fibrosis of the penis shaft, resulting in a bend upon erection |

| | |
|---|---|
| **BPH** | **B**enign **P**rostatic **H**yperplasia |
| **Epispadias** | Abnormal urethral opening on the dorsal surface of the penis |
| **Hypospadiasis** | Abnormal urethral opening on the ventral surface of the penis; may occur in anterior, middle, or posterior of penis |
| **Impotence** | Inability to achieve an erection |
| **Sterility** | Inability to reproduce |
| **Appendix testis** | Common redundant testicular tissue |
| **VUR** | **V**esico**U**reteral **R**eflux |

## UROLOGIC DIFFERENTIAL DIAGNOSIS

**What are the layers of the scrotum?**

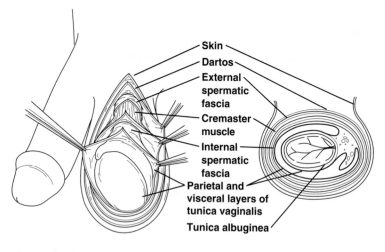

- Skin
- Dartos
- External spermatic fascia
- Cremaster muscle
- Internal spermatic fascia
- Parietal and visceral layers of tunica vaginalis
- Tunica albuginea

**What is the differential diagnosis of scrotal mass?**

Cancer, torsion, epididymitis, hydrocele, spermatocele, varicocele, inguinal hernia, testicular appendage, swollen testicle after trauma, nontesticular tumor (para-testicular tumor: e.g., rhabdomyosarcoma, leiomyosarcoma, liposarcoma)

| | |
|---|---|
| **What are the causes of hematuria?** | Bladder cancer, trauma, UTI, cystitis from chemotherapy or radiation, stones, kidney lesion, BPH |
| **What is the most common cause of severe gross hematuria without trauma or chemotherapy/radiation?** | Bladder cancer |
| **What is the differential diagnosis for bladder outlet obstruction?** | BPH, stone, foreign body, urethral stricture, urethral valve |
| **What is the differential diagnosis for ureteral obstruction?** | Stone, tumor, iatrogenic (suture), stricture, gravid uterus, radiation injury, retroperitoneal fibrosis |
| **What is the differential diagnosis for kidney tumor?** | Renal cell carcinoma, sarcoma, adenoma, angiomyolipoma, hemangiopericytoma, oncocytoma |

## RENAL CELL CARCINOMA (RCC)

| | |
|---|---|
| **What is it?** | Most common solid renal tumor (90%); originates from proximal renal tubular epithelium |
| **What is the epidemiology?** | Primarily a tumor of adults 40 to 60 years of age with a 3:1 male:female ratio; 5% of cancers in adults |
| **What percentage of the tumors are bilateral?** | 1% |
| **What are the risk factors?** | Male sex, tobacco, von Hippel-Lindau syndrome, polycystic kidney |
| **What are the symptoms?** | Pain (40%), hematuria (35%), weight loss (35%), flank mass (25%), HTN (20%) |
| **What is the classic TRIAD of renal cell carcinoma?** | 1. Flank pain<br>2. Hematuria<br>3. Palpable mass (**triad** occurs in only 10% to 15% of cases) |

| | |
|---|---|
| **How are most cases diagnosed these days?** | Found incidentally on an imaging study (CT, MRI, U/S) for another reason |
| **What radiologic tests are performed?** | 1. IVP<br>2. Abdominal CT with contrast |
| **Define the stages (AJCC):** | |
| **I** | Tumor <2.5 cm, no nodes, no metastases |
| **II** | Tumor >2.5 cm limited to kidney, no nodes, no metastases |
| **III** | Tumor extends into IVC or main renal vein; positive regional lymph nodes but <2 cm in diameter and no metastases |
| **IV** | Distant metastasis or positive lymph node >2 cm in diameter or tumor extends past Gerota's fascia |
| **What is the metastatic workup?** | CXR, IVP, CT, LFTs, calcium |
| **What gland is removed with a radical nephrectomy?** | Adrenal gland |
| **What are the sites of metastases?** | Lung, liver, brain, bone; tumor thrombus entering renal vein or IVC is not uncommon |
| **What is the unique route of spread?** | Tumor thrombus into **IVC lumen** |
| **What is the treatment?** | Radical nephrectomy (excision of the kidney and adrenal, including Gerota's fascia) for stages I through IV |
| **What is the unique treatment for metastatic spread?** | 1. Alpha-interferon<br>2. LAK cells (lymphokine-activated killer) and IL-2 (interleukin-2) |
| **What is a syndrome of RCC and liver disease?** | Stauffer's syndrome |

## BLADDER CANCER

| | |
|---|---|
| **What is the incidence?** | Second most common urologic malignancy<br>Male:female ratio of 3:1<br>White patients are more commonly affected than are African American patients. |
| **What is the most common histology?** | Transitional cell carcinoma (TCC)—90%; remaining cases are squamous or adenocarcinomas |
| **What are the risk factors?** | Smoking, industrial carcinogens (aromatic amines), schistosomiasis, truck drivers, petroleum workers |
| **What are the symptoms?** | **Hematuria,** with or without irritative symptoms (e.g., dysuria), frequency |
| **What is the classic presentation of bladder cancer?** | "Painless hematuria" |
| **What tests are included in the workup?** | Urinalysis and culture, IVP, cystoscopy with cytology and biopsy |
| **Define the stages (according to the Jewett/Marshall system):** | |
| **O** | Superficial, limited to mucosa; also known as carcinoma in situ (CIS) |
| **A** | Involves lamina propria |
| **B** | Muscle invasion |
| **C** | Extends to perivesicular fat |
| **D** | Abdominal organ metastasis (contiguous), lymph node metastasis, distant metastasis |

**What is the treatment according to stage:**

**Stage O?**

Bladder chemotherapy (intravesical chemotherapy)

**Stage A?**

TURB

**Stages B and C?**

Radical cystectomy, lymph node dissection, removal of prostate/uterus/ovaries/anterior vaginal wall, and urinary diversion (e.g., ileal conduit)

**Stage D?**

+/− Cystectomy and **systemic chemotherapy**

**What are the indications for a partial cystectomy?**

Superficial, isolated tumor, apical with 3 cm margin from any orifices

**What is TURB?**

**T**rans-**U**rethral **R**esection of the **B**ladder

## PROSTATE CANCER

**What is the incidence?**

**Most common** GU cancer (>100,000 new cases per year in the United States); most common carcinoma in men in the United States; second most common cause of death in men in the United States

**What is the epidemiology?**

"A disease of elderly men" present in one-third of men 70 to 79 years of age and in two-thirds of men 80 to 89 years of age at autopsy; African American patients have a 50% higher incidence than do white patients.

**What is the histology?**

Adenocarcinoma (95%)

**What are the symptoms?**

Often asymptomatic; usually presents as a nodule found on routine rectal examination; in 70% of cases, cancer begins in the periphery of the gland and moves centrally; thus, obstructive symptoms occur late.

| | |
|---|---|
| **What percentage of patients have metastasis at diagnosis?** | 40% of patients have metastatic disease at presentation, with symptoms of bone pain and weight loss. |
| **What are the common sites of metastasis?** | Osteoblastic bony lesions, lung, liver, adrenal |
| **What provides lymphatic drainage?** | Obturator and hypogastric nodes |
| **What is the significance of Batson's plexus?** | Spinal cord venous plexus; route of isolated skull/brain metastasis |
| **What are the steps in early detection and surveillance?** | 1. Prostate-specific antigen (PSA)—most sensitive and specific marker<br>2. Acid phosphatase—often elevated in metastatic prostate cancer; used mostly to detect recurrences<br>3. Digital rectal examination (DRE) |
| **When should men get a PSA-level check?** | Controversial:<br>1. All men >50 years old<br>2. >40 years old if first-degree family history or black patient |
| **What percentage of patients with prostate cancer will have an elevated PSA?** | Approximately 60% |
| **How is the diagnosis made?** | Transrectal biopsy |
| **What are the indications for transrectal biopsy with normal rectal examination?** | PSA > 10 or abnormal transrectal ultrasound |
| **Staging (AJCC):**<br>    **Stage I** | Clinically inapparent tumor, no nodes, no metastases |
|     **Stage II** | Tumor within prostate, no nodes, no metastases |

| | |
|---|---|
| **Stage III** | Tumor through prostate capsule, no nodes, no metastases |
| **Stage IV** | Tumor extends into adjacent structures or + nodes or + metastases. |
| **What does a "radical prostatectomy" remove?** | 1. Prostate gland<br>2. Seminal vesicles<br>3. Ampullae of the vasa deferentia |
| **What is "hormonal" therapy?** | 1. Bilateral orchiectomy or<br>2. Luteinizing hormone-releasing hormone (LHRH) agonists |
| **How do LHRH agonists work?** | Decrease LH release from pituitary, which then decreases testosterone production in the testes |
| **What are the generalized treatment options according to stage:** | |
| **Stage I?** | Prostatectomy, +/− lymph node dissection |
| **Stage II?** | Prostatectomy, +/− lymph node dissection |
| **Stage III?** | Radiation therapy +/− lymph node dissection |
| **Stage IV?** | Hormonal treatment +/− radiation therapy |
| **Which tumors can be observed?** | Nonpalpable, small (<5% of gland), low grade, stage AI, found incidentally |

## BENIGN PROSTATIC HYPERPLASIA

| | |
|---|---|
| **What is it also known as?** | BPH |
| **What is it?** | Disease of elderly men (average age is 60 to 65 years); prostate gradually enlarges, creating symptoms of urinary outflow obstruction |

**What is the size of a normal prostate?** Between 20 and 25 gm

**Where does BPH occur?** Periurethrally (*Note*: prostate cancer occurs in the periphery of the gland.)

**What are the symptoms?** Obstructive-type symptoms: hesitancy, weak stream, nocturia, intermittency, UTI, urinary retention

**How is the diagnosis made?** History, DRE, elevated postvoid residual (PVR), urinalysis, cystoscopy, U/S

**What lab tests should be performed?** Urinalysis, PSA, BUN, CR

**What is the differential diagnosis?** **Prostate cancer** (e.g., nodular)—biopsy
Neurogenic bladder—history of neurologic disease
Acute prostatitis—hot, tender gland
Urethral stricture—RUG, history of STD
Stone
UTI

**What are the treatment options?** Pharmacologic—α-1 blockade
Hormonal—antiandrogens
Surgical—TURP, TUIP, open prostate resection
Transurethral balloon dilation

**Why do α-adrenergic blockers work?**
1. Relax sphincter
2. Relax prostate capsule

**What is Proscar®?** Finasteride: 5-α-reductase inhibitor; blocks transformation of testosterone to dihydrotestosterone; may shrink and slow progression of BPH

**What is Hytrin®?** Terazosin: α-blocker; may increase urine outflow by relaxing prostatic smooth muscles

| | |
|---|---|
| **What are the indications for surgery?** | Due to obstruction:<br>    Urinary retention<br>    Hydronephrosis<br>    UTIs<br>    Severe symptoms |
| **What is TURP?** | **T**rans**U**rethral **R**esection of **P**rostate: resection of prostate tissue via a scope |
| **What is TUIP?** | **T**rans**U**rethral **I**ncision of **P**rostate |
| **What percentage of tissue removed for BPH will have malignant tissue on histology?** | Up to 10%! |
| **What are the possible complications of TURP?** | Immediate:<br>    Failure to void<br>    Bleeding<br>    Clot retention<br>    UTI<br>    Incontinence |

## TESTICULAR CANCER

| | |
|---|---|
| **What is the incidence?** | Rare; 2 to 3 new cases per 100,000 men per year in the United States |
| **What is its claim to fame?** | Most common solid tumor of young adult men (20 to 40 years) |
| **What are the risk factors?** | Cryptorchidism (6% of testicular tumors develop in patients with a history of cryptorchidism) |
| **What is cryptorchidism?** | Failure of the testicle to descend into the scrotum |
| **Does orchiopexy as an adult remove the risk of testicular cancer?** | NO |
| **What are the symptoms?** | Most patients present with a painless lump, swelling, or firmness of the testicle; they often notice it after incidental trauma to the groin. |

**What percentage of patients present with an acute hydrocele?**
10%

**What percentage present with symptoms of metastatic disease (back pain, anorexia)?**
Approximately 10%

**What are the classifications?**
Germ cell tumors (95%):
    Seminomatous (35%)
    Nonseminomatous (65%)
    Embryonal cell carcinoma
        Teratoma
        Mixed cell
        Choriocarcinoma
Nongerminal (5%):
    Leydig cell
    Sertoli cell
    Gonadoblastoma

**What is the major classification based on therapy?**
Seminomas and nonseminoma tumors

**What are the tumor markers for testicular tumors?**
1. Beta-human chorionic gonadotropin ($\beta$-HCG)
2. Alpha-fetoprotein (AFP)

**What are the tumor markers by tumor type?**
$\beta$-HCG—increased in choriocarcinoma (100%), embryonal carcinoma (50%), and rarely in pure seminomas (10%); (half of nonseminomatous tumors)
AFP—increased in embryonal carcinoma and yolk sac tumors (half of nonseminomatous tumors)

**Which tumors almost *never* have an elevated AFP?**
Choriocarcinoma and seminoma

**In which tumor is $\beta$-HCG almost always found elevated?**
Choriocarcinoma

**How often is $\beta$-HCG elevated in patients with pure seminoma?**
Only about 10% of the time!

| | |
|---|---|
| **How often is β-HCG elevated with nonseminoma?** | ≈ 65% |
| **What other tumor markers may be elevated and useful for recurrence surveillance?** | LDH, CEA, human chorionic somatomammotropic (HCS), gamma-glutamyl transpeptidase (GGT), placental alkaline phosphate (PLAP) |
| **What are the steps in workup?** | P.E., scrotal U/S, check tumor markers, CXR, CT (chest/pelvis/abd) |

**Define the stages according to TMN staging (AJCC):**

| | |
|---|---|
| Stage I | Confined to testis, into tunica albuginea or epididymis, no nodes, no metastases |
| Stage II | **Positive** nodes, no metastases, any tumor |
| Stage III | Distant metastases (any nodal status, any size tumor) |

| | |
|---|---|
| **What is the initial treatment for all testicular tumors?** | **Inguinal** orchiectomy (removal of testicle through a groin incision) |

**What is the treatment of *seminoma* at the various stages:**

| | |
|---|---|
| Stage I and II? | Inguinal orchiectomy and **radiation** to retroperitoneal nodal basins |
| Stage III? | Orchiectomy and chemotherapy |

**What is the treatment of *non*seminomatous disease at the various stages:**

| | |
|---|---|
| Stages I and II? | Orchiectomy and retroperitoneal lymph node **dissection** versus close follow-up for retroperitoneal nodal involvement |
| Stage III? | Orchiectomy and chemotherapy |

| | |
|---|---|
| **What percentage of stage I seminomas are cured after treatment?** | 95% |

| | |
|---|---|
| **Which type is most radiosensitive?** | Seminoma (think: **S**eminoma = **S**ensitive to radiation) |
| **Why not remove testis with cancer through a scrotal incision?** | It could result in tumor seeding of the scrotum. |
| **What is the major side effect of retroperitoneal lymph node dissection?** | Impotence |

## TESTICULAR TORSION

| | |
|---|---|
| **What is it?** | Torsion (twist) of the spermatic cord, resulting in venous outflow obstruction, and subsequent arterial occlusion → infarction of the testicle |
| **What is the classic history?** | Acute onset of scrotal pain usually after vigorous activity or minor trauma |
| **What is a "bell clapper" deformity?** | Bilateral nonattachment of the testicles by the gubernaculum to the scrotum (free like the clappers of a bell) |

| | |
|---|---|
| **What are the symptoms?** | Pain in the scrotum, suprapubic pain |
| **What are the signs?** | Very tender, swollen, elevated testicle; nonillumination; absence of cremasteric reflex |
| **What is the differential diagnosis?** | Testicular trauma, inguinal hernia, epididymitis, appendage torsion |

| | |
|---|---|
| **How is the diagnosis made?** | Surgical exploration, U/S (solid mass) and Doppler flow study, cold Tc-99m scan (nuclear study) |
| **What is the treatment?** | Surgical detorsion and bilateral orchiopexy to the scrotum |
| **How much time is available from the onset of symptoms to detorse the testicle?** | Less than 6 hours will bring about the best results; >90% salvage rate |
| **What are the chances of testicle salvage after 24 hours?** | <10% |

## EPIDIDYMITIS

| | |
|---|---|
| **What is it?** | Infection of the epididymis |
| **What are the signs/symptoms?** | Swollen, tender testicle; dysuria; scrotal ache/pain; fever; chills; scrotal mass |
| **What is the cause?** | Bacteria from the urethra |
| **What are the common bugs in the following types of patients:** | |
| **Elderly patients/children?** | *Escherichia coli* |
| **Young men?** | STD bacteria: Gonorrhea, Chlamydia |
| **What is the major differential diagnosis** | Testicular torsion |
| **What is the work up?** | U/A, urine culture, swab if STD suspected, +/− U/S with Doppler or nuclear study to rule out torsion |
| **What is the treatment?** | Antibiotics |

## PRIAPISM

| | |
|---|---|
| **What is priapism?** | Persistent penile erection |

| | |
|---|---|
| **What are its causes?** | Low flow: leukemia, drugs (e.g., prazosin), sickle-cell disease, impotence treatment gone wrong<br>High flow: pudendal artery fistula, usually from trauma |
| **What is first-line treatment?** | 1. Aspiration of blood from corporus cavernosum<br>2. Alpha-adrenergic agent |

## IMPOTENCE

| | |
|---|---|
| **What is it?** | Inability to achieve an erection |
| **What are the six major causes?** | 1. **Vascular:** decreased blood flow or leak of blood from the corpus cavernosus (most common cause)<br>2. **Endocrine:** low testosterone<br>3. **Anatomic:** structural abnormality of the erectile apparatus (e.g., Peyronie's disease)<br>4. **Neurologic:** damage to nerves (e.g., postoperative, IDDM)<br>5. **Medications** (e.g., clonidine)<br>6. **Psychologic:** performance anxiety, etc. (very rare) |
| **What lab tests should be performed?** | Fasting GLC (rule out diabetes and thus diabetic neuropathy)<br>Serum testosterone<br>Serum prolactin |
| **What test evaluates for vascular causation of impotence?** | **Intracavernous vasoactive injection:** injection of papaverine or PGE1 into the cavernous cavity of the penis; a full erection subsequently rules out a vascular cause of the impotence |
| **What other diagnostic tests are often useful?** | U/S with Doppler flow studies, cavernous pressures, arteriography (pudendal), penile monitoring for erection |
| **What is the treatment?** | Depends on the cause: vacuum pump, penile prosthesis, vasoactive injections (inject PGE1, papaverine, sildenafil, phentolamine), psychologic therapy, testosterone injections, Viagra® |

## CALCULUS DISEASE

**What is the incidence?**

One in ten people will have stones.

**What are the risk factors?**

Poor fluid intake, IBD, hypercalcemia ("CHIMPANZEES"), renal tubular acidosis, small bowel bypass

**What are the types of stones?**

1. Calcium oxalate/calcium PO4 (75%)—secondary to hypercalciuria (increased intestinal absorption, decreased renal reabsorption, increased bone reabsorption)
2. Struvite (MgAmPh)(15%)—infection stones; seen in UTI with urea-splitting bacteria (Proteus); may cause staghorn calculi; high urine pH
3. Uric acid (7%)—stones are radiolucent (think: **U**ric = **U**nseen); seen in gout, Lesch-Nyhan, chronic diarrhea, cancer; low urine pH
4. Cystine (1%)—genetic predisposition

**What type of stones are not seen on AXR?**

Uric acid (think: **U**ric = **U**nseen)

**What stone is associated with UTIs?**

Struvite stones (think: **S**truvite = **S**epsis)

**What stones are seen in IBD/bowel bypass?**

Calcium oxalate

**What are the symptoms?**

Severe pain; patient cannot sit still: renal colic (typically pain in the kidney/ureter that radiates to the testis or penis), hematuria (remember, patients with peritoneal signs are motionless)

**What are the classic findings/symptoms?**

Flank pain, stone on AXR, hematuria

**Diagnosis?**

KUB (90% radiopaque), IVP, urinalysis and culture, BUN/Cr, CBC

| | |
|---|---|
| **What is the significance of hematuria and pyuria?** | Stone with concomitant infection |
| **Treatment?** | Narcotics for pain, vigorous hydration, observation<br>Further options: ESWL (lithotripsy), ureteroscopy, percutaneous lithotripsy, open surgery; metabolic workup for recurrence |
| **What are the indications for intervention?** | Urinary tract obstruction<br>Persistent infection<br>Impaired renal function |
| **What are the contraindications of outpatient treatment?** | Pregnancy, diabetes, obstruction, severe dehydration, severe pain, urosepsis/fever, pyelonephritis, previous urologic surgery, one functioning kidney |
| **What are the three common sites of obstruction?** | 1. Ureteropelvic junction (UPJ)<br>2. Ureterovesicular junction (UVJ)<br>3. Intersection of the ureter and the iliac vessels |

## INCONTINENCE

| | |
|---|---|
| **What are the common types of incontinence?** | Stress incontinence, overflow incontinence, urge incontinence |
| **Define the following terms:**<br>   **Stress incontinence** | Loss of urine associated with coughing, lifting, exercise, etc.; seen most often in women, secondary to relaxation of pelvic floor following multiple deliveries |
|    **Overflow incontinence** | Failure of the bladder to empty properly; may be caused by bladder outlet obstruction (BPH or stricture) or detrusor hypotonicity |
|    **Urge incontinence** | Loss of urine secondary to detrusor instability in patients with stroke, dementia, Parkinson's disease, etc. |
|    **Mixed incontinence** | Stress **and** urge incontinence combined |

| | |
|---|---|
| **Enuresis** | Bedwetting in children |
| **How is the diagnosis made?** | History (including meds), physical examination (including pelvic/rectal examination), urinalysis, postvoid residual (PR), urodynamics, cystoscopy/ vesicocystourethrogram (VCUG) may be necessary |
| **What is the "Marshall test"?** | Woman with urinary stress incontinence placed in the lithotomy position with a full bladder leaks urine when asked to cough. |

**What is the treatment of the following disorders:**

| | |
|---|---|
| **Stress incontinence?** | Bladder neck suspension |
| **Urge incontinence?** | Pharmacotherapy (anticholinergics, α-agonists) |
| **Overflow incontinence?** | Self-catheterization, surgical relief of obstruction, alpha blockers |

## UTI

| | |
|---|---|
| **What is it?** | Urinary tract infection |
| **What is the etiology?** | Ascending infection, instrumentation, sex in females |
| **What are the common organisms?** | 1. *E. coli* (90%)<br>2. *Proteus*<br>3. *Klebsiella, Pseudomonas* |
| **What are the predisposing factors?** | Stones, obstruction, reflux, diabetes mellitus, pregnancy, indwelling catheter/ stent |
| **What are the symptoms?** | Lower UTI—frequency, urgency, dysuria, nocturia<br>Upper UTI—back/flank pain, fever, chills |
| **How is the diagnosis made?** | Symptoms, urinalysis (>10 WBCs/HPF, >$10^5$ CFU) |

| When should workup be performed? | After first infection in male patients (unless Foley is in place) After first pyelonephritis in prepubescent female patients |
| --- | --- |
| What is the treatment? | Lower: 1 to 4 days of oral antibiotics Upper: 3 to 7 days of IV antibiotics |

## WARD QUESTIONS

| Why should orchiopexy be performed? | Decreases the susceptibility to blunt trauma Increases the ease of follow-up examinations |
| --- | --- |
| In which area of the prostate does BPH arise? | Periurethral |
| In which area of the prostate does prostate cancer arise? | Periphery |
| What type of bony lesions are seen in metastatic prostate cancer? | Osteoblastic (radiopaque) |
| What percentage of renal cell carcinoma shows evidence of metastatic disease at presentation? | Approximately 33% |
| What is the most common site of distant metastasis in renal cell carcinoma? | Lung |
| What is the most common solid renal tumor of childhood? | Wilms' tumor |
| What type of renal stone is radiolucent? | Uric acid (think: **U**ric = **U**nseen) |
| What are posterior urethral valves? | The most common obstructive urethral lesion in infants and newborns; occurs only in males; found at the distal prostatic urethra |

| | |
|---|---|
| **What is the most common intraoperative bladder tumor?** | A Foley catheter—don't fall victim! |
| **What provides drainage of the left gonadal (e.g., testicular) vein?** | Left renal vein |
| **What provides drainage of the right gonadal vein?** | IVC |
| **What are the signs of urethral injury in the trauma patient?** | "High-riding, ballottable" prostate, blood at the urethral meatus, severe pelvic fracture, ecchymosis of scrotum |
| **What is the evaluation for urethral injury in the trauma patient?** | RUG (**R**etrograde **U**rethro**G**ram) |
| **What is the evaluation for a transected ureter intraoperatively?** | IV indigo carmine and then look for leak of blue urine in the operative field |
| **What aid is used to help identify the ureters in a previously radiated retroperitoneum?** | Ureteral stents |
| **How can a small traumatic EXTRAperitoneal bladder rupture be treated?** | Foley catheter |
| **How should a traumatic INTRAperitoneal bladder rupture be treated?** | Operative repair |
| **What percentage of patients with an injured ureter will have no blood on urinalysis?** | 33% |
| **What is the classic history for papillary necrosis?** | Patient with diabetes taking NSAIDs or patient with sickle cell trait |

**What unique bleeding problem can be seen with prostate surgery?**

Release of TPA and urokinase (treat with ε-aminocaproic acid)

**What is the scrotal "blue dot" sign?**

Torsed appendix testis

**What is Peyronie's disease?**

Curved penile orientation with erection due to fibrosis of corpora cavernosa

# Rapid Fire Power Review

## TOP 100 CLINICAL SURGICAL MICROVIGNETTES

1. **Elderly woman, SBO, and air in biliary tract** — Gallstone ileus

2. **Elderly woman with pain down inner aspect of thigh** — Obturator hernia (Howship-Romberg sign)

3. **Abdominal pain, hypotension, and abdominal pulsatile mass** — Ruptured abdominal aortic aneurysm (AAA)

4. **Abdominal pain "out of proportion" to abdominal exam** — Mesenteric ischemia

5. **Arm pain and syncope with arm movement** — Subclavian steal syndrome

6. **Increasing creatinine on ACE inhibitor** — Renal artery stenosis

7. **Child with MIDLINE neck mass** — Thyroglossal duct cyst

8. **Child with LATERAL neck mass** — Branchial cleft cyst

9. **Crush injury and dark urine** — Myoglobinuria

10. **Emesis, chest pain radiating to back, and mediastinal air** — Boerhaave's

11. **Lower GI bleed + technetium pertechnetate scan** — Meckel's diverticulum

12. **Flushing, diarrhea, and right sided heart failure** — Carcinoid

13. **Pneumaturia and LLQ pain** — Colovesicular fistula

14. **Desmoid tumor, osteoma, and colon cancer** — Gardner's syndrome

15. **Epigastric pain radiating to back and flank ecchymosis** — Hemorrhagic pancreatitis

16. **Pancreatitis and palpable epigastric mass** — Pancreatic pseudocyst

17. **Liver abscess with "anchovy paste"** — Amebic abscess

18. **RUQ pain, travel, and exposure to sheep** — Hydatid cyst

19. **Caput medusa** — Portal hypertension

20. **45-year-old woman with RUQ pain for 12 hours, fever, and leukocytosis** — Acute cholecystitis

21. **Elderly man with large nontender palpable gallbladder** — Pancreatic cancer (Courvoisier's sign)

22. **Female taking birth control pills with liver mass** — Hepatic adenoma

23. **Liver tumor with "central scar"** — Focal nodular hyperplasia

24. **Pancreatic mass, gallstones, diabetes, and diarrhea** — Somatostatinoma

25. **RUQ bruit and CHF in young adult** — Liver hemangioma

| | |
|---|---|
| 26. **Excruciating pain with bowel movement** | Anal fissure |
| 27. **Abdominal pain, diarrhea, and anal fistulae** | Crohn's disease |
| 28. **ECG with "peaked" T waves** | Hyperkalemia |
| 29. **Buccal mucosa with pigmentation** | Peutz-Jeghers syndrome |
| 30. **LLQ pain, fever, and change in bowel habits** | Diverticulitis |
| 31. **Elevated urine 5-HIAA** | Carcinoid |
| 32. **Institutionalized, abdominal pain, vomiting, and distention, with proximal colonic dilation** | Sigmoid volvulus |
| 33. **Infant with projectile vomiting** | Pyloric stenosis |
| 34. **Newborn with failure to pass meconium in first 24 hours** | Hirschsprung's |
| 35. **Infant with bilious vomiting** | Malrotation |
| 36. **Newborn with abdominal defect and umbilical cord on sac** | Omphalocele |
| 37. **Teenager with knee pain and "onion skinning" on x-ray** | Ewing's sarcoma |
| 38. **Pulmonary capillary wedge pressure <18, CXR with bilateral pulmonary infiltrates, and PaO$_2$:FiO$_2$ ratio <200** | Acute respiratory distress syndrome (ARDS) |

39. **Increased peak airway pressure, low urine output, and urinary bladder >25 mmHg** — Abdominal compartment syndrome

40. **Newborn with inability to "pass an NGT"** — Esophageal atresia

41. **Traumatic blinding in one eye followed by blindness in the contralateral eye 2 weeks later** — Sympathetic ophthalmia

42. **Mitotic pupil, ptosis, and anhydrosis** — Horner's syndrome

43. **Traumatic head injury, conscious in ER followed by unconsciousness** — Epidural hematoma ("lucid interval")

44. **"Worst headache of my life"** — Subarachnoid hemorrhage

45. **Hematuria, flank pain, and abdominal mass (palpable)** — Renal cell carcinoma

46. **60-year-old white man with painless hematuria** — Bladder cancer

47. **RUQ pain, jaundice, and fever** — Cholangitis

48. **Epigastric pain radiating to back, with nausea and vomiting** — Pancreatitis

49. **Chest pain radiating to back and described as a "tearing" pain** — Aortic dissection

50. 40-year-old man with tachycardia/hypertension and confusion on postoperative day #2 — Alcohol withdrawal

51. Marfanoid body habitus and mucosal neuromas — MEN II-B

52. Psammoma bodies — Papillary thyroid cancer

53. Sulphur granules — Actinomyces infection

54. Thyroid tumor with AMYLOID tissue — Thyroid medullary cancer

55. PALPABLE neck tumor and hypercalcemia — Parathyroid cancer

56. Hypertension, diaphoresis (episodic), and palpitations — Pheochromocytoma

57. Jejunal ulcers — Zollinger-Ellison syndrome

58. Pituitary tumor, pancreatic tumor, and parathyroid tumor — MEN- I

59. Necrotizing migratory erythema — Glucagonoma

60. Medullary thyroid cancer, pheochromocytoma, and hyperparathyroidism — MEN-IIa

61. Hypokalemia refractory to IV potassium supplementation — Hypomagnesemia

62. Newborn with pneumatosis — Necrotizing enterocolitis (NEC)

63. Child with abdominal mass that crosses midline — Neuroblastoma

64. **Child <4 years of age with abdominal tumor that does NOT cross midline**

Wilms tumor

65. **"Currant jelly" stools and abdominal colic**

Intussusception

66. **Femur fracture, respiratory failure, petechiae, and mental status changes**

Fat embolism

67. **Hearing loss, tinnitus, and vertigo**

Ménière's disease

68. **Adolescent boy with nasal obstruction and recurrent epistaxis**

Juvenile nasopharyngeal angiofibroma

69. **Child <5 years of age sitting upright and drooling, with "hot potato" voice**

Epiglottitis

70. **Angina, syncope, and CHF**

Aortic stenosis

71. **Tobacco use, asbestos exposure, and pleuritic chest pain**

Mesothelioma

72. **Supracondylar fracture and contracture of forearm flexors**

Volkmann's contracture

73. **Tibia fracture, "pain out of proportion," pain on passive foot movement, and palpable pulses**

Compartment syndrome

74. **25-year-old man with liver mass with fibrous septae and NO history of cirrhosis or hepatitis**

**Fibrolamellar** hepatocellular carcinoma

75. **ECG with flattening of T waves and U waves** — Hypokalemia

76. **Central pontine myelinosis** — Too-rapid correction of hyponatremia

77. **Polydipsia, polyuria, and constipation** — Hypercalcemia

78. **Factor VIII deficiency** — Hemophilia A

79. **Abdominal pain, fever, hypotension, HYPERkalemia, and HYPOnatremia** — Adrenal insufficiency (Addisonian crisis)

80. **Massive urine output and HYPERnatremia** — Diabetes insipidus

81. **Increased urine osmolality, HYPOnatremia, and low serum osmolality** — SIADH

82. **IV antibiotics, fever, diarrhea** — *Clostridium difficile* pseudomembranous colitis

83. **Bleeding gums and wound dehiscence** — Vitamin C deficiency

84. **Fever, central line, and HYPERglycemia** — Central line infection

85. **Appendectomy followed by fever and abdominal pain on post-operative day #7** — Peritoneal abscess

86. **Advancing crepitus, fever, and blood blisters** — Necrotizing fasciitis

87. **High *intra*operative fever** — Malignant hyperthermia

88. **Confusion, ataxia, and ophthalmoplegia** — Wernicke's encephalopathy

89. **Tracheal deviation, decreased breath sounds, and hyperresonance**

    Tension pneumothorax

90. **Hypotension, decreased heart sounds, and JVD**

    Pericardial tamponade

91. **Four ribs broken in two places and pulmonary contusion**

    Flail chest

92. **Otorrhea (clear) and Battle's sign**

    Basilar skull fracture

93. **Ulcer and decreased pain with food**

    Duodenal ulcer

94. **Vomiting, retching, and epigastric pain**

    Mallory-Weiss tear

95. **Fever on postoperative day #1, with "bronze" weeping, tender wound**

    Clostridial wound infection

96. **Hematochezia and tenesmus**

    Rectal cancer

97. **Upper GI bleed, jaundice, and RUQ pain**

    Hemobilia

98. **Gallstones, epigastric pain radiating to back, and nausea**

    Gallstone pancreatitis

99. **18-year-old woman with bloody nipple discharge**

    Ductal papilloma

100. **Irritability, diaphoresis, weakness, tremulousness, and palpitations**

    Insulinoma

# Figure Credits

**Chapter 10 (carotid endarterectomy)**
Lawrence PF, Bell RM, Dayton MT. *Essentials of General Surgery.* 3rd ed. Philadelphia, PA: Lippincott Williams & Wilkins; 2000:545.

**Chapter 30 (craniocaudal view and MLO view mammograms)**
Gay SB, Woodcock RJ Jr. *Radiology Recall.* Philadelphia, PA: Lippincott Williams & Wilkins; 2000:522.

**Chapter 30 (free air seen on chest radiograph)**
Lawrence PF, Bell RM, Dayton MT. *Essentials of General Surgery.* 3rd ed. Philadelphia, PA: Lippincott Williams & Wilkins; 2000:267, Fig 7-19A.

**Chapter 38 (anatomy of the larynx)**
Doherty GM, Meko JB, Olson JA, et al. *The Washington Manual of Surgery,* 2nd ed. Philadelphia, PA: Lippincott Williams & Wilkins; 1999: 635, Fig 42-6.

**Chapter 40 (Sengstaken-Blakemore balloon)**
Lawrence PF, Bell RM, Dayton MT. *Essentials of General Surgery.* 3rd ed. Philadelphia, PA: Lippincott Williams & Wilkins; 2000:353, Fig 18-8.

**Chapter 38 (pneumothorax)**
Daffner RH. *Clinical Radiology. The Essentials.* 2nd ed. Baltimore, MD: Williams & Wilkins; 1999:154, Fig 4-91B.

**Chapter 38 (widened mediastinum)**
Greenfield LJ, Mulholland MW, Oldham KT, et al. *Surgery. Scientific Principles and Practice.* 3rd ed. Philadelphia, PA: Lippincott Williams & Wilkins; 2001:330, Fig 11-40.

**Chapter 56 (rectus abdominis flap reconstruction)**
Greenfield LJ, Mulholland M, Oldham KT, et al. *Surgery: Scientific Principles And Practices.* 2nd ed. Philadelphia, PA: Lippincott-Raven; 1997:2238, Fig 114-4.

**Chapter 57 (gastrinoma triangle)**
Greenfield LJ, Mulholland M, Oldham KT, et al. *Surgery: Scientific Principles And Practice.* 2nd ed. Philadelphia, PA: Lippincott-Raven; 1997:924, Fig 34-8.

**Chapter 56 (mammogram showing breast cancer)**
Daffner RH. *Clinical Radiology: The Essentials.* 2nd ed. Baltimore, MD: Williams & Wilkins; 1999:245, Fig 6-9A.

**Chapter 66 (endovascular repair)**
Zelenock GB, Huber TS, Messina LM, et al. *Mastery of Vascular and Endovas-cular Surgery.* Philadelphia, PA: Lippincott Williams & Wilkins; 2005.

**Chapter 74 (Colles' fracture)**
McKenney MG, Mangonon PC, Moylan JA. *Understanding Surgical Disease: The Miami Manual of Surgery.* Philadelphia PA: Lippincott-Raven; 1998:355, Fig 4.

**Chapter 75 (Kocher's point)**
Spector SA. *Clinical Companion in Surgery.* Philadelphia, PA: Lippincott Williams & Wilkins; 1999:430, Fig 33-1.

# Index

## A

Abbreviations, 15–18
Abdominal abscess, 208
Abdominal aortic aneurysms
  colonic ischemia in, 507–508
  definition of, 503
  diagnosis of, 505
  endovascular repair of, 506, 509
  epidemiology of, 504
  general questions about, 41, 208
  repair of, 506, 509
  risk factors for, 504
  rupture of, 505
  signs and symptoms of, 504
  treatment of, 506–507
Abdominal compartment syndrome, 153–154
Abdominal pain, 203–204, 206
Abdominal radiology, 185–190
Abdominal trauma, 37, 238, 243
Abdominal wall, 105, 213, 216
Abdominal wound dehiscence, 154
Abdominal x-rays
  appendicitis evaluations, 295
  description of, 39, 185–190
Abdominoperineal resection, 83
Abduction, 700
ABI, 497
ABO crossmatching, 687
Abrasion, 582
Abscess, 18
  abdominal, 208
  Bezold's, 602
  breast, 418
  definition of, 170
  diverticular, 321
  drainage of, 71
  lidocaine and, 191
  liver, 353–355
  lung, 632
  pancreatic, 391–392
  pelvic, 174
  perirectal, 329–330
  peritoneal, 174, 188

  peritonsillar, 614
  spinal epidural, 747–748
  "stitch," 174
  subcutaneous, 174
Absorbable suture, 53
Absorption atelectasis, 157
A-C (Assist-Control), 491
Accessory spleen, 460
Acetaminophen, 135
Achalasia, 649–650
Achilles tendon rupture, 716
Achlorhydria, 19
Acholic stool, 19
Acid burns, 245
Acid-base findings, 109
ACL, 699
Acral lentiginous melanoma, 475
ACTH, 419–422
Actinic keratosis, 473
*Actinomyces,* 178–179
Acute abdomen, 203–209
Acute acalculous cholecystitis, 375–376
Acute appendicitis, 38, 187
Acute arterial occlusion, 501–503
Acute cholecystitis, 189, 374–375
Acute mesenteric ischemia, 510–511
Acute pancreatitis, 263, 384–387
Acute respiratory distress syndrome, 32, 487
Acute rhinitis, 609
Acute sinusitis, 609–610
Acute suppurative otitis media, 601–602
Acute suppurative thyroiditis, 452
Addisonian crisis, 146–147
Addison's disease, 429
Adduction, 700
Adeno-, 19
Adenomatous polyp, 315
ADH, 147
Adhesion, 19
Adjuvant RX, 197
Admission orders, 12–14
Adnexa, 19
Adrenal adenoma, 422

Adrenal carcinoma, 422
Adrenal crisis, 182
Adrenal glands
  Addison's disease, 429
  anatomy of, 419
  Conn's syndrome, 427–429
  Cushing's syndrome, 33, 420–423
  glucagonoma, 431–432
  incidentaloma, 423–424
  insulinoma, 430–431
  multiple endocrine neoplasia, 436–439
  pheochromocytoma, 424–427
  physiology of, 419
  somatostatinoma, 432
  Zollinger-Ellison syndrome, 432–436
Adrenal vein, 419
α-Adrenergic blockers, 763
Adson forceps, 42
Adson maneuver, 630
Adson pickup, 44
Advanced trauma life support, 226, 242
Advancement flap, 584
Adventitia, 19
Aerobic metabolism, 486
Afferent, 19
Afferent loop syndrome, 32
AFO, 700
Afterload, 486, 657
A-gram, 338, 496
AI, 656
AIDS, 207
Air leaks, 97
Air-fluid level, 186
Airway management, 226–227
Albumin, 135
Albumin-furosemide "sandwich," 122
Albuterol, 135
Alcohol withdrawal, 156
Alcoholism, 358
Aldosterone, 428
-algia, 19
Alkali burns, 245
Alkaline phosphatase, 347, 366
Allen test, 148–149
Allen's test, 26
Allergic rhinitis, 609
Allis clamp, 48
Allografts, 248, 680, 700
Alpha-fetoprotein, 765

Amaurosis fugax, 19, 512
Ameba infection, 178
Amelanotic melanoma, 475
American Joint Committee for Cancer
    staging, 467, 477, 758, 761–762
Aminoglutethimide, 422
Amoebic infections, 130
Amphotericin, 131
Ampulla, 19
Amputations, 501
Amyand's hernia, 212
Anaerobic infections, 129
Anaerobic metabolism, 486
Anal fissure, 37, 330–331
Anal melanoma, 327–328
Analgesic, 19
Anaphylactic shock, 169
Anaplastic carcinoma, 449
Anastomosis, 19
Anatomic snuffbox, 590, 711
Anemia, 461
Anergy, 19
Anesthesia
  definition of, 190
  general questions about, 190–195
  malignant hyperthermia, 193
Aneurysm(s)
  abdominal aortic (see Abdominal aortic
      aneurysms)
  popliteal artery, 518–519
  splenic artery, 518
  thoracic aortic, 673–674
Aneurysmal bone cyst, 723
Angio-, 19
Angiocatheters, 171
Angiosarcoma, 349
Animal bites, 589
Anion gap, 482
Ankle to brachial index, 497
Ann Arbor staging, 469
Annular pancreas, 399, 569
Anomaly, 19
Anorectal fistulas, 329
Anosmia, 593
Anterior chamber, 234
Anterior cord syndrome, 737
Anterior drawer test, 715
Anterior mediastinum, 643–644
Anterior spinal syndrome, 104, 508, 674

Anteroposterior radiograph, 184
Antibiotics
    burns treated with, 251–252
    colorectal carcinoma surgery, 313
    general questions about, 129–131
    perforated appendix treated with, 296
    prophylactic, 176–177, 183
    topical, 251
Anticoagulation, 661
Antidiuretic hormone, 147
Antihypertensives, 80, 135
Antiseptic acid, 40
Antithrombin III deficiency, 126
Antithymocyte globulin, 684
Antrectomy, 89, 264
Anuria, 151
Anus
    anatomy of, 325
    cancer of, 325–328
    fistula in ano, 328–330
    hemorrhoids, 332–334
    imperforate, 548
    malformations of, 548
    perianal warts, 331–332
Aortic dissection, 674–679
Aortic injury
    thoracic, 37, 237–238
    traumatic, 185
Aortic insufficiency, 664–665
Aortic stenosis, 663–664
Aortoenteric fistula, 508
Aortograms, 238
Aphthous ulcer, 196
Apley's law, 577
Apnea, 19
Appearance, 2
Appendectomy, 41, 85, 136, 297–298
Appendicitis
    in adults, 38, 187, 207, 292–298
    in children, 558–559, 579
Appendix
    anatomy of, 292
    general questions about, 104
    tumors of, 299
Appendix testis, 756
ARDS, 32, 487
Army-Navy retractor, 51
AROM, 700
Arterial blood gases, 71

Arterial insufficiency ulcer, 196
Arterial lines, 148
Arterial oxygen content, 482
Arteries, 106
Arteriovenous malformation, 743
Artery, 493
Arthritis, 723–724
Arthrodesis, 702
Arthroplasty, 702
Artificial heart valves, 41, 667
AS, 656
ASD, 656
Aspirated foreign body, 529
Aspiration pneumonia, 141–142
Aspiration pneumonitis, 142
Aspirin, 125, 135, 498
Assist-control ventilation, 491
Astrocytoma, 740–742
Atelectasis, 19, 137, 180, 182
ATGAM, 684
Atherosclerosis, 493–494
ATLS, 226, 242
Atrial fibrillation, 149, 662, 677
Augmentin, 130
Austin Flint murmur, 679
Autografts, 248, 680
A-V block, 678
AVN, 700
Avulsion fracture, 706
Axilla, 400–402
Axillary artery to the femoral artery, 88
Axillary dissection, 400, 410
Axillary nerve, 713
Azathioprine, 683
Aztreonam (Azactam), 131

**B**

B cells, 681
$B_{12}$ deficiency, 145
Babcock clamp, 46
Backwash ileitis, 340
Bacteremia, 169
Bacteria, 178
Bacterial translocation, 179
Balance's sign, 460
Balanitis, 755
Balanoposthitis, 755
Ballance's sign, 26
Bandage scissors, 44

Bariatric, 19
Bariatric surgery, 280–281
Barium enema, 319, 343
Barlow's maneuver, 727
Barrett's esophagus, 26, 272, 653
Basal cell carcinoma, 472
Basal energy expenditure, 160
Basilar skull fracture, 234, 730
Bassini herniorrhaphy, 82
Bassini procedure, 215
Batson's plexus, 761
Battle's sign, 26
Beck's triad, 27, 230
Beckwith-Wiedemann syndrome, 570
Bell clapper's deformity, 753, 767
Bell's palsy, 604
Belsey Mark IV, 273, 653
Benign, 197
Benign prostatic hyperplasia,
    762–764, 773
Bennett's fracture, 707
Benzodiazepines, 136, 195
Bergman's triad, 27
Berry aneurysm, 743
Beta, 20
Betadine, 9
Bezold's abscess, 602
Bible cyst, 591
Bicarbonate, 163
Bifurcation, 20
Bile, 110, 201, 366
Bile acids, 199
Bile duct
    cholangiocarcinoma of, 382
    obstruction of, 208, 370–371
Bile salts, 20, 161
Bili-, 20
Biliary atresia, 565–566
Biliary colic, 368, 372, 375
Biliary surgery, 369–370
Biliary system, 188
Biliary tract
    anatomy of, 364–366
    cholangiocarcinoma, 368, 381–382
    cholangitis, 376–377
    cholecystitis (see Cholecystitis)
    cholelithiasis, 371–373
    diagnostic studies of, 369
    gallstone ileus, 378–379

    obstructive jaundice, 370–371
    pathophysiology of, 367–369
    physiology of, 366–367
    sclerosing cholangitis, 377–378
Bilious vomiting, 575
Billroth I, 81–82, 265
Billroth II, 81–82, 265
Biloma, 368
Biopsy
    breast cancer, 406–407
    mammotome, 406
    needle loc, 406
    sentinel node, 410, 478
Bird's beak sign, 187
Bites, 178, 245, 589
Bladder cancer, 759–760
Bladder candidiasis, 171
Bladder fistula, 307
Bladder outlet obstruction, 757
Bladder rupture, 242, 774
Bladder tumors, 773–774
Blepharoplasty, 579
Blind loop syndrome, 33, 145
Blood transfusions, 36, 123, 125
Blood types, 123
Blount's disease, 728
Blowout fracture, 625
Blue dot sign, 542, 775
Blue toe syndrome, 500, 520
Blumer's shelf, 27, 276
Blunt esophagectomy, 656
Blunt trauma, 238, 575
BMI, 280
Boas' sign, 27
Bochdalek's hernia, 212, 535–536
Body fluid compartments, 106
Boerhaave's syndrome, 33, 268–269
"Bogata Bag," 154
Boil, 20
Bolus, 112–113
Bone cysts, 723
Bone tumors, 719–721, 729
Bony orbit, 595
Borchardt's triad, 27
Bouchard's nodes, 723
Boutonniere deformity, 590
Bovie, 20, 127–128
Bovine electrocautery, 49
Bowel obstruction

large, 37
pediatric, 537, 577
small, 143–144, 285–288, 300, 577
"Bowel prep," 181
Bowen's disease, 326, 473
Boxer's fracture, 589, 707–708
BPH, 756
Brachial plexus, 713
Brachytherapy, 197
Brain tumors
cerebellar astrocytomas, 741–742
general questions about, 739–740
gliomas, 740
medulloblastoma, 742
meningiomas, 741
Branchial cleft anomalies, 527
Breast
anatomy of, 400–402
benign diseases of, 415–419
lymphatic drainage of, 402
Paget's disease of, 414
suspensory ligaments, 402
Breast abscess, 418
Breast cancer
adjuvant therapy for, 411–412
biopsy evaluations, 406–407, 410
chemotherapy for, 412
DCIS, 412–413
description of, 35, 39
general questions about, 403–412
invasive, 413–415
LCIS, 413–415
male, 415
mammograms, 189–190, 405–406
metastases, 408
modified radical mastectomy for, 409
radiation therapy for, 408–409
risk factors for, 403–404
screening for, 405–406
signs and symptoms of, 404
staging of, 408
susceptibility genes, 403
tamoxifen for, 410–411
treatment of, 408–410
types of, 404–405
Breast cyst, 417
Breast mass, 407
Breast milk, 402, 522
Breast reconstruction, 410–411, 414

Breathing, 228–231
Breslow classification, 477
Bronchogenic carcinoma, 635–639
Brooke ileostomy, 82, 283
Brown's sign, 628
Brown-Séquard syndrome, 738
Bsoas' sign, 372
Budd-Chiari syndrome, 33, 360
Buerger's disease, 520
Bullous myringitis, 600
BUN/Cr ratio, 152
Bupivacaine, 192
Burn(s), 245–253, 581
Burn shock, 249

# C

CA-19-9, 396
CABG, 656, 659–660
CAD, 656
Calcaneus fracture, 713
Calcium, 163, 201, 454
Calculus, 20, 770–771
Calories, 159
Calot's node, 104
Calot's triangle, 103, 365–366
Canal cancer, 327
Cancer (*see also* Carcinoma)
anal, 325–328
bladder, 759–760
gastric, 275–279
general questions about, 197–198
head and neck, 627
nasal cavity, 611–612
oral cavity, 615
paranasal sinus, 611–612, 627
prostate, 760–762, 773
testicular, 764–767
Candidiasis, 171
Cantle's line, 345
Captopril provocation test, 517
Caput medusae, 359–360
Carafate (*see* Sucralfate)
Carbohydrates, 160
Carbon dioxide retention, 488
Carbon monoxide inhalation, 252
Carbuncle, 20, 179
Carcinoembryonic antigen, 41, 82
Carcinoid syndrome, 27, 33, 301–302
Carcinoid triad, 27

Carcinoid tumors, 300–304, 641–642
Carcinoma (*see also* Cancer)
  bronchogenic, 635–639
  esophageal, 654–656
  gallbladder, 380–381
  hepatocellular, 352–353
  pancreatic, 395–398
  parathyroid, 458–460
  renal cell, 757–758, 773
Cardiac index, 481, 657
Cardiac output, 481, 490, 657–658, 661
Cardiac tamponade, 27, 230
Cardiac tumors, 673
Cardiogenic shock, 167–168
Cardiopulmonary bypass, 661–663
Cardiovascular complications,
  148–150
Cardiovascular surgery
  abbreviations, 656–657
  aortic insufficiency, 664–665
  aortic stenosis, 663–664
  artificial valve placement, 667
  cardiopulmonary bypass, 661–663
  congenital heart disease (*see*
    Congenital heart disease)
  coronary artery bypass grafting, 656,
    659–660
  coronary artery disease, 658–659
  general questions about, 656–658
  infectious endocarditis, 667–668
  mitral regurgitation, 666
  mitral stenosis, 665–666
  postpericardiotomy syndrome, 660
Carotid endarterectomy, 76
Carotid vascular disease, 512–515
Carpal tunnel syndrome, 591–593
Cast saw, 718
Cat bites, 589
Catgut sutures, 53
Catheter
  Coudé, 100, 753
  epidural, 193
  femoral vein, 232
  Fogarty, 502
  Foley, 22, 67, 100–101, 194, 232,
    236, 753
  Hickman, 101
  intravenous, 65
  suprapubic, 753

  Swan-Ganz, 488
  Tenckhoff, 102
Cation, 113–114
Cauda equina syndrome, 746
Caustic esophageal strictures, 653–654
Cauterization, 20
CBC differential, 205
C-C mammogram, 189
CEA, 82, 311
Cecal volvulus, 323–324
Cecum, 104, 552
Cefazolin, 130
Cefoxitin, 130
Ceftazidime, 130
Celiac trunk, 346
Celiotomy, 20, 240
Cellulitis, 169
Central cord syndrome, 737
Central diabetes insipidus, 148
Central line infections, 171
Central lines, 101
Central pontine myelinolysis, 117
Central venous pressure, 481
Cephal-, 20
Cephalosporins, 130
Cerebellar astrocytomas, 741–742
Cerebral contusion, 735
Cerebrovascular accident, 150, 513
Cervical disc disease, 746–747
Cervical spine
  bony fracture of, 237
  injury to, 184
  ligamentous injury, 237
  studies for evaluating, 237
Chance fracture, 738
Charcot's joint, 717, 724
Charcot's triad, 27
Chemotherapy, 412
Chest pain, 149
Chest radiology, 183–185
Chest tubes, 93–98
Chest wall tumors, 630–631
Chest x-rays, 183–185
Chief cells, 199, 271
Chilaiditi's sign, 188
Child abuse, 576
Children (*see also* Pediatric surgery)
  abdomen in, 537–538
  annular pancreas in, 569

anorectal malformations in, 548
appendicitis in, 558–559, 579
aspirated foreign body in, 529
biliary atresia in, 565–566
biliary tract disorders in, 564–569
blood volumes in, 523
branchial cleft anomalies in, 527
chest deformities in, 529–536
choledochal cyst in, 566–568
cholelithiasis in, 568
congenital diaphragmatic hernia in, 535–536
congenital hip dislocation, 727–728
cystic hygroma in, 528–529
duodenal atresia in, 545
esophageal atresia in (see Esophageal atresia)
gastroesophageal reflux disease in, 542–543
gastroschisis in, 556–557
hepatoblastoma in, 574, 579
Hirschsprung's disease, 549–552
inguinal hernias in, 220, 538–542
intussusception in, 560–561, 578
lung mass in, 529
malrotation, 552–553, 578
Meckel's diverticulum in, 561–562
meconium ileus in, 546–547
meconium peritonitis in, 547
meconium plug syndrome in, 547
midgut volvulus, 552–553
neck masses in, 525–529
necrotizing enterocolitis in, 563–564
neuroblastoma in, 570–573, 579
omphalocele, 553–557
orthopaedic disorders, 724–729
pulmonary sequestration in, 536–537
pyloric stenosis in, 543–545
rhabdomyosarcoma in, 573–574
stridor in, 527–528
thyroglossal duct cyst in, 525–527
traumatic injuries in, 575
tumors in, 569–574, 577
umbilical hernia in, 542
Child's classification, 347–348
Chimerism, 680
Chloride, 107, 108
Chol-, 20
Cholangiocarcinoma, 368, 381–382

Cholangitis
general questions about, 27, 36, 368, 376–377
sclerosing, 377–378
Cholecyst-, 20
Cholecystectomy, 85, 365, 369–370
Cholecystenteric fistula, 306
Cholecystitis
acute, 374–375
acute acalculous, 375–376
general questions about, 207, 368
Cholecystokinin, 200, 366
Cholecystostomy tube, 93
Choledochal cyst, 566–568
Choledocho-, 20
Choledochojejunostomy, 79, 85, 369
Choledocholithiasis, 368, 373
Cholelithiasis
in adults, 38, 208, 367, 371–373
in children, 568
Cholestasis, 130
Cholesteatoma, 599–600
Chromium deficiency, 161
Chronic mesenteric ischemia, 510
Chronic obstructive pulmonary disease, 138
Chronic otitis media, 602
Chronic pancreas, 388–390
Chronic sinusitis, 610–611
Chvostek's sign, 27, 118
Chyme, 20
CI, 481
Cigarette smoking, 80
Cimetidine, 134
Ciprofloxacin (Cipro), 131, 137
Circulating nurse, 7
Circulation
fetal, 523–525
trauma assessments of, 231–232
Circumcision, 576
Cirrhosis, 358
Clark's classification, 476
Claudication, 496, 498
Clay shoveler's fracture, 708, 738
"Clean" wound, 172
Clean-contaminated wound, 172
Cleido-, 20
Clindamycin, 130
Clips, 128

Clonidine "rebound," 137
Closed fracture, 704
Closed reduction, 700
Clostridial myositis, 175
*Clostridium difficile,* 155
Clotting factors, 125
$CO_2$ insufflation, 224
Coarctation of the aorta, 670–671
Cobblestoning, 343
Colic, 20, 203
Collateral circulation, 670
Collection chamber, 95
Colles' fracture, 706–707
Colloid fluids, 21, 122
Colon
  anatomy of, 307–308
  bleeding from, 337
  colorectal carcinoma, 309–314
  diverticular disease of, 318–324
  familial polyposis syndrome, 316
  Gardner's syndrome, 317
  general questions about, 105, 201
  penetrating injuries to, 243
  Peutz-Jeghers' syndrome, 317–318
  polyps of, 315–316
Colon cancer, 38, 197
Colon surgery, 80, 136
Colonic fistulas, 305–306
Colonic ischemia, 507–508
Colonic villous adenomas, 39
Colonic volvulus, 37, 321
Colonoscopy, 21, 319, 337
Colony-forming units, 170
Colorectal carcinoma, 309–314
Colostomy, 21, 79, 282–283
Comminuted fracture, 704
Common bile duct
  description of, 189
  obstruction of, 36
Common carotid artery, 514
Communicating hydrocele, 540, 753
Communicating hydrocephalus, 748
Compartment syndrome, 33, 503,
  711–712, 727
Complete blood count, 127
Compliance, 486, 657
Computed tomography
  abdominal, 188
  pelvic, 188

  peritoneal abscess findings, 174
  reading of, 185
  trauma evaluations, 239
Congenital diaphragmatic hernia,
  535–536
Congenital heart disease
  coarctation of the aorta, 670–671
  Ebstein's anomaly, 672
  IHSS, 670
  patent ductus arteriosus, 669
  tetralogy of Fallot, 669–670
  transposition of the great
    vessels, 672
  vascular rings, 672
  ventricular septal defect, 668–669
Congenital hip dislocation, 727–728
Congenital pyloric stenosis, 543–545
Conjoint tendon, 219
Conn's syndrome, 427–429
Consent form, 79
Constipation, 21, 143, 538
Contaminated wound, 172
Continuous positive airway
  pressure, 491
Contractility, 486
Contrast allergy, 189
Contusion
  cerebral, 735
  definition of, 582
Cooper's hernia, 212
Cooper's ligament, 82
Cor pulmonale, 21
Cord lipoma, 217, 542
Cordis, 101
Core biopsy, 467
Coronary arteries, 658
Coronary artery bypass grafting, 41, 88,
  656, 659–660
Coronary artery disease, 658–659
Coronary ligament, 345
Coronary veins, 105
Corrigan's pulse, 664
Corticosteroids, 682–683
Cortisol, 420, 683
Coudé catheter, 100, 753
Coumadin (*see* Warfarin)
Courvoisier's gallbladder, 383
Courvoisier's law, 27–28
Courvoisier's sign, 396

CPAP, 491
CPB, 656
CPP, 731
Cranial nerves, 593–595
Craniosynostosis, 750–751
Cremaster muscle, 216
CRH, 419
Cricoid pressure, 191
Cricothyroidotomy, 83, 242, 626
Crigler-Najjar syndrome, 565
Crocodile tears, 628
Crohn's disease, 287, 299, 338–344
Cronkhite-Canada syndrome, 318
Cross, 124
Croup, 618–619, 628
Cryoprecipitate, 123
Cryptorchidism, 540, 576, 755, 764
Crystalloid fluids, 249
Cullen's sign, 28, 391
Curettage, 21
Curling's ulcer, 196, 261
Cushing's disease, 422
Cushing's reflex, 731
Cushing's syndrome, 33, 420–423
Cushing's triad, 28
Cushing's ulcer, 196, 261
Cut-off sign, 187
Cutting needles, 55
CVA, 513
CVP, 481
Cyanotic heart disease, 673
Cyclosporine, 683–684
Cyst
    aneurysmal bone, 723
    bible, 591
    breast, 417
    choledochal, 566–568
    definition of, 21
    dermoid, 645
    epidermal, 72, 472
    sebaceous, 72, 473
    thyroglossal duct, 525–527
Cystic fibrosis, 547
Cystic hygroma, 528–529
Cystogram, 752
Cystosarcoma phyllodes, 416
Cystoscope, 752
Cytomegalovirus, 698
Cytotec (*see* Misoprostol)

**D**
DAI, 735
Daily notes, 13–14
Dakin solution, 42, 91
Damage control surgery, 244
Dance's sign, 28, 576
Dantrolene (Dantrium), 135
DCIS, 412–413
De Quervain's thyroiditis, 452
Dead space, 487
Deaver retractor, 50
DeBakey classifications, 674–675
DeBakey forceps, 42
DeBakey pickups, 8, 43
Decompression, 232
Decortication, 632
Decubitus ulcer, 196
Deep venous thrombosis, 138–139,
    180, 182
Degenerative arthritis, 723
Delayed primary closure, 90
Demerol, 136, 192–193
Depolarizing agents, 191
Dermatomes, 105, 207, 729
Dermis, 72
Dermoid cyst, 645
Dexamethasone, 683
Dexamethasone suppression test, 420
Dextrose, 111
Diabetes insipidus, 148
Diabetic ketoacidosis, 146
Diagnostic peritoneal lavage, 238–239
Dialysis, 152
Diaphragm, 105, 243
Diaphragmatic hernia, congenital,
    535–536
Diaphysis, 702
Diarrhea
    postvagotomy, 145
    in pseudomembranous colitis, 176
    in Zollinger-Ellison syndrome, 433
DIC, 152–153
Dieulafoy's ulcer, 196, 261
Diffuse axonal injury, 735
Diffuse esophageal spasm, 650–651
Diflucan (*see* Fluconazole)
DiGeorge's syndrome, 454
Digital arteries, 588
Digitalis, 116, 122

DIOS, 547
Direct bilirubin, 21
Direct inguinal hernia, 212–213
Dirty wound, 172
Disability, 233
Dislocation
  definition of, 702
  elbow, 714
  hip, 714
  knee, 714–715
  shoulder, 713–714
Dissecting aortic aneurysm, 677
Disseminated intravascular coagulation,
  152–153
Dissociative agent, 191
Disulfiram-like reaction, 130
Diverticular abscess, 321
Diverticular disease, 318–324
Diverticulitis, 208, 320–321
Diverticulosis, 318–319
Dobbhoff tube, 100
Dobutamine, 485
Dog bites, 245
Dopamine, 484
Double-barrel colostomy, 282
Double bubble sign, 578
DPL, 238–239
Drains, 91–93
DRE, 754
Dressings, 251
Drop finger, 589
Dry gangrene, 500
Ductus arteriosus, 524
Ductus venosus, 524
Duhamel procedure, 551
Duke stages, 311–312
Dumping syndrome, 33, 145–146, 259
Duodenal artery, 36
Duodenal atresia, 545
Duodenal hematoma, 575
Duodenum
  anatomy of, 284
  injury to, 244
  perforation of, 262
  ulcers of, 103, 252, 257–261
Dupuytren's contracture, 591, 717
-dynia, 21
Dys-, 21
Dyspareunia, 21

Dysphagia, 21, 593
Dyspnea, 149
Dysuria, 754

**E**
Eagle-Barrett's syndrome, 576
Ear disorders
  acute suppurative otitis media,
    601–602, 626
  Bell's palsy, 604
  bullous myringitis, 600
  cholesteatoma, 599–600
  facial nerve paralysis, 603–604, 626
  glomus tumors, 607
  malignant otitis externa, 597–598
  Ménière's disease, 607, 627
  otitis externa, 597, 625
  otitis media, 601–602, 626
  otosclerosis, 602–603
  sensorineural hearing loss, 605
  tumors, 598–599
  tympanic membrane perforation, 599
  vertigo, 606
Earrings, 6
Ebstein's anomaly, 672
Ecchymosis, 21
Echinococcal cysts, 355
ECMO, 525
-ectomy, 21, 78
Ectopic ACTH, 420
EEA stapler, 47–48
Efferent, 21
Eisenmenger's syndrome, 668
Ejection fraction, 657, 666
Elbow dislocation, 714
Electrical burns, 245
Electrocardiogram, 80, 121–122, 149
Electrolyte deficiency, 36
Electrolyte imbalances
  description of, 113–114
  hypercalcemia, 117–118
  hyperglycemia, 120
  hyperkalemia, 114–115, 121
  hypermagnesemia, 119
  hypernatremia, 116
  hyperphosphatemia, 121
  hypocalcemia, 118–119
  hypoglycemia, 120
  hypokalemia, 115–116

hypomagnesemia, 119–120
hyponatremia, 116–117
hypophosphatemia, 120–121
"pseudohyponatremia," 117
Electrolyte-mediated ileus, 122
Electrolytes, 202, 252
Embolism
description of, 502
mesenteric, 511
paradoxical, 520
pulmonary, 138–141, 180, 190
"Saddle," 140
Emergency abdominal surgery, 36
Emergent thoracotomy, 231
Empiric, 170
Empyema, 632
End colostomy, 282
Endartectomy, 21
Endocarditis, 181, 667–668
Endocrine complications, 146–148
Endocrine systems
adrenal glands (*see* Adrenal glands)
parathyroid glands (*see* Parathyroid
glands)
thyroid gland (*see* Thyroid gland)
Endotracheal tube, 493
Endovascular repair, 495, 506
End-to-end anastomosis stapler, 47–48
End-to-side portocaval shunt, 363
Enteral feeding, 162
Enteritis, 22
Enterocutaneous fistula, 305
Enterohepatic circulation, 199, 366
Enterolysis, 22, 85
Entrapment, 625
Enuresis, 755, 772
Epidermal cyst, 72, 472
Epidermis, 72
Epididymis, 541
Epididymitis, 754, 768
Epidural abscess, 747–748
Epidural analgesia, 193
Epidural anesthesia, 190
Epidural catheter, 193
Epidural hematoma, 37, 733–734
Epigastric hernia, 212
Epigastric pain, 206
Epiglottitis, 619, 628
Epinephrine, 192, 194, 426, 485

Epispadias, 756
Epistaxis, 608
Epithelialization, 581
ERCP, 369, 373, 390
Eschar, 22
Esophageal atresia
with tracheoesophageal fistula,
532–535
without tracheoesophageal fistula, 532
Esophageal carcinoma, 654–656
Esophageal diseases
achalasia, 649–650
anatomy, 648–649
caustic esophageal strictures, 653–654
diffuse esophageal spasm, 650–651
nutcracker esophagus, 651–652
Zenker's diverticulum, 649
Esophageal laceration, 37
Esophageal perforation, 36
Esophageal reflux, 652–653
Esophageal spasm, 650–651
Esophageal varices, 267–268, 358–361
Esophagus, 202
anatomy of, 648–649
Barrett's, 26, 272, 653
nutcracker, 651–652
ETOH withdrawal, 181
Euvolemia, 117
Eversion, 700
Ewing's sarcoma, 721–723
Excisional biopsy, 22, 90, 467
Exploratory laparotomy, 87
Extended lymph node dissection, 279
External oblique aponeurosis, 219
Extra-anatomic bypass graft, 508
Extracellular fluid, 106, 107
Extracorporeal membrane
oxygenation, 525
Extralobar, 537, 642
Extremity fractures, 244
Exudate, 631

**F**
Face lift, 579
Facial fractures, 623–625
Facial nerve paralysis, 603–604, 626
Faintness, 6
Falciform ligament, 345
False aneurysm, 494

Familial hypocalciuric hypercalcemia, 456
Familial polyposis syndrome, 316
Famotidine, 135
Fascia, 22
Fascial dehiscence, 154
FAST, 238
Fat emboli syndrome, 27
Fats, 160
Fat-soluble vitamins, 161
Fatty acid deficiency, 161
Fecalith, 39, 187, 295
Felon, 179, 588
FEM DISTAL bypass, 499–500
Femoral artery to popliteal artery bypass, 87
Femoral canal, 219
Femoral fracture, 711
Femoral hernia, 212, 219
Femoral vein, 65–66
Femoral vein catheter, 232
Femoral vessels, 103
FEM-POP bypass, 499
FENA, 151–152, 483
FESS, 611
Fetal circulation, 523–525
FEV1, 639
Fever, 157, 180–182
Fibrin glue, 128
Fibroadenoma, 416–417
Fibrocystic disease, 417
Fibrous dysplasia, 721
Figure-of-eight suture, 128
FiO$_2$, 158, 487
First degree burns, 245, 247
First-degree A-V block, 678
First-degree hemorrhoid, 332–333
Fistula
    anorectal, 329
    aortoenteric, 508
    bladder, 307
    cholecystenteric, 306
    colonic, 305–306
    definition of, 22
    enterocutaneous, 305
    external pancreatic, 306
    general questions about, 304
    pancreatic, 399
    pancreatic enteric, 306
    tracheoesophageal, 532–535
Fistula in ano, 328–330

Fitz-Hugh-Curtis syndrome, 33, 179
Fixation, 700
Flagyl (*see* Metronidazole)
Flail chest, 229–230
Flaps, 583–585
Flexor digitorum profundus, 587–588
Flexor digitorum superficialis, 588
Fluconazole, 131
Fludrocortisone, 147
Fluid resuscitation
    in burns, 248–250
    in pediatric patients, 575
    in trauma, 232
Fluids, 106–113
Focal nodular hyperplasia, 350–351
Fogarty catheter, 502
Foley catheter, 22, 67, 100–101, 194, 232, 236, 753
Follicular adenocarcinoma, 446–447
Foot dorsiflexion, 700
Forceps, 42–43
Forearm compartment syndrome, 712
Foregut, 103
Foreign body aspiration, 529
Fothergill's sign, 28
Fournier's gangrene, 178, 753
Fourth degree burns, 246
Fourth-degree hemorrhoid, 334
Fox's sign, 28, 391
Fractional excretion of sodium, 483
Fractures, 704–709
    avulsion, 706
    basilar skull, 234, 730
    Bennett's, 707
    boxer's, 589, 707–708
    calcaneal, 713
    chance, 738
    in children, 724
    clay shoveler's, 708, 738
    closed, 704
    Colles', 706–707
    comminuted, 704
    extremity, 244
    facial, 623–625
    femoral, 711
    Galeazzi, 708
    greenstick, 706
    hangman's, 708, 738
    humeral, 711

impacted, 705
intra-articular, 706
Jefferson's, 738
Jones', 707
laryngeal, 242
Le Fort, 623–624
longitudinal, 705
mandibular, 234, 623, 625
maxillofacial, 232
midface, 623–625
Monteggia, 708
night stick, 708, 717
oblique, 705
odontoid, 738–739
open, 704, 709–710
pathologic, 705
pelvic, 236, 239, 242–243
periarticular, 706
pilon, 709
Pott's, 709
simple, 704
skull, 234, 730, 736
Smith's, 707
spiral, 705
stress, 705
tibial plateau, 708
torus, 706
transcervical, 708
transverse, 704
tripod, 624–625
FRED, 224
Free air, 188, 205
Free flap, 584
Free peritoneal air, 38
Frequency, 22, 754
Fresh frozen plasma, 123
Frey procedure, 389
Frey's syndrome, 627
FROM, 699
FTSG, 579, 583
Fungal sinusitis, 610
Furosemide, 135
Furuncle, 22, 178
FWB, 699

**G**

G cells, 199, 271
Galactorrhea, 416
Galeazzi fracture, 708

Gallbladder
    carcinoma of, 380–381
    general questions about, 188–189,
        200, 365
    hydrops of, 382
Gallbladder emptying, 366
Gallstone ileus, 378–379
Gallstone pancreatitis, 390
Gallstones, 39, 187, 202, 369, 371–372
Gamekeeper's thumb, 591
Ganciclovir, 698
Gangrene, 500
Gardner's syndrome, 33, 317
Gas-bloat syndrome, 275
Gastrectomy, 79, 278
Gastric bypass, 280–281
Gastric cancer, 38, 275–279
Gastric decompression, 232
Gastric dilatation, 142
Gastric mucosa, 270
Gastric parietal cells, 199, 271
Gastric resection, 41
Gastric secretions, 110
Gastric ulcers, 40, 195, 252, 259–261, 263
Gastric varices, 463
Gastric volvulus, 27, 279
Gastrin, 200–201, 433–434
Gastrinoma triangle, 104
Gastrocolic reflex, 202
Gastroenteritis, 207
Gastroesophageal reflux disease,
        271–275, 542–543
Gastrografin enema, 323
Gastrointestinal anastomosis stapler, 47, 58
Gastrointestinal bleeding
    description of, 182
    lower, 334–338
    upper (see Upper gastrointestinal
        bleeding)
Gastrointestinal carcinoids, 36, 303
Gastrointestinal hormones, 199–202
Gastrointestinal lymphoma, 470
Gastrointestinal tract, 102
Gastrojejunostomy, 79
Gastropexy, 22
Gastroschisis, 556–557
Gastrostomy, 79, 282, 284
GCS, 233
General anesthesia, 191

Gentamicin, 131
GERD, 542–543
Gerota's fascia, 102
GET/GETA, 191
GIA stapler, 47, 58
Gilbert's syndrome, 382, 564
Glasgow Coma Scale, 233, 730–732
Gliomas, 740
Globus, 593
Glomus tumors, 607
Glottic lesions, 620–621
Gloves, 7, 40
Glucagonoma, 400, 431–432
Glucose-6-phosphate deficiency, 462
Gomco clamp, 753
Goodsall's rule, 28–29, 328–329
Gout, 724
Gown, 6–7
Graham patch, 85, 262–263
Gram-negative infections, 130
Granulation tissue, 582
Graves' disease, 450–451
"Great imitator," 207
Great vessels
    aortic dissection, 673–679
    diseases of, 673–679
    injuries to, 235
Greenfield filter, 140
Greenstick fracture, 706
Grey Turner's sign, 29, 391
Groin hernias, 213–219
Grynfeltt's hernia, 210
G-tube, 92
Gubernaculum, 102
Gunshot wounds, 240, 244
Gut sutures, 53
Gynecologic pain, 206
Gynecomastia, 418–419

**H**

Haldol, 134
Halo sign, 236
Halothane, 195
Hamartoma, 349
Hamburger sign, 559
Hamman's sign/crunch, 29, 269
Hand
    bones of, 585
    carpal tunnel syndrome, 591–593
    general questions about, 585–586
    intrinsic muscles of, 585
    No Man's Land, 585–586
    sensory supply to, 586–591
    splinting of, 591
    trauma zones of, 586
Hangman's fracture, 708, 738
Haplotype, 681
Harmonic scalpel, 128
Hartmann's pouch, 88, 282, 365
Hartmann's procedure, 83
Hashimoto's thyroiditis, 452
Hasson technique, 224
ß-HCG, 765–766
Head and neck
    anatomy, 593–597
    cancer of, 627
    cranial nerves, 593–595
    ear (see Ear disorders)
    general questions about, 593
    nose, 608–612
Head trauma
    cerebral contusion, 735
    epidural hematoma, 733–734
    general questions about, 729–730
    Glasgow Coma Scale, 730–732
    subdural hematoma, 734–735
    traumatic subarachnoid hemorrhage,
      735
Hearing loss, 605
Heart transplantation, 41, 695–696
Heart-lung transplantation, 41
Heberden's nodes, 723
Heel spur, 717
Heerfordt's syndrome, 626
Heimlich valve, 98
Heineke-Mikulicz pyloroplasty, 86
Hemangioma, 22, 576
    hepatic, 351
Hemangiomas, 576
Hematemesis, 22, 266
Hematochezia, 254, 310
Hematocrit, 39, 123, 125
Hematoma, 22
    epidural, 733–734
    subdural, 734–735
    wound, 154
Hematuria, 755, 757, 771
Hemicolectomy, 89

Hemobilia, 356
Hemodynamic monitoring, 488–490
Hemoglobin, 123
Hemophilia A, 125–126
Hemophilia B, 126
Hemoptysis, 22, 632–633
Hemorrhage
  description of, 237
  intracerebral, 744–745
  subarachnoid, 735, 743–744
Hemorrhagic pancreatitis, 390–391
Hemorrhoidal vein, 357
Hemorrhoidectomy, 334
Hemorrhoids, 332–334, 360
Hemostasis, 127–128
Hemothorax, 22, 230–231
Heparin, 132–133
Heparin rebound, 662
Heparin-induced thrombocytopenic
    thrombosis syndrome, 33
Hepatic lobectomy, 348–349
Hepaticojejunostomy, 83, 369
Hepato-, 22
Hepatoblastoma, 574, 579
Hepatocellular adenoma, 349–350
Hepatocellular carcinoma, 352–353
Hepatocytes, 347
Hepatoma, 197, 349
Hernia
  congenital diaphragmatic, 535–536
  definition of, 37, 209
  femoral, 219
  general questions about, 209–213
  groin, 213–219
  hiatal (see Hiatal hernias)
  incarcerated, 209, 220
  inguinal (see Inguinal hernias)
  reducible, 209
  repair of, 215–219
  review questions for, 220
Hernia sac, 216–217, 540
Herniorrhaphy, 22, 79
Herpes simplex virus, 698
Hesitancy, 23, 755
Hesselbach's hernia, 212
Hesselbach's triangle, 103, 213, 217–218,
    538
Heterotopic, 680
5-HIAA, 302

Hiatal hernia
  definition of, 212
  esophageal, 221–222
  paraesophageal, 222
Hiatus, 23
Hickman catheter, 101
HIDA/PRIDA scan, 369, 376
Hidradenitis, 23
High ligation procedure, 215
Highly selective vagotomy, 84
Hill procedure, 274
Hindgut, 103
Hip dislocation, 714, 727–728
Hirschsprung's disease, 549–552
Histocompatibility antigens, 680
History, 9–10
HITT syndrome, 33
HIV, 124
HLA crossmatching, 687
HLA matching, 681
Hodgkin's disease, 468–470
Homans' sign, 29, 139
Horizontal mattress stitch, 56
Hormones, 199–202
Horner's syndrome, 571, 636, 752
Howship-Romberg sign, 29, 220
Human bites, 178, 245, 589
Humeral fracture, 711
Hungry bone syndrome, 459
Hürthle cell thyroid cancer, 447–448
Hutchinson's freckle, 475–476
Hydatid liver cysts, 355–356
Hydrocele, 540, 753
Hydrocephalus, 748–749
Hyperacute rejection, 687
Hyperaldosteronism, 428–429
Hypercalcemia, 117–118, 454,
    456–458
Hypercoagulable states, 127
Hyperglycemia, 113, 120
Hyperkalemia, 114–115, 121
Hypermagnesemia, 119
Hypernatremia, 116
Hyperparathyroidism, 455–458
Hyperphosphatemia, 121
Hypersplenism, 463
Hypertension, 156
  portal, 102, 357–364, 464
  surgically correctable, 464–465

Hyperthyroidism, 450
Hypertrophic pulmonary
    osteoarthropathy, 639, 641
Hypertrophic scar, 582
Hyperventilation, 732
Hypervolemia, 117
Hypoalbuminemia, 118
Hypocalcemia, 118–119, 387, 459
Hypochloremic alkalosis, 108
Hypogastric artery, 105
Hypoglossal nerve, 595
Hypoglycemia, 120
Hypokalemia, 109, 115–116
Hypokalemic hypochloremic metabolic
    acidosis, 109
Hypomagnesemia, 119–120
Hyponatremia, 116–117
Hypoparathyroidism, 459
Hypophosphatemia, 120–121
Hypospadias, 756
Hyposplenism, 463
Hypotension, 155
Hypovolemia, 108, 113, 116
Hypovolemic shock, 164–166, 231, 242
Hypoxia, 156
Hytrin, 763

**I**

$^{123}$I scintiscan, 443
IABP, 656, 679
ICP, 731
Icterus, 23
ID tag, 6
I:E, 492
IHSS, 670
Ileal conduit, 283
Ileoanal pull-through, 89
Ileostomy, 23, 283–284
Ileum, 105, 285
Ileus
    electrolyte-mediated, 122
    gallstone, 378–379
    general questions about, 23, 36,
        143–144, 186
Iliac veins, 139
Ilioinguinal nerve, 216, 542
IMA, 657
IMA artery, 441
$^{131}$I-MIBG, 425–426

Imipenem and cilastatin, 131
Immunology, 680–681
Immunosuppression
    agents used in, 682–685
    description of, 173
Impacted fracture, 705
Imperforate anus, 548
Impotence, 756, 769
IMV, 491
In situ, 197
Incarcerated hernia, 209, 220
Incentive spirometry, 157
Incidental appendectomy, 297
Incidentaloma, 423–424
Incision and drainage, 86
Incisional biopsy, 23, 90, 467
Incisional hernia, 211
Incisions, 72–77
Incontinence, 755, 771–772
Indirect bilirubinemia, 565
Indirect inguinal hernia, 212, 214–215,
    538
Induction therapy, 682
Induration, 23
Infarction, 678
Infections
    ameba, 178
    central line, 171
    clostridial myositis, 175
    general questions, 169–170
    necrotizing fasciitis, 175
    orthopaedic, 718–719
    parotitis, 177
    prophylactic antibiotics for, 176–177
    pseudomembranous colitis, 176
    suppurative hidradenitis, 175–176
    urinary tract, 37, 170–171, 180, 755,
        772–773
    wound, 171–174, 180–182
Infectious endocarditis, 667–668
Inferior mesenteric vein, 357
Inferior vena cava filter, 141
Inflammation, 169, 581
Inflammatory bowel disease, 338–344, 377
Infliximab, 343
Inguinal canal, 213, 217
Inguinal hernias
    in children, 220, 538–542
    direct, 212–213

indirect, 212, 214–215, 538
laparoscopic repair of, 215
repair of, 76, 215–219, 540–542
Inhalational anesthesia, 193
Inhalational injury, 249, 251
Inner ear, 597
Inotropes, 122
INR, 123, 133–134
Insensible fluid losses, 110
Inspissated, 23
Instrument tray, 8
Instruments, surgical, 42–52
Insulin, 80, 163
Insulinoma, 32, 430–431
Intensive care note, 14–15
Intensive care unit
basics of, 480–481
drugs used in, 484–486
formulas, 481–484
hemodynamic monitoring in, 488–490
physiology, 486–488
Interlobar, 536, 642
Intermittent claudication, 496, 498
Intermittent mandatory ventilation, 491
Internal carotid artery, 514–515, 596
Internal hernia, 210
Intestinal lymphoma, 470
Intestinal transplantation, 696
Intra-abdominal injury, 235, 242, 245
Intra-abdominal pressure, 153
Intra-aortic balloon pump, 679
Intra-articular fracture, 706
Intracellular fluid, 107
Intracerebral hemorrhage, 744–745, 751
Intracranial pressure, 731–732
Intraparietal hernia, 212
Intravenous access, 232
Intravenous catheter, 65
Intrinsic factor, 199, 271
Intubation, 191
Intussusception, 23, 560–561, 578
Inversion, 700
Involuntary guarding, 203
IOC, 225, 369, 373, 375
Iris scissors, 44
Irish's node, 276
Iron, 161, 201
Ischemia, 678
Islet cell tumor, 400

Isograft, 680
Isoproterenol, 485
Isotonic fluids, 112
-itis, 23
ITP, 463–464
Ivor-Lewis procedure, 655
IVP, 755

**J**
J tube, 144
Jackson-Pratt drain, 92
Jaundice
obstructive, 144, 367, 370–371
physiologic, 564
Jefferson's fracture, 738
Jejunal interposition loop, 146
Jejunostomy, 282
Jejunum, 105, 284
Jewett/Marshall staging system, 759–760
Jones' fracture, 707
J-tube, 92
Juvenile nasopharyngeal angiofibroma, 612
Juvenile polyps, 318

**K**
Kanavel's signs, 589
Kasabach-Merritt syndrome, 351
Kasai, 566
Kehr's sign, 29, 460
Kelly clamp, 45
Kelly's sign, 29
Keloid, 582
Ketoacidosis, diabetic, 146
Ketoconazole, 422
Kidney stones, 39, 186, 189, 205
Kidney transplantation, 74, 688–691, 694
Kidney tumors, 757
Kienbock's disease, 717
Kissing ulcer, 259
Kjellberg, 733
Klatskin tumor, 368, 381
Knee
anatomy of, 715–716
dislocation of, 714–715
ligaments of, 715
Knots, 60–65
Kocher clamp, 49
Kocher incisions, 73, 370
Kocher maneuver, 83, 265

Kocher's point, 731
Kock pouch, 282
Krukenberg's tumor, 29, 276
KUB, 187
Kulchitsky cells, 300
Kussmaul's sign, 230

# L

Laceration, 582
Lactated Ringer's, 110
Lactational mastitis, 418
LAD, 657
Ladd's bands, 552
Ladd's procedure, 553
Langer's lines, 579
Lap appy, 23, 85
Lap chole, 23, 76, 85, 369–370, 373, 375
Lap Nissen, 273–275, 653
Lap Toupet, 653
Laparoscope, 223
Laparoscopy
    appendectomy, 295, 297–298
    camera use during, 224–225
    definition of, 223
    description of, 23
    gastric cancer treated with, 277
    general questions about, 223–225
    splenectomy, 225
Laparotomy, 23, 39, 113, 163, 188
Laparotomy pad, 8
Laplace's law, 29
Large bowel obstruction, 37
Laryngeal fracture, 242
Laryngomalacia, 528
Laryngotracheobronchitis (*see* Croup)
Larynx
    anatomy of, 617
    functions of, 626
    malignant lesions of, 619–620
Lasix, 483 (*see* Furosemide)
Lateral pectoral nerve, 401
LBBB, 678
LCIS, 413–415
Le Fort fractures, 623–624
Left gonadal vein, 774
Left lateral decubitus, 77
Left testicular vein, 102
Left vagus nerve, 103
Legg-Calvé-Perthes disease, 728

Leiomyoma, 23
Leiomyosarcoma, 23
Lentigo maligna melanoma, 475
Leriche's syndrome, 34, 498–499
Lethal triad, 244
Levothyroxine, 442
Lichtenstein herniorrhaphy, 83
Lichtenstein procedure, 215
Lidocaine, 191–192, 194
Lieno-, 102
Lithotomy position, 77
Little League elbow, 729
Littre's hernia, 210, 541
Liver
    abscesses of, 353–355
    anatomy of, 345–348
    blood supply to, 202, 346
    carcinoid syndrome and, 302
    cysts of, 355–356
    hemobilia of, 356
    hydatid liver cysts, 355–356
    lobes of, 104
    metastases to, 314, 435–436
    transplantation of, 41, 75, 353, 691–693
    venous supply to, 346
Liver cancer, 348
Liver disease, 347
Liver tumors, 37
    benign, 348–349
    focal nodular hyperplasia, 350–351
    general questions about, 348–349
    hemangioma, 351
    hepatocellular adenoma, 349–350
    hepatocellular carcinoma, 352–353
LLQ pain, 208
LOA, 287
Local anesthesia, 190–191
Long thoracic nerve, 401, 410
Longitudinal fracture, 705
Loop colostomy, 282–283
Low anterior resection, 83
Lower extremity amputations, 501
Lower extremity arterial insufficiency
    ulcer, 196
Lower gastrointestinal bleeding,
    334–338, 537
Low-molecular-weight heparin, 133
Lucid interval, 751
Lumbar disc herniation, 745–746

Lumbar hernia, 210
Lumpectomy, 409
Lumpectomy and radiation, 86
Lung abscess, 632
Lung diseases
    bronchogenic carcinoma, 635–639
    carcinoid tumors, 641–642
    pulmonary sequestration, 536–537,
        642–643
    solitary pulmonary nodules,
        640–641
Lung transplantation, 41, 697–698
Lymph nodes, 103
Lymphocytotoxic crossmatching, 687
Lymphoma, 468–470, 646, 699
Lynch's syndrome, 309
Lysis of adhesions, 85

# M

Mackler's triad, 269
Macrophages, 682
Mafenide acetate, 251
Maintenance fluids, 111–113
Major histocompatibility complex, 681
Male breast cancer, 415
Male gynecomastia, 418–419
Malignant, 197
Malignant hyperthermia, 193
Malignant melanoma, 471
Malignant mesothelioma, 634
Malignant otitis externa, 597–598
Malignant thyroid nodules, 444–445
Malleable retractor, 52
Mallet finger, 590
Mallory-Weiss syndrome, 34, 266–267
Maloney dilator, 654
Malrotation, 552–553, 578
Mammograms, 189–190, 405–406
Mammoplasty, 580
Mammotome biopsy, 406
Mandibular fractures, 234, 623, 625
MAP, 482, 657
Marcaine (*see* Bupivacaine)
Margin cancer, 327
Marginal ulcer, 196, 261
Marjolin's ulcer, 196, 472
Marshall test, 772
Massive hemothorax, 230–231
MAST, 245

Mastectomy
    modified radical, 409
    simple, 413
Mastitis, 418
Mattress stitches, 56
Maxillofacial fracture, 232
Mayo scissors, 47
Mayo tray, 8
McBurney's incisions, 73, 297
McBurney's point, 30, 104, 293
McBurney's sign, 30
MCL, 699
McMurray's sign, 716
McVay herniorrhaphy, 82
McVay procedure, 215
Mean arterial pressure, 482, 657
Mechanical ventilation, 490–493
Meckel's diverticulum, 30, 39, 289–291,
        561–562
Meckel's scan, 291, 562
Meconium ileus, 546–547
Meconium peritonitis, 547
Meconium plug syndrome, 547
Medial pectoral nerve, 401
Median arcuate ligament syndrome,
        511–512
Median nerve, 587, 713
Median sternotomy, 75
Mediastinal diseases
    anatomy, 643–644
    lymphoma, 646
    superior vena cava syndrome, 647–648
    teratomas, 645
    thymoma, 644–645
    tumors, 644–646
Mediastinal tumors, 530
Mediastinitis, 646–647
Medications
    antibiotics, 129–131
    heparin, 132–133
    narcotics, 136
    steroids, 132, 162
    warfarin, 133–134
Medullary carcinoma, 448
Medulloblastoma, 742
Melanoma
    acral lentiginous, 475
    amelanotic, 475
    anal, 327–328

Melanoma (*Cont.*)
  digital, 478
  general questions about, 25, 35
  lentigo maligna, 475
  metastases, 477–478
  nodular, 475
  risk factors for, 474
  skin, 473–479
  staging of, 476–479
  superficial spreading, 475
  treatment of, 478
MELD score, 692
Melena, 23, 254, 310
Mendelson's syndrome, 34, 142
MEN-I syndrome, 433, 436–437
MEN-IIA syndrome, 437–438
MEN-IIB syndrome, 438–439
Ménière's disease, 607, 627
Meningiomas, 741
Meningitis, 751
Meniscus, 716
Mental status, 156, 236
Meperidine, 192
Mesenteric adenitis, 297
Mesenteric embolus, 511
Mesenteric fibrosis, 288
Mesenteric ischemia, 135, 510–511
Mesenteric lymphadenitis, 558
Mesothelioma, 634–635
Metabolic acidosis, 108, 484
Metabolic alkalosis, 109, 484
Metachronous tumors, 197
Metallic skin staples, 57
Metaphysis, 702
Metastases
  breast cancer, 408
  colorectal carcinoma, 311–312, 314
  hepatocellular carcinoma, 352
  liver, 314
  melanoma, 477–478
  oral cavity cancer, 615
  sarcoma, 466
  Zollinger-Ellison syndrome, 435–436
Methimazole, 451
Methylprednisolone, 683
Metoclopramide, 134
Metronidazole, 131
Metyrapone, 423
Metzenbaum scissors, 46

Microcytic anemia, 124
MIDCAB, 662
Middle ear, 597
Middle lobe syndrome, 632
Middle mediastinum, 643
Midface fractures, 623–625
Midgut, 103
Midgut volvulus, 552–553
Midline laparotomy incisions, 73
Mikulicz's syndrome, 626
Milk leg, 519
Milk line, 402
Millard-Gubler syndrome, 752
Minute ventilation, 490
Mirizzi's syndrome, 34, 383
Misoprostol, 135
Mitotane, 423
Mitral regurgitation, 666
Mitral stenosis, 665–666
Mittelschmerz, 30
Mixed incontinence, 771
Mixed venous oxygen saturation, 483, 486
Modified neck dissection, 622–623
Modified radical mastectomy, 86, 409
MODS, 482
MOF, 484
Mohs surgery, 473
Mondor's disease, 416, 679
Monocryl sutures, 54
Monroe-Kelly hypothesis, 731
Monteggia fracture, 708
Morbid obesity, 280
Morgagni's hernia, 212
Morphine, 192
Morrison's pouch, 103
Motion pain, 203
MR, 657
MRCP, 382
Mucous neck cells, 199, 271
Mucus fistula, 83, 282
Multiple organ dysfunction syndrome, 482
Multiple organ failure, 484
Munchausen syndrome, 34
Murphy's sign, 30, 374
Muscle fibers, 202
Musculocutaneous nerve, 713
Myasthenia gravis, 644
Mycobacterial infections, 578
Mycophenolate mofetil, 685

Myocardial infarction, 149–150, 658
Myofibroblasts, 581
Myoglobinuria, 245

# N
Nafcillin (Nafcil), 131
Nail polish, 6
Narcotics, 136
Nasal cannula, 159
Nasal cavity cancer, 611–612
Nasal septum, 595
Nasoduodenal tube, 184
Nasogastric decompression, 250
Nasogastric tubes, 68–72, 98–100, 122, 142, 184, 244
Nasotracheal intubation, 227
Neck dissection, 622–623
Neck mass, 525–529, 621–622, 628
Necrotic, 24
Necrotizing enterocolitis, 563–564
Necrotizing fasciitis, 175
Necrotizing migratory erythema, 432
Needle loc biopsy, 406
Needle-driver, 45
Negative feedback loop, 442
Nelson's syndrome, 423
Neoadjuvant RX, 197
Nephrogenic diabetes insipidus, 148
Nephrolithiasis, 208
Neuhauser's sign, 546
Neural tube defects, 749–750
Neuroblastoma, 570–573, 579
Neurogenic shock, 168–169
Neurogenic tumors, 644–646
Neuromuscular blocking agents, 194
Neurosurgery
    head trauma (see Head trauma)
    pediatric, 748–752
    spinal cord trauma, 736–739
    spine disorders (see Spine disorders)
    vascular, 743–745
Night stick fracture, 708, 717
NIGRO protocol, 327
Nissen fundoplication, 85, 273–275, 653
Nitroglycerine, 485
Nitrous oxide, 192
No Man's Land, 585–586
Nobel Prize winners, 41–42
Nocturia, 755

Nodular melanoma, 475
Nonabsorbable suture, 53–54
Noncommunicating hydrocele, 540, 754
Noncommunicating hydrocephalus, 748
Nondepolarizing muscle blockers, 194
Nonrebreather mask, 158
Nonseminoma, 766
Non-small cell carcinoma, 637–639
Nonsteroidal anti-inflammatory drugs, 195
Non-union, 702
Norepinephrine, 485
Normal saline, 110
Nose disorders, 608–612
Nosocomial infection, 170
Nursemaid's elbow, 728
Nutcracker esophagus, 651–652
Nutrition, 159–163, 521–522
Nylon sutures, 54
Nystatin, 131

# O
Obesity, 280
Oblique fracture, 705
OBR, 143
Obstipation, 24
Obstructive jaundice, 370–371
Obturator hernia, 210
Obturator sign, 30, 293
Octreotide, 135, 303
Odontoid fracture, 738–739
Odynophagia, 24, 593
Ogilvie's syndrome, 34
OKT3, 684
Oliguria, 151
Omphalocele, 553–557
Oncology, 197–198
Ondansetron, 134
OPCAB, 663
Open fracture, 704, 709–710
Open pneumothorax, 229
Open reduction, 700
Operating room, 5–9
Operative note, 11–12
Operative wounds, 172–174
Opiates, 202
OPSS, 462
Oral cavity
    cancer of, 615
    salivary gland tumors, 616–617

Oral hypoglycemic agents, 80
Orbit, 595
Orchidopexy, 576
Orchiopexy, 773
Orchitis, 754
Organ preservation, 688
Organs of Zuckerkandl, 427
ORIF, 699
-orraphy, 24, 78
Orthopaedic infections
  osteomyelitis, 718–719
  septic arthritis, 719
Orthopaedic surgery
  Achilles tendon rupture, 716
  arthritis, 723–724
  dislocations, 713–715
  general questions about, 717–718
  knee, 714–716
  pediatric, 724–729
  rotator cuff, 716–717
  terminology associated with, 699–702
  trauma, 703, 709–713
Orthopaedic tumors
  Ewing's sarcoma, 721–723
  general questions about, 719–721
  osteosarcoma, 721–722
Orthotopic, 680
Ortolani's sign, 728
Osgood-Schlatter's disease, 729
Ossicles, 597
Osteoarthritis, 723
Osteomyelitis, 718–719, 722
Osteosarcoma, 721–722
Osteotomy, 702
Ostomies, 282–284
-ostomy, 24, 78
Otalgia, 593
Otitis externa, 597, 625
  malignant, 597–598
Otitis media, acute suppurative,
  601–602, 626
-otomy, 24, 78
Otorrhea, 593
Otosclerosis, 602–603
Overflow incontinence, 771–772
Oxygen delivery, 483
Oxygenation, 490
Oxygen-induced hypoventilation, 157
Oxyhemoglobin dissociation curve, 125

# P

Packed red blood cells, 123
Paget's disease
  of the anus, 326
  of the breast, 414
Pancoast's tumor, 636
Pancreas
  abscess of, 391–392
  anatomy of, 383–384
  annular, 399, 569
  chronic, 388–390
  endocrine sufficiency, 388
  exocrine, 384
  fistula, 399
  general questions about, 399–400
  glucagonoma tumors, 400
  head of, 383–384, 395
  insulinoma, 399
  necrosis of, 392
  pseudocyst of, 392–395
  secretions, 110
  somatostatinoma, 400
  transplantation of, 41, 693–695
  traumatic injuries to, 243
Pancreatic carcinoma, 395–398
Pancreatic divisum, 399
Pancreatic ducts, 383
Pancreatic enteric fistula, 306
Pancreatic exocrine sufficiency, 388
Pancreaticoduodenectomy, 89
Pancreatitis
  acute, 263, 384–387
  gallstone, 390
  general questions about, 9, 36, 207
  hemorrhagic, 390–391
  postoperative, 143
Pannus, 724
Pantaloon hernia, 210–211
$PaO_2$, 487
Papillary adenocarcinoma, 445–446
Papillary necrosis, 774
Paradoxic alkalotic aciduria, 109
Paradoxical embolus, 520
Paraesophageal hiatal hernia, 222
Parafollicular cells, 442
Paralytic ileus, 288
Paraneoplastic syndromes, 198, 636
Paraphimosis, 755
Parasternal wounds, 244

Parastomal hernia, 211
Parathyroid glands
    anatomy of, 453–454
    carcinoma of, 458–460
    embryology of, 454
    physiology of, 454
Parathyroidectomy, 459
Paratopic, 680
Parietal cells, 199, 271
Parkland formula, 249
Paronychia, 589
Parotid gland, 595, 626
Parotitis, 177
Parrot's beak sign, 187
Partial cystectomy, 760
Partial shunt, 362
Passaro's triangle, 434–435
Patent ductus arteriosus, 669
Patent urachus, 577
Pathologic fracture, 705
Patient-controlled analgesia,
    194–195
PCA pump, 194–195
PCL, 699
PCWP, 481–482, 488–490
Pectoralis major, 103
Pectoralis minor, 103
Pectus carinatum, 531
Pectus excavatum, 530–531
Pediatric surgery (see also Children)
    general questions about, 521
    intravenous fluids, 521–522
    neurosurgery, 748–752
    nutrition, 521–522
    orthopaedic, 724–729
Pediatric trauma, 575
PEEP, 491–492
Pellagra, 300–301
Pelvic abscess, 174
Pelvic fractures, 236, 239, 242–243
Pemberton's sign, 451
Penetrating abdominal trauma, 37
Penetrating neck injuries, 240–241
Penicillin allergy, 135
Penrose drain, 92
Pentalogy of Cantrell, 556
Pentoxifylline, 498
Pepcid (see Famotidine)
Pepsin, 199, 271

Peptic ulcer
    definition of, 195
    perforated, 262–263
Peptic ulcer disease, 256
Perc nephrostomy, 752
Percocet, 131
Percutaneous, 24
Percutaneous endoscopic gastrostomy,
    86–87
Perianal warts, 331–332
Periarticular fracture, 706
Pericarditis, 660, 678
Peripheral vascular disease, 495–500
Peripheral vertigo, 606
Perirectal abscess, 329–330
Peritoneal abscess, 174, 188
Peritoneal fat stripe, 187
Peritoneal fluid, 186
Peritoneal lavage, 178
Peritoneal signs, 203
Peritoneal tap, 239, 564
Peritonitis, 204, 547
Peritonsillar abscess, 614
Periumbilical pain, 293
Petit's hernia, 210
Peutz-Jeghers syndrome, 34, 317–318
-pexy, 24
Peyer patches, 202
Peyronie's disease, 755, 775
PF ratio, 487
Pfannenstiel incision, 74
Pharyngotonsillitis, 613–614
Phenergan (see Promethazine)
Phenoxybenzamine, 426
Pheochromocytoma, 31, 424–427, 438
Phimosis, 755
Phleb-, 24
Phlebolith, 24
Phlegmasia cerulea dolens, 519
Phlegmon, 24
Physical examination, 9–10
Physiologic jaundice, 564
Physis, 702
Pierre-Robin syndrome, 577
Piggyback technique, 692
Pilon fracture, 709
Pituitary tumors, 742
Plantarflexion, 700
Plastic surgery, 579–584

-plasty, 78
Platelet count, 124
Platelets, 123–124, 125, 135
Pleural diseases, 631–635
Pleural effusion, 138, 184, 631–632
Pleural fluid, 184
Pleuravac, 95
Plica, 24
Plicae circulares, 24, 105, 285
Plicae semilunares, 24
Plug and patch hernia, 83
Plug and patch procedure, 215
Plummer-Vinson syndrome, 34
Pneumatosis intestinalis, 187
Pneumaturia, 24, 755
Pneumonia
    aspiration, 141–142
    general questions about, 37, 182
    ventilator-associated, 183
Pneumoperitoneum, 223
Pneumothorax
    chest x-ray findings, 184
    general questions about, 24, 97, 157,
        228–229
    spontaneous, 633
Poland's syndrome, 578
Polydactyly, 580
Polyposis syndromes
    familial, 316
    Gardner's syndrome, 317
Polyps, 315–316
Polysporin, 251
Polyuria, 755
Popliteal artery aneurysm, 518–519
Pop-off suture, 59
Porcelain gallbladder, 40, 380, 382
Port-A-Cath, 101
Portal hypertension, 102, 357–364,
    464
Portal vein, 358
Positive end-expiratory pressure, 491–492
Posterior cord syndrome, 738
Posterior fossa tumor, 627
Posterior mediastinum, 643–644
Posterior neck triangles, 596
Posterior urethral valves, 773
Posteroanterior radiograph, 184
Posthitis, 753
Postoperative fever, 180–182

Postoperative notes, 12–13
Postoperative pancreatitis, 143
Postoperative respiratory failure, 138
Postpericardiotomy syndrome, 660
Postpyloric tube feedings, 386
Post-transplant lymphoproliferative
    disease, 699
Post-traumatic arthritis, 723
Postvagotomy diarrhea, 145
Potassium, 107
Pott's disease, 709
Pott's fracture, 709
Pouch of Douglas, 104
Pouchitis, 344
Poupart's ligament, 82, 216, 540
Povidone-iodine, 9
PPI, 134
Prednisone, 683
Prehn's sign, 754
Preload, 486, 657
Premature ventricular contractions, 678
Preoperative note, 11
Pressure support, 491
Priapism, 738, 755, 768–769
Primary hyperaldosteronism, 428
Primary intention, 54
Primary wound closure, 90–91
Pringle maneuver, 86
Progress note, 13–14
Prolactinoma, 742
Prolene sutures, 54
PROM, 700
Promethazine, 134–135
Pronation, 700
Prone, 77
Properitoneal hernia, 212
Prophylactic, 170
Prophylactic antibiotics, 176–177, 183
Proscar, 763
Prostate cancer, 760–762, 773
Prostate-specific antigen, 761
Prosthetic heart valve, 181, 667
Protamine, 132–133
Protein, 159, 160
Protein C deficiency, 126
Protein S deficiency, 126
Proton pump inhibitors, 134
Pseudoaneurysm, 494
Pseudocapsule, 468

Pseudocyst
    description of, 24
    pancreatic, 392–395
Pseudogout, 724
Pseudohermaphroditism, 754
Pseudohyperkalemia, 115
"Pseudohyponatremia," 117
Pseudomembranous colitis,
    155, 176
*Pseudomonas,* 178
Pseudomyxoma peritonei, 299
Pseudopolyps, 343
Psoas shadow, 187
Psoas sign, 30, 293
PT, 122, 127
PTC, 369
PTCA, 657
PTH, 454
PTT, 122
PTU, 451
Puestow procedure, 84, 399
Pulmonary capillary wedge pressure,
    481–482, 488–490
Pulmonary embolism, 138–141,
    180, 190
Pulmonary sequestration, 536–537,
    642–643
Pulmonary vascular obstructive
    disease, 668
Pulmonary vascular resistance, 482
Pulse volume recordings, 497
Pursestring stitch, 57
Pus, 25
PVC, 678
PVR, 482, 497, 755
PWB, 699
Pyloric stenosis, 543–545, 578
Pyloroplasty, 79, 264
Pylorus, 104
Pyrosis, 271
Pyuria, 755, 771

# R

Raccoon eyes, 31
Radial nerve, 587, 713
Radiation therapy, 408–409
Radical neck dissection, 622
Radical nephrectomy, 758
Radical prostatectomy, 762

Radiology
    abdomen, 185–190
    chest, 183–185
Ramsay Hunt's syndrome, 628
Ranitidine, 134
Ranson's criteria, 386–387
Ranula, 627
Rapid-sequence anesthesia intubation, 191
Raynaud's phenomenon, 519
RBBB, 678
Rebound tenderness, 203
Rectal cancer (*see* Colorectal carcinoma)
Rectal disease, 207
Rectal examination, 235
Rectal pain, 208
Rectum (*see also* Anus)
    anatomy of, 307–308
    blood supply to, 308
    polyps of, 315–316
    venous supply to, 308
Red blood cells, 125
RED reaction syndrome, 34
Reducible hernia, 209
Reduction, 700
Refeeding syndrome, 34, 163
Referred pain, 207
Regional anesthesia, 190
Reglan (*see* Metoclopramide)
Rejection of transplant
    description of, 687–688
    heart, 695–696
    intestinal, 696
    kidney, 690–691, 694
    liver, 692–693
    lung, 697
Relaxing incision, 218
Renal artery stenosis, 135, 516–518
Renal cell carcinoma, 757–758, 773
Renal failure, 151–152, 689
Renal vein renin ratio, 517
Rendu-Osler-Weber syndrome, 34
Renin, 428, 517
Replogle tube, 577
Respiratory acidosis, 109, 484
Respiratory alkalosis, 109, 484
Respiratory care, 157–159
Respiratory failure, postoperative, 138
Rest pain, 496
Retention suture, 59

Retractors, 50–52
Retrocecal appendix, 296, 298
Retrograde pyelogram, 752
Retroperitoneal appendix, 296, 298
Retroperitoneal varices, 360
Reverse Trendelenburg position, 78
Reynold's pentad, 31
Rhabdomyosarcoma, 573–574
Rheumatoid arthritis, 724
Rhinoplasty, 580
Richardson retractor, 52
Richter's hernia, 211
Riedel's thyroiditis, 453
Right gonadal vein, 774
Right lateral decubitus, 77
Right renal vain, 105
Right testicular vein, 102
Right-angle clamp, 45
RIND, 512
Rings, 6
Rinne test, 605
RLQ pain, 208
Rocky-Davis incision, 74, 297
ROM, 699
Ross procedure, 667
Rotational flap, 584
Rotator cuff, 716–717
Rotter's nodes, 402
Rounds, 3
Roux-en-Y limb, 82
Rovsing's sign, 31, 293
RQ, 160
Rubor, 25
RUG, 752
Rule of nines, 246–247
Rule of twos, 291, 562
Ruptured abdominal aortic aneurysms, 208
RUQ pain, 208

**S**

Sacral sparing, 736
"Saddle" embolus, 140
Saint's triad, 31
Saliva, 110
Salivary glands
    parotid gland, 595, 626
    stones of, 626
    submandibular gland, 595
    tumors of, 616–617, 627

Salter classification, 724–727
Sarcomas
    Ewing's sarcoma, 721–723
    osteosarcoma, 721–722
    rhabdomyosarcoma, 573–574
    soft tissue, 465–468
Scalpel blades, 49
Schwartze's sign, 603
Sciatic hernia, 211
Sciatica, 746
Scissors, 42–43
Sclerosing cholangitis, 377–378
Scoliosis, 728
Scrotal mass, 756
Scrotum, 216, 541, 756
Scrub nurse, 7
Seagesser's sign, 460
Seatbelt sign, 235
Sebaceous cyst, 72, 473
Seborrheic keratosis, 473
Second degree burns, 246–248
Secondary hyperaldosteronism, 429
Secondary intention, 54
Secondary wound closure, 90
Second-degree A-V block, 678
Second-degree hemorrhoid, 333
Secretin, 200
Seizures, 136
Seldinger technique, 83
Selective exploration, 241
Selective shunt, 362–363
Seminoma, 766
Sengstaken-Blakemore tamponade
    balloon, 267–268, 361
Sensorineural hearing loss, 605
Sentinel loops, 187
Sentinel node biopsy, 410, 478
Sentinel pile, 331
Sepsis, 169
Septic arthritis, 719
Septic shock, 166–167, 169
Seroma, 155
Serotonin, 302
Seton, 329
Shin splints, 717
Shock, 36
    anaphylactic, 169
    cardiogenic, 167–168
    definition of, 164

hypovolemic, 164–166, 231, 242
neurogenic, 168–169
septic, 166–167, 169
signs of, 164
spinal, 168–169, 736
Short bowel syndrome, 143
Short-gut syndrome, 143
Shortness of breath, 156
Shoulder dislocation, 713–714
Shouldice herniorrhaphy, 83
Shouldice procedure, 215
Shunt fraction, 487
Shunt series, 749
Shunts, 362–364
SIADH, 34, 117, 147
Side-to-side portocaval shunt, 363
Sigmoid volvulus, 322–323
Sigmoidoscopy, 319
Silk glove sign, 31, 220, 539
Silk sutures, 54
Silver sulfadiazine, 251
Simple fracture, 704
Simple interrupted stitch, 55
Simple mastectomy, 85, 413
Simple running stitch, 56
SIMV, 491
Sinus cancer, 611–612, 627
Sinuses, 596
Sinusitis, 609–611
Sipple's syndrome, 35
Sirolimus, 685
SIRS, 169, 484
Sister Mary Joseph's sign, 32, 276
Sitz bath, 330
Skin cancer, 471–473
Skin grafts, 583
Skin lesions, 471–473
Skin sutures, 61
Skull fractures, 234, 730, 736
Sliding esophageal hiatal hernia, 221
Sliding hernia, 210
Slipped capital femoral epiphysis, 728
Small bowel, 105
    anatomy of, 284–285
    layers of, 104
    Meckel's diverticulum, 289–291
    obstruction of, 143–144, 186, 285–288,
        300, 577
    secretions, 110

traumatic injuries to, 243
tumors of, 288–289
Smith's fracture, 707
Smoke inhalation, 248–249
Sneezing, 6
Soave procedure, 551
Sodium, 107, 108
Sodium nitroprusside, 485–486
Soft tissue sarcomas, 465–468
Solitary pulmonary nodules, 640–641
Somatostatin, 201
Somatostatinoma, 432
Space of Retzius, 104, 755
Spermatic cord, 103, 213, 216–217,
        540, 542
Spermatocele, 754
Sphincterotomy, 370
Spigelian hernia, 210
Spina bifida occulta, 750
Spinal anesthesia, 190, 193
Spinal cord trauma, 736–739
Spinal dysraphism, 749–750
Spinal immobilization, 226
Spinal shock, 168–169, 736
Spine disorders
    cervical disc disease, 746–747
    epidural abscess, 747–748
    lumbar disc herniation, 745–746
Spiral fracture, 705, 727
Spironolactone, 429
Spleen
    accessory, 460
    anatomy of, 459–460
    rupture of, 460
Splenectomy, 181, 225, 279, 461–462
Splenic artery aneurysm, 518
Splenic vein thrombosis, 387, 463
Splenomegaly, 463
Splenorrhaphy, 461
Split liver transplant, 692
Spontaneous pneumothorax, 633
Spurling's sign, 747
Squamous cell carcinoma, 471–472, 621
Stab wounds, 240, 244
Stamm gastrostomy, 84
Stanford classifications, 675–676
Staples, 66
Starling curve, 486
Steatorrhea, 25

Stenosis, 25
Step off, 625
Sterile field, 7, 25
Sterility, 756
Steri-Strips, 66
Steroids, 132, 162
"Stitch" abscess, 174
Stitches, 66
Stoma, 282
Stomach
  anatomy of, 270
  gastric cancer, 275–279
  gastric volvulus, 279
  gastroesophageal reflux disease, 271–275
  physiology of, 271
Strangulated hernia, 210
Strap muscles, 596
Stress fracture, 705
Stress gastritis, 265–266
Stress incontinence, 771–772
Stridor, 527–528
Stroke (*see* Cerebrovascular accident)
Stroke volume, 481, 657
STSGs, 245, 248, 252, 580, 583
Subacute thyroiditis, 452
Subarachnoid hemorrhage, 735, 743–744
Subclavian steal syndrome, 515–516
Subcutaneous abscess, 174
Subcutaneous air, 235
Subcuticular stitch, 57
Subdural hematoma, 734–735
Subluxation, 702
Submandibular gland, 595
Subtotal gastrectomy, 278
Subungual tumor, 589
Succinylcholine, 122, 191, 194
Succus, 25
Sucking chest wound, 228
Sucralfate, 134
Suction-control chamber, 96
Suffixes, 78–79
Superficial spreading melanoma, 475
Superinfection, 170
Superior mesenteric artery syndrome, 287
Superior vena cava syndrome, 35, 647–648
Supination, 700
Supine, 77

Suppurative hidradenitis, 175–176
Supraglottic lesions, 620
Suprapubic catheter, 753
Suprapubic pain, 207
Surgeon's knot, 60
Surgery clerkship, 1–9
Surgical gown, 6–7
Surgical hemostasis, 127–128
Surgical history, 40–42
Surgical instruments, 42–52
Surgical notes, 9–15
Surgical positions, 77–78
Surgical prophylaxis, 182–183
Surgicel, 128
Suspensory breast ligaments, 402
Suture ligament, 59
Sutures, 8–9
  description of, 52–54
  figure-of-eight, 128
  techniques for, 55–59
  wound closure, 54–59
SV, 481
SVR, 482, 657, 662
Swan-Ganz catheter, 488
Sweetheart retractor, 51
Swenson procedure, 550
Swimmer's ear (*see* Otitis externa)
Synchronous intermittent mandatory ventilation, 491
Synchronous tumors, 197
Syndactyly, 580
Syndrome of inappropriate antidiuretic hormone, 34
Synthetic mesocaval H-graft, 363
Synthetic portocaval H-graft, 363
Syringomyelia, 752
Systemic inflammatory response syndrome, 484
Systemic vascular resistance, 482, 657

**T**
T3, 442
T4, 442
T cells, 681
Tachycardia, 156
Tacrolimus, 684–685
Tagamet (*see* Cimetidine)
Tail of Spence, 402
Takayasu's arteritis, 520

Tamoxifen, 410–411
Tamponade physiology, 661
Taper-point needle, 55
TAPP procedure, 215
TBSA, 245
Tenckhoff catheter, 102
Tenesmus, 25
Tennis elbow, 717
Tenosynovitis, 589
Tension pneumothorax, 228
TEPA procedure, 215
Teratomas, 645
Terminal ileum, 201, 285
Tertiary intention, 54
Testicles, 216, 541
Testicular cancer, 764–767
Testicular torsion, 767–768
Tetanus, 179, 181
Tetralogy of Fallot, 669–670
THA, 699
Thermodilution, 490
Third degree burns, 246–248
Third spacing, 108–110
Third-degree A-V block, 679
Third-degree hemorrhoid, 333
Third-nerve palsy, 752
Thoracic aortic aneurysm, 673–674
Thoracic aortic injury, 37, 237–238
Thoracic duct, 104
Thoracic great vessel injury, 235
Thoracic outlet syndrome, 35, 629–630
Thoracic pain, 206
Thoracic surgery
    chest wall tumors, 630–631
    esophagus (*see* Esophageal diseases)
    hemoptysis, 632–633
    lung abscess, 632
    lung diseases (*see* Lung diseases)
    mediastinum (*see* Mediastinal diseases)
    mesothelioma, 634–635
    pleural diseases, 631–635
    spontaneous pneumothorax, 633
    thoracic outlet syndrome, 629–630
Thoracic trauma, 234
Thoracodorsal nerve, 401
Thoracostomy tube, 93
Thoracotomy, 25, 75
THR, 699
3-for-1 rule, 241

Thrombocytopenia, 124, 461
Thrombophlebitis, 180
Thrombosis, 32
Thumbprinting, 187
Thymoma, 644–645
Thyroglossal duct cyst, 525–527
Thyroid carcinoma
    anaplastic, 449
    follicular adenocarcinoma, 446–447
    general questions about, 445
    Hürthle cell, 447–448
    medullary, 448
    papillary adenocarcinoma, 445–446
Thyroid gland
    anatomy of, 439–442
    benign disease of, 450–451
    blood supply to, 440
    general questions about, 449–453
    physiology of, 442
    toxic multinodular goiter, 451
    venous drainage of, 440–441
Thyroid isthmus, 441
Thyroid nodule
    general questions about, 442–444
    malignant, 444–445
Thyroidectomy, 441, 449–450
Thyroiditis, 451–453
TIA, 512
Tibial pin, 701
Tibial plateau fracture, 708
Tidal volume, 490
Tidling, 97
Tietze's syndrome, 35, 631
Tinel's test, 630
TIPS, 362
Tissue perfusion, 164
TKA, 699
TKR, 699
TMN staging, 197, 312, 766
TMR, 662–663
Tobin index, 493
Tonicity, 111
Tonsil clamp, 46
Tonsillectomy, 614
Toradol, 136
TORCHES, 575
Torus fracture, 706
Total gastrectomy, 278
Total parenteral nutrition, 41, 162–163, 387

Toupet procedure, 274
Toxic multinodular goiter, 451
Toxic shock syndrome, 35
Tracheobronchomalacia, 528
Tracheoesophageal fistula, 532–535
Tracheostomy, 90, 626
TRAM flap, 411, 584
Transcervical fracture, 708
Transect, 25
Transfusion hemolysis, 36, 124, 125
Transfusion reaction, 125
Transient ischemic attack, 512
Transplant surgery
    cells, 681
    complications of, 698–699
    donor/recipient matching, 687
    heart, 695–696
    immunology, 680–681
    immunosuppression, 682–686
    infection secondary to, 698
    intestinal, 696
    kidney, 688–691
    liver, 691–693
    lung, 697–698
    malignancies secondary to, 699
    organ preservation, 688
    pancreas, 693–695
    rejection, 687–688
    terminology, 680
Transposition of the great vessels, 672
Transudate, 631
Transurethral resection of the prostate, 87
Transverse fracture, 704
Trauma
    airway management, 226–227
    breathing assessments, 228–231
    circulation assessments, 231–232
    disability assessments, 233
    general questions about, 226, 241–245
    orthopaedic, 703, 709–713
    pediatric, 575
    penetrating neck, 240–241
    primary survey, 226–234
    secondary survey, 234–236
    studies for evaluating, 236–240
Traumatic aortic injury, 185
Traumatic myositis, 718
Traumatic subarachnoid hemorrhage, 735
Trendelenburg operation, 141

Trendelenburg position, 25, 78, 166
TRH, 442
Triangular ligaments of the liver, 345
Trigeminal nerve, 595
Triple A repair, 88
"Triple" antibiotics, 178
Tripod fracture, 624–625
Trisegmentectomy, 349
Trismus, 593
"Trophic" tube feeds, 163
Trousseau's sign, 32, 118
Trousseau's syndrome, 35
True aneurysm, 494
Truncal vagotomy, 89, 258–259, 264
TRUS, 754
TSH, 442
TTP, 464
T-tube, 93
Tube(s)
    chest, 93–98
    nasogastric, 68–72, 98–100, 122, 142,
        184, 244
Tube check, 284
Tube feedings, 163
Tubular adenoma, 316
Tubulovillous adenoma, 316
TUIP, 764
Tullio's phenomenon, 606
Tumor(s) *(see also specific tumor)*
    appendiceal, 299
    brain *(see Brain tumors)*
    carcinoid, 300–304, 641–642
    cardiac, 673
    central nervous system, 739
    chest wall, 630–631
    external ear, 598–599
    glomus, 607
    hepatoblastoma, 574, 579
    liver, 37
    mediastinal, 644–646
    neuroblastoma, 570–573, 579
    neurogenic, 644–646
    pediatric, 569–574, 577
    pituitary, 742
    rhabdomyosarcoma, 573–574
    salivary gland, 616–617
    small bowel, 288–289
    staging of, 311–312
    Wilms', 569–570, 578

Tumor markers, 197
TURB, 760
Turcot's syndrome, 318
Turf toe, 717
TURP, 221, 755, 764
Two-hand knot, 63
Two-hand tie, 63
Tympanic membrane perforation, 599
Type, 124

## U

U wave, 115
Ulcerative colitis, 338–344
Ulcers, 195–196
Ulnar nerve, 586, 713
Umbilical arteries, 523–524
Umbilical hernia, 212, 542, 576
Umbilical veins, 523–524
Umbilicus, 105
Unhappy triad, 716
Unicameral bone cyst, 723
Unstable fracture, 701
Upper gastrointestinal bleeding, 38
  Boerhaave's syndrome, 33, 268–269
  duodenal ulcers, 103, 252, 257–261
  esophageal variceal bleeding, 267–268
  gastric ulcers, 40, 195, 252, 259–261, 263
  general questions about, 254–256
  Mallory-Weiss syndrome, 266–267
  pediatric, 537
  peptic ulcer disease, 256
  perforated peptic ulcer as cause of,
    262–263
  stress gastritis, 265–266
  surgical treatments for, 263–265
Urachus, 524, 577
Ureteral obstruction, 757
Ureteral stents, 752
Urethra, 68, 239
Urethral injury, 236, 774
Urge incontinence, 771–772
Urgency, 25, 754
Urinary retention, 154
Urinary tract infections, 37, 170–171,
  180, 755, 772–773
Urine osmolality, 152
Urine output, 156
  in burn patients, 250
  pediatric, 522

reporting of, 480
in trauma patients, 241
Urology
  benign prostatic hyperplasia, 762–764,
    773
  bladder cancer, 759–760
  calculus disease, 770–771
  differential diagnosis, 756–757
  epididymitis, 754, 768
  impotence, 769
  incontinence, 771–772
  priapism, 738, 755, 768–769
  prostate cancer, 760–762, 773
  renal cell carcinoma, 757–758, 773
  terminology associated with, 752–756
  testicular cancer, 764–767
  testicular torsion, 767–768
  urinary tract infections, 37, 170–171,
    180, 755, 772–773
Uterine pain, 208

## V

VAD, 657, 679
Vagotomy, 264
Vagus nerve, 103
Valentino's sign, 32, 293
Valgus, 702
Vancomycin, 131
Varices
  esophageal, 267–268, 358–361
  gastric, 463
  retroperitoneal, 360
Varicocele, 754
Varus, 701
Vascular anastomosis, 41
Vascular prosthetic graft, 136
Vascular rings, 528, 672
Vascular surgery
  abdominal aortic aneurysms (see
    Abdominal aortic aneurysms)
  acute arterial occlusion, 501–503
  carotid vascular disease, 512–515
  general questions about, 493–495
  lower extremity amputations, 501
  median arcuate ligament syndrome,
    511–512
  mesenteric ischemia, 510–511
  peripheral vascular disease, 495–500
  renal artery stenosis, 516–518

Vascular surgery (*Cont.*)
    splenic artery aneurysm, 518
    subclavian steal syndrome, 515–516
Vasopressin, 267
Vasopressors, 166
VATS, 629
Vein graft, 500
Venous stasis ulcer, 196
Ventilation, 490
Ventilator-associated pneumonia, 183
Ventral hernia, 211
Ventricular aneurysm, 678
Ventricular assist device, 679
Ventricular septal defect, 668–669
Venturi mask, 158
Veress needle, 224
Vertical mattress stitch, 56
Vertigo, 606
Vicryl suture, 53
Villous adenoma, 316
Virchow's node, 32, 276
Virchow's triad, 32, 139
Vitamin A deficiency, 161
Vitamin B$_{12}$, 201
    • absorption of, 161
    deficiency of, 145, 161
Vitamin C deficiency, 161
Vitamin D, 454
Vitamin K deficiency, 161
Vitamin K-dependent clotting factors, 163
Vitelline duct, 525
Volarflexion, 700
Volatile anesthesia, 193
Volkmann's contracture, 712, 717
Voluntary guarding, 203
Volvulus
    cecal, 323–324
    colonic, 321
    gastric, 27, 279
    midgut, 552–553
    sigmoid, 322–323
Vomiting bilious, 553
von Willebrand's disease, 126
VSD, 657
VUR, 756
VY advancement flap, 585

**W**

Warfarin, 127, 133–134
Warren shunt, 362–363

Water loss, 107
Water seal, 97
Water-seal chamber, 96
WBAT, 699
WDHA syndrome, 399
Weber test, 605
Weitlaner retractor, 51
Wenckebach phenomenon, 679
Wermer's syndrome, 35
Wernicke's encephalopathy, 181–182
Westermark's sign, 32, 140
Wet gangrene, 500
Wet-to-dry dressing, 25, 91
Wheezing, 138
Whipple procedure, 89–90, 397–398
Whipple's triad, 32, 430
White lines of Toldt, 104, 308
Whole blood, 123
Wilms' tumor, 569–570, 578
Wolff-Parkinson-White syndrome,
    678
Wound(s)
    dehiscence of, 91, 154
    general questions, 90–91
    healing of, 91, 162, 580–582
    operative, 172–174
Wound contraction, 581–582
Wound hematoma, 154
Wound infections
    burn, 250, 252
    general questions about, 154, 171–174,
        180–182
Wound seroma, 155
Wrist dorsiflexion, 700

**X**

Xenograft, 680
Xigris, 127
XRT, 197

**Y**

Yankauer suction, 50

**Z**

Zantac (*see* Ranitidine)
Zenker's diverticulum, 649
Zinc deficiency, 161
Zofran (*see* Ondansetron)
Zollinger-Ellison syndrome, 35, 432–436
Z-plasty, 584